ENGLISH IN
PAEDIATRICS 2

ENGLISH IN PAEDIATRICS 2

Textbook for mothers, babysitters, nurses, and paediatricians

Irena Baumruková

ISBN: Softcover   978-1-6641-1285-8
                  eBook   978-1-6641-1284-1

Print information available on the last page.

Rev. date: 10/20/2020

To order additional copies of this book, contact:
Xlibris
UK TFN: 0800 0148620 (Toll Free inside the UK)
UK Local: 02036 956328 (+44 20 3695 6328 from outside the UK)
www.Xlibrispublishing.co.uk
Orders@Xlibrispublishing.co.uk
784453

PREFACE

The textbook English in Paediatrics is designed for mothers and carers as well as medical students, paediatric nurses and paediatricians who wish to live, study and/or work in English-speaking countries or need to study original English texts. The teachers can choose from reading texts and different types of useful exercises according to the language level (basic to advanced) and professional interests of their students.

In the first units you can find information about pyloric stenosis; acute appendicitis; irritable bowel syndrome; serious life-threatening infections (infectious mononucleosis, HIV); food allergy and food intolerance; respiratory disorders; tonsillectomy and adenoidectomy; acute upper airways' obstruction; asthma; cystic fibrosis; cardiac disorders; kidney and urinary tract disorders; enuresis; haematuria; and dialysis. Later you will learn about genital disorders; liver disorders; cystic fibrosis; cirrhosis and portal hypertension. malignant disease; radiotherapy; haematological disorders; and bleeding disorders. Next units deal with these topics: child and adolescent mental health; disobedience, defiance, and tantrums; antisocial behaviour and drug misuse; After that you will get to know about chronic fatigue syndrome; dermatological disorders; atopic eczema; diabetes and endocrinology; thyroid disorders; musculoskeletal disorders; neurological disorders; motor disorders. The book also includes texts, concerning adolescent medicine; impact of chronic conditions; health-risk behaviour; childhood injuries; various influences on child health promotion; documentation of nursing care; and defining characteristics to select an appropriate nursing diagnosis. The students may read about family home care; communication and health assessments of the child and family; initiating a comprehensive family assessment; performing paediatric physical examination; paediatric symptom checklist; health problems of the newborn; conditions caused by defects in physical development; emergency treatment of shock; as well as about the child with respiratory dysfunction; the child with gastrointestinal dysfunction, and the child with renal dysfunction.

The previous book deals with these topics: Unit 1 — Pregnancy and birth; A pregnancy calendar; The start of life; Your growing baby; Changes in you; Week 40. Unit 2 — Antenatal care; Initial talk; Table of screening and diagnostic tests; Common complaints; "Small for dates" babies; Eating for a healthy baby; Taking supplements; Practical preparations. Unit 3 — Labour and birth; Internal examinations; The birth; Pain relief; Special procedures; Breech birth. Unit 4 — Your new baby; First impressions after delivery; Checks on the baby; Getting back to normal; Caring for your baby- the first weeks of life; Handling your baby; Feeding your baby. Unit 5 — Breastfeeding your baby; Bottle feeding your baby; Introducing solid food; Warning; Crying and your baby; Sleep and your baby; All about medicines. Unit 6 — Bathing and washing your baby; Nappies and nappy care; Growing and learning, becoming a person; Age: 15 months. Unit 7 — Your child's health; The first three months; Chilling; Overheating; Vomiting; Diagnostic guide; First signs of illness; The child with a temperature; Epilepsy; Going to hospital. Unit 8 — Caring of a sick child; Colds and flu; Having your child immunized; Infectious illnesses; Chickenpox; Whooping cough. Unit 9 — Eye problems; Ear problems; Mouth infections; Throat infections; Coughs and chest infections; Bronchiolitis. Unit 10 — Stomach pain; Constipation, vomiting, and diarrhoea; Bladder, kidney, and genital problems; Skin problems; Hives; Atopic eczema; Sunburn; Warts and verrucas; Lice and nits. Unit 11 — Your child's safety; First aid; Cardiopulmonary resuscitation for a baby up to 12 months; Choking; Drowning; Burns and scalds; Serious bleeding; Nose bleeds; Bruises and swelling; Foreign object in the eye; Minor bites and stings. Unit 12 — The child in society; Socioeconomic status; National and international environment. Unit 13 — History and examination; General enquiry and systems review; Developmental skills; Cardiovascular system; Causes of hepatomegaly; Splenomegaly; Neurology, neurodevelopment; Bones and joints; Eyes, Ears and throat. Unit 14 — Investigations during consultation; Normal child development, hearing and vision; Pattern of child development; Developmental milestones; Analysing child development. Unit 15 — Developmental problems and the child with special needs; Developmental problems; Abnormal motor development; Slow acquisition of cognitive skills; general learning difficulty; Hearing impairment; Visual impairment; Care of the sick child and young person; Pain in children; Ethics. Unit 16 — Paediatric emergencies; Features of paediatric emergencies; Management of the seriously injured child; Anaphylaxis; Neurological emergencies; SIDS; Accidents and poisoning; Choking, suffocation and strangulation; Burns and scalds. Unit 17 — Child protection; Examples of injuries and a guide as how likely it is due to an inflicted injury; Genetics. Unit 18 — Congenital infections; Newborn life support – sequence of resuscitation; Birthweight, gestational age, and birthweight centile; Lesions in newborn infants that resolve spontaneously. Neonatal medicine; Medical problems of preterm infants; Circulation; Infection. Unit 19 — Growth and puberty; Measurement; Assessment of a child with short stature; Formula feeding; Obesity; Early childhood caries; Features of gastrointestinal disorders.

CONTENTS

Pyloric stenosis; Acute appendicitis; Irritable bowel syndrome; Fluid management of dehydration due to gastroenteritis; Causes of nutrient malabsorption; Infection and immunity

Text 1
Pyloric stenosis

In pyloric stenosis, there is hypertrophy of the pyloric muscle causing gastric outlet obstruction.

Clinical features are:
- vomiting, ultimately becoming projectile
- hunger after vomiting until dehydration leads to loss of interest in feeding
- weight loss if presentation is delayed

Diagnosis

The baby is given a milk feed, which will calm the hungry infant, allowing examination. The pyloric mass, which feels like an olive, is usually palpable in the right upper quadrant. If the stomach is overdistended with air, it will need to be emptied by a nasogastric tube.

Management

Definitive treatment by pyloromyotomy can be performed. This involves division of the hypertrophied muscle down to, but not including the mucosa.

Crying

Some babies cry for prolonged periods in spite of feeding and comforting and this is distressing for all concerned. It can engender a feeling of anxiety, helplessness and depression in parents and carers. In some instances, tense, anxious or irritable caregivers are more likely to have fretful babies. A cause for the crying is identified in a minority of infants. If of sudden onset, it may be due to a urinary tract, middle ear or meningeal infection; pain from an unrecognized fracture; oesophagitis; or torsion of the testis. Severe nappy rash and constipation may produce a miserable, crying infant. Eruption of teeth is painful in some infants.

However, teething does not cause vomiting, diarrhoea, high fever or seizures. Reducing overstimulation from jigging and winding and encouraging a quiet environment and holding the baby close may help many babies.

Infant 'colic'

Paroxysmal, inconsolable crying or screaming often accompanied by drawing up of the knees and passage of excessive flatus takes place several times a day. It typically occurs in the first few weeks of life. The condition is benign but is very frustrating and worrying for parents. If severe and persistent, it may be due to a cow's milk protein allergy.

Acute abdominal pain

The differential diagnosis of acute abdominal pain in children is extremely wide, encompassing surgical causes and medical conditions. In young children it is essential not to delay the diagnosis and treatment of acute appendicitis, as progression to perforation can be rapid. Of the surgical causes, appendicitis is by far the most common. The testes, hernial orifices and hip joints must always be checked.

Causes of acute abdominal pain
Extra abdominal
- Upper respiratory tract infection
- Lower lobe pneumonia
- Torsion of the testis
- Hip and spine

Intraabdominal
Surgical
- Acute appendicitis
- Intestinal obstruction including intussusception
- Inguinal hernia
- Peritonitis
- Inflamed Meckel diverticulum
- Pancreatitis
- Trauma

Medical
- Non-specific abdominal pain
- Gastroenteritis
- Urinary tract
- urinary tract infection

- acute pyelonephritis
- hydronephrosis
- renal calculus
- Henoch-Schönlein purpura
- Diabetic ketoacidosis
- Sickle cell disease
- Hepatitis
- Inflammatory bowel disease
- Constipation
- Recurrent abdominal pain of childhood
- Gynaecological in pubertal females
- Psychological
- Lead poisoning
- Acute porphyria (rare)
- Unknown

Exercise 1
Answer the following questions. Prepare short talks and/or dialogues on these topics

1. Describe clinical features of pyloric stenosis, the diagnosis and management.
2. Which are the most common causes of crying?
3. Characterize acute abdominal, extra abdominal, intraabdominal, surgical, and medical pains.

Translation 1

1. In pyloric stenosis, there is hypertrophy of the pyloric muscle causing gastric outlet obstruction. 2. The pyloric mass, which feels like an olive, is usually palpable in the right upper quadrant. 3. Definitive treatment by pyloromyotomy can be performed. 4. Some babies cry for prolonged periods in spite of feeding and comforting and this is distressing for all concerned. 5 If crying is of sudden onset, it may be due to a urinary tract, middle ear or meningeal infection; pain from an unrecognized fracture; oesophagitis; or torsion of the testis. 6. Teething does not cause vomiting, diarrhoea, high fever or seizures. 7. In colic paroxysmal, inconsolable crying or screaming often accompanied by drawing up of the knees and passage of excessive flatus takes place several times a day. 8. In young children it is essential not to delay the diagnosis and treatment of acute appendicitis, as progression to perforation can be rapid. 9. Of the surgical causes, appendicitis is by far the most common. 10. Causes of surgical pain are: appendicitis, intestinal

obstruction, inguinal hernia, peritonitis, inflamed Meckel diverticulum, pancreatitis, or trauma. 11. Causes of medical pain are: gastroenteritis, urinary tract infection, acute pyelonephritis, hydronephrosis, renal calculus, Henoch-Schönlein purpura, diabetic ketoacidosis, sickle cell disease, hepatitis, inflammatory bowel disease, constipation, gynaecological problems, or lead poisoning.

Text 2
Acute appendicitis
The clinical features of acute uncomplicated appendicitis are:

Symptoms
- Anorexia
- Vomiting
- Abdominal pain, initially central and colicky but then localizing to the right iliac fossa.

Signs
- Fever
- Abdominal pain aggravated on walking, coughing, jumping, bumps on the road during a car journey
- Persistent tenderness with guarding in the right iliac fossa

Appendicectomy is straightforward in uncomplicated appendicitis. Complicated appendicitis includes the presence of an appendix mass, an abscess, or perforation. It may be reasonable to elect for conservative management with intravenous antibiotics, with appendicectomy being performed after several weeks.

Intussusception
Intussusception describes the invagination of proximal bowel into a distal segment. Presentation is typical with:
- Paroxysmal, severe colicky pain with pallor
- May refuse feeds, may vomit, which may become bile stained
- A sausage shaped mass — often palpable in the abdomen
- Passage of a characteristic redcurrant jelly stool comprising blood-stained mucus.
- Abdominal distension and shock.

Exercise 2
Study the following summary and then interpret basic information in English.

1. Pyloric stenosis
More common in boys and in those with a family history.
Signs are visible gastric peristalsis, palpable abdominal mass on test feed, and possible dehydration.
Associated with hyponatraemia, hypokalaemia, and hypochloremic alkalosis.
Diagnosis may be confirmed by ultrasound.
Treated by surgery after rehydration and correction of electrolyte imbalance.
2. Acute abdominal pain in older children and adolescents
Exclude medical causes, in particular lower lobe pneumonia, diabetic ketoacidosis, hepatitis, and pyelonephritis.
Check for strangulated hernia or torsion of the testis in boys.
On palpating the abdomen in children with acute appendicitis, guarding and rebound tenderness are often absent but pain may be demonstrated on coughing, walking or jumping.
To distinguish between acute appendicitis and non-specific abdominal pain may require close monitoring, joint management between paediatricians and paediatric surgeons and evaluation in hospital.
3. Intussusception
Usually occurs between 3 months and 2 years of age.
Clinical features are paroxysmal, colicky pain with pallor, abdominal mass and redcurrant jelly stool.
Shock is an important complication and requires urgent treatment.
Reduction is attempted by rectal air insufflation unless peritonitis is present.
Surgery is required if reduction with air is unsuccessful or for peritonitis.
4. Meckel diverticulum
Generally asymptomatic, but may present with bleeding (which may be life-threatening) or intussusception or volvulus.
Treatment is by surgical resection.
5. Malrotation
Uncommon but important to diagnose.
Usually presents in the first 1—3 days of life with intestinal obstruction.
May present at any age with volvulus causing obstruction and ischaemic bowel.
Clinical features are bilious vomiting, abdominal pain and tenderness from peritonitis or ischaemic bowel.
An urgent upper gastrointestinal contrast study is indicated if there is bilious vomiting.
Treatment is urgent surgical correction.

Recurrent abdominal pain

Recurrent abdominal pain is a common problem. It is often defined as pain sufficient to interrupt normal activities and lasts for at least 3 months. The pain is characteristically periumbilical and the children are otherwise entirely well. Constipation is a frequent cause and must be excluded. In some children, it may be a manifestation of stress or it may become part of a vicious cycle of anxiety with escalating pain. There is evidence that anxiety may lead to altered bowel motility, which may be perceived by the child as pain. Many children will have distinct symptom constellations resulting from functional abnormalities of gut motility, irritable bowel syndrome, constipation, coeliac disease, abdominal migraine and functional dyspepsia.

Management

The aim is to identify any serious cause without subjecting the child to unnecessary investigation. To do this, a full history and thorough examination is required, which includes inspection of the perineum for anal fissures. A urine microscopy and culture are mandatory as urinary tract infections may cause pain. An abdominal ultrasound is particularly helpful in excluding gall stones and pelvic-ureteric junction obstruction. It is also necessary to make a distinction between 'serious' and 'dangerous'. These disorders can be serious, if for example, they lead to substantial loss of schooling, but they are not dangerous.

Exercise 3
Answer the following questions. Prepare short talks and/or dialogues on these topics

1. What are the clinical features of acute uncomplicated appendicitis?
2. Describe intussusception.
3. Characterize recurrent abdominal pain and its management.

Translation 2

1. The clinical features of acute uncomplicated appendicitis are: anorexia, vomiting, abdominal pain, and fever. 2. Appendicectomy is straightforward in uncomplicated appendicitis. 3. Intussusception describes the invagination of proximal bowel into a distal segment. 4. Presentation is typical with: paroxysmal, severe colicky pain with pallor, the child may refuse feeds, vomit may become bile stained, and there is passage of a characteristic redcurrant jelly stool comprising blood-stained mucus. 5. Recurrent abdominal pain is often defined as pain sufficient to interrupt normal activities and lasts for at least 3 months. 6. There is evidence that

anxiety may lead to altered bowel motility, which may be perceived by the child as pain. 7. Many children will have irritable bowel syndrome, constipation, coeliac disease, abdominal migraine and functional dyspepsia. 8. A urine microscopy and culture is mandatory as urinary tract infections may cause pain. 9. An abdominal ultrasound is particularly helpful in excluding gall stones and pelvic-ureteric junction obstruction.

Text 3
Irritable bowel syndrome

This disorder is associated with altered gastrointestinal motility and an abnormal sensation of intra-abdominal events. There is often a positive family history and a characteristic set of symptoms:
- non-specific abdominal pain
- explosive, loose, or mucousy stools
- bloating
- feeling of incomplete defecation
- constipation (often alternating with normal or loose stools).

Causes and assessment of the child with recurrent abdominal pain
Gastrointestinal
- Irritable bowel syndrome
- Constipation
- Non-ulcer dyspepsia
- Abdominal migraine
- Gastritis and peptic ulceration
- Eosinophilic oesophagitis
- Inflammatory bowel disease
- Malrotation

Gynaecological
- Dysmenorrhoea
- Ovarian cyst
- Pelvic inflammatory disease

Hepatobiliary/pancreatic
- Hepatitis
- Gall stones
- Pancreatitis

Urinary tract
- Urinary tract infection

- Pelvic-ureteric junction (PUJ) obstruction

Psychosocial — bullying, abuse, stress, etc. — a small proportion
Symptoms and signs that suggest organic disease
- Epigastric pain at night, haematemesis (duodenal ulcer)
- Diarrhoea, weight loss, growth failure, blood in stools (inflammatory bowel disease)
- Vomiting (pancreatitis)
- Jaundice (liver disease)
- Dysuria, secondary enuresis (urinary tract infection)
- Bilious vomiting and abdominal distension (malrotation)

Gastroenteritis

It is a cause of significant morbidity, particularly in younger children. In gastroenteritis, death is from dehydration; its prevention or correction is the mainstay of management. Rapid intravenous therapy is indicated in shock from gastroenteritis. However, it may be harmful in head injury, malnutrition or diabetic ketoacidosis.

Conditions that can mimic gastroenteritis

Systemic infection	Septicaemia, meningitis
Local infection	Respiratory tract infection, otitis media, hepatitis A, urinary tract infection
Surgical disorders	Pyloric stenosis, intussusception, acute appendicitis, necrotizing enterocolitis, Hirschsprung disease
Metabolic disorder	Diabetic ketoacidosis
Renal disorder	Haemolytic uremic syndrome
Other	Coeliac disease, cow's milk protein allergy, lactose intolerance, adrenalin sufficiency

Dehydration

The following children are at increased risk of dehydration:
- infants, particularly those under 6 months of age or those born with low birthweight
- if they have passed six or more diarrhoeal stools in the previous 24 hours
- if they have vomited three or more times in the previous 24 hours

- if they have been unable to tolerate extra fluids
- if they have malnutrition

The history and examination are used to assess the degree of dehydration as:
- no clinically detectable dehydration
- clinical dehydration
- shock — must be identified without delay

Clinical features of shock from dehydration in an infant
- Decreased level of consciousness
- Sunken fontanelle
- Dry mucous membranes
- Eyes sunken and tearless
- Tachypnoea
- Prolonged capillary refill time
- Tachycardia
- Weak peripheral pulses
- Reduced tissue turgor
- Pale or mottled skin
- Hypotension
- Sudden weight loss
- Reduced urine output
- Cold extremities

Clinical assessment of dehydration

	Clinical dehydration	Shock
General appearance	Appears unwell or deteriorating	Appears unwell or deteriorating
Conscious level	Altered responsiveness, e.g. irritable, lethargic	Decreased level of consciousness
Urine output	Decreased	Decreased
Skin colour	Normal	Pale or mottled
Extremities	Warm	Cold
Eyes	Sunken	Grossly sunken
Mucous membranes	Dry	Dry
Heart rate	Tachycardia	Tachycardia
Breathing	Tachypnoea	Tachypnoea
Peripheral pulses	Normal	Weak
Capillary refill time	Normal	Prolonged (<2 s)

Skin turgor	Reduced	Reduced
Blood pressure	Normal	Hypotension (indicates decompensated)

Exercise 4
Answer the following questions. Prepare short talks and/or dialogues on these topics

1. Explain causes and assessment of the child with recurrent abdominal pain (gastrointestinal, gynaecological, hepatobiliary/ pancreatic, urinary tract, psychosocial).
2. Describe symptoms and signs that suggest organic disease.
3. Characterize gastroenteritis and conditions that can mimic gastroenteritis.
4. Speak about children who are at increased risk of dehydration.
5. What are clinical features of shock from dehydration in an infant?
6. Describe clinical assessment of dehydration and shock.

Translation 3
1. Irritable bowel syndrome is associated with altered gastrointestinal motility. 2. There is often a positive family history and a characteristic set of symptoms: abdominal pain, explosive, loose, or mucousy stools, bloating, feeling of incomplete defecation, and constipation. 3. Gastrointestinal causes in the child with recurrent abdominal pain are: irritable bowel syndrome, constipation, non-ulcer dyspepsia, abdominal migraine, gastritis and peptic ulceration, Eosinophilic oesophagitis, inflammatory bowel disease, and malrotation. 4. Gynaecological causes are: dysmenorrhoea, ovarian cyst, or pelvic inflammatory disease. 5. Other causes are: hepatitis, gall stones, pancreatitis, urinary tract infection, pelvic-ureteric junction obstruction. 6. Symptoms and signs that suggest organic disease include: epigastric pain at night, haematemesis, diarrhoea, jaundice, weight loss, growth failure, blood in stools, vomiting, dysuria, bilious vomiting and abdominal distension. 7. Conditions that can mimic gastroenteritis are: septicaemia, meningitis, respiratory tract infection, otitis media, hepatitis A, urinary tract infection, pyloric stenosis, intussusception, acute appendicitis, necrotizing enterocolitis, Hirschsprung disease, diabetic ketoacidosis, haemolytic uremic syndrome, Coeliac disease, cow's milk protein allergy, lactose intolerance, or adrenal insufficiency.

Exercise 5

Match the column A with the column B. Try to learn the expressions and/or sentences by heart.

A

1. The history and examination are used to assess the degree of dehydration as: ...
2. Clinical features of shock from dehydration in an infant include: ...
3. Clinical assessment of dehydration includes: ...

B

a. *... general appearance, conscious level, urine output, skin colour, cold extremities, eyes, mucous membranes, heart rate, breathing, peripheral pulses, capillary refill time, skin turgor, and blood pressure.*

b. *... no clinically detectable dehydration, clinical dehydration, shock – must be identified without delay.*

c. *... decreased level of consciousness, sunken fontanelle, dry mucous membranes, eyes sunken and tearless, tachypnoea, prolonged capillary refill time, tachycardia, weak peripheral pulses, reduced tissue turgor, pale or mottled skin, hypotension, sudden weight loss, reduced urine output, cold extremities.*

Text 4

Fluid management of dehydration due to gastroenteritis

No clinical dehydration

Prevent dehydration

- Continue breastfeeding and other milk feeds
- Encourage fluid intake to compensate for increased gastrointestinal losses
- Discourage fruit juices and carbonated drinks
- Oral rehydration solution (ORS) and supplemental fluid if at increased risk of dehydration

Clinical dehydration

⇓

Oral rehydration solution

- Give fluid deficit replacement (50mL/kg) over 4 hours as well as maintenance fluid requirement. Give ORS often and in small amounts.
- Continue breastfeeding.
- Consider supplementing ORS with usual fluids if inadequate intake of ORS.
- If inadequate fluid intake or vomits persistently, consider giving ORS via nasogastric tube.

Shock

⇓

Intravenous therapy

- Give bolus of 0.9% sodium chloride solution. Repeat if necessary. If remains shocked, consider consulting paediatric intensive care specialist.

Intravenous therapy for rehydration

- Replace fluid deficit over 24 hours in most cases and give maintenance fluids.
- Unless a recent weight measurement is available, clinical estimation of hydration status is difficult.
- Monitor plasma for electrolytes, urea, creatinine, and glucose. Consider intravenous potassium supplementation.
- Continue breastfeeding if possible.

⇓

After rehydration

- Give full strength milk and reintroduce usual solid food.
- Avoid fruit juices and carbonated drinks.
- Advise parents — diligent handwashing, towels used by infected child not to be shared, do not return to childcare facility or school until 48 hours after last episode.

Malabsorption

Disorders affecting the digestion or absorption of nutrients manifests as:

- abnormal stools
- poor weight gain or faltering growth
- specific nutrient deficiencies

The true malabsorption stool is difficult to flush down the toilet and has an odour that pervades the whole house. Some disorders affecting the small intestinal mucosa or pancreas may lead to the malabsorption of many nutrients.

Coeliac disease

Coeliac disease is an enteropathy in which the gliadin fraction of gluten and other related prolamins in wheat, barley, and rye provoke a damaging immunological response in the proximal small intestinal mucosa. Villi become progressively shorter and then absent, leaving a flat mucosa. The classical presentation is of a profound malabsorptive syndrome at 8 — 24 months of age after the introduction of wheat-containing weaning foods. There is faltering growth, abdominal distension and buttock wasting, abnormal stools, and general irritability.

Management

All products containing wheat, rye, and barley are removed from the diet and this results in resolution of symptoms. Supervision by a dietician is essential. The gluten-free diet should be adhered to for life. Non-adherence to the diet risks the development of micronutrient deficiency, especially osteopenia, and there is increased risk in bowel malignancy, especially small bowel lymphoma.

Exercise 6
Answer the following questions. Prepare short talks and/or dialogues on these topics

1. Explain fluid management of dehydration due to gastroenteritis.
2. Describe intravenous therapy for rehydration.
3. What is meant by the term malabsorption?
4. Characterize coeliac disease.

Translation 4

1. To prevent dehydration continue breastfeeding and other milk feeds, encourage fluid intake and discourage fruit juices and carbonated drinks. 2. Give oral rehydration solution often and in small amounts, consider giving ORS via nasogastric tube. 3. If the baby remains shocked, consider

consulting paediatric intensive care specialist. 4. Replace fluid deficit over 24 hours, monitor plasma for electrolytes, urea, creatinine, and glucose. 5. Consider intravenous potassium supplementation. 6. Advise parents diligent handwashing, towels used by infected child not to be shared. 7. Disorders affecting the digestion or absorption of nutrients manifests as: abnormal stools, poor weight gain or faltering growth, and specific nutrient deficiencies. 8. Some disorders affecting the small intestinal mucosa or pancreas may lead to the malabsorption of many nutrients.

Exercise 7
Match the column A with the column B. Try to learn the expressions and/or sentences by heart.

A

1. Coeliac disease is an enteropathy in which the gliadin fraction of gluten and other related prolamins ...
2. The classical presentation is of a profound malabsorptive syndrome ...
3. All products containing wheat, rye, and barley ...
4. Non-adherence to the diet risks the development of micronutrient deficiency, ...

B

a. ... *at 8-24 months of age after the introduction of wheat-containing weaning foods.*
b. ... *in wheat, barley, and rye provoke a damaging immunological response in the proximal small intestinal mucosa.*
c. ... *especially osteopenia, and there is increased risk in bowel malignancy, especially small bowel lymphoma*
d. ... *are removed from the diet and the gluten-free diet should be adhered to for life.*

Text 5
Causes of nutrient malabsorption

Cholestatic liver disease or biliary atresia

Bile salts no longer enter duodenum in the bile. This leads to effective solubilization of the products of triglyceride hydrolysis. Fat and fat-soluble malabsorption result.

Exocrine pancreatic dysfunction, e.g. cystic fibrosis
Absent lipase, proteases, and amylase lead to defective digestion on triglyceride, protein, and starch ('pan-nutrient malabsorption')

Small-intestinal mucosal disease
- Loss of absorptive surface area, e.g. coeliac disease
- Specific enzyme defects, e.g. transient lactase deficiency following gastroenteritis, but is uncommon
- Specific transport defects, e.g. glucose-galactose malabsorption (severe life-threatening diarrhoea with first milk feed), acrodermatitis enteropathica (zinc malabsorption, also erythematous rash around mouth and anus)

Lymphatic leakage or obstruction
Chylomicrons (containing absorbed lipids) unable to reach thoracic duct and the systemic circulation, e.g. intestinal lymphangiectasia (abnormal lymphatics)

Short bowel syndrome
Small-intestinal resection, due to congenital anomalies or necrotizing enterocolitis, leads to nutrient, water and electrolyte malabsorption

Loss of terminal ileal function e.g. resection or Crohn's disease
Absent bile acid and vitamin B_{12} absorption

Chronic non-specific diarrhoea
This condition is the most common cause of persistent loose stools in preschool children. The stools are of varying consistency, sometimes well formed, sometimes explosive and loose. The presence of undigested vegetables in the stools is common. Affected children are well and thriving. The diarrhoea may result from undiagnosed coeliac disease or excessive ingestion of fruit juice, especially apple juice. Occasionally the cause is temporary cow's milk allergy.

Exercise 8
Study the following summary and then interpret basic information in English.

1. Gastroenteritis
Results in death from dehydration of hundreds of thousands of children worldwide every year.

Is mostly viral, but it can be caused by Campylobacter, Shigella, and Salmonella and other organisms.
Infants are particularly susceptible to dehydration.
Dehydration is assessed as no clinical dehydration, clinical dehydration or shock according to symptoms and signs.
Oral rehydration solution is the mainstay of treatment and usually effective; intravenous fluid is only required for shock or ongoing vomiting or clinical deterioration.
2. Coeliac disease
A gluten sensitive enteropathy.
Classical presentation is at 8-24 months of age with abnormal stools, faltering growth, abdominal distension, muscle wasting, and irritability.
Other, more subtle, modes of presentation — e.g. short stature, anaemia, abdominal pain and screening, e.g. children with diabetes mellitus, are now much more common.
Diagnosis — positive serology, flat mucosa on duodenal biopsy and resolution of symptoms and catch-up growth upon gluten withdrawal.
Treatment — gluten-free diet for life.
3. Chronic diarrhoea
In an infant with faltering growth, consider coeliac disease and cow's milk protein allergy.
Following bowel resection, cholestatic liver disease or exocrine pancreatic dysfunction, consider malabsorption.
In an otherwise well toddler with undigested vegetables in stool, consider chronic non-specific diarrhoea.

Inflammatory bowel disease

The incidence of inflammatory bowel disease in children has increased markedly in the last two decades. Crohn's disease is more common than ulcerative colitis. Crohn's disease can affect any part of the gastrointestinal tract from mouth to anus, whereas in ulcerative colitis the inflammation is confined to the colon. Inflammatory bowel disease may cause poor general health, restrict growth, and have an adverse effect on psychological well-being.

Crohn's disease

Lethargy and general ill health without gastrointestinal symptoms can be mistaken for psychological problems. It may also mimic anorexia nervosa.

Presentation of Crohn's disease in children and adolescents
Growth failure

Puberty delayed

Classical presentation (25%):
- abdominal pain
- diarrhoea
- weight loss

General ill health:
- fever
- lethargy
- weight loss

Extra intestinal manifestations:
- oral lesions or perianal skin tags
- uveitis
- arthralgia
- erythema nodosum

Ulcerative colitis

Ulcerative colitis is a recurrent, inflammatory and ulcerating disease involving the mucosa of the colon. Characteristically, the disease presents with rectal bleeding, diarrhoea and colicky pain. Weight loss and growth failure may occur.

Constipation

Constipation is an extremely common reason for consultation in children. Parents may use the term to describe decreased frequency of defecation, the degree of hardness of the stool or painful defecation. After 1 year of age, most children have a daily bowel action. A pragmatic definition of constipation is the infrequent passage of dry, hardened faeces often accompanied by straining or pain and bleeding associated with hard stools. The constipation may have been precipitated by dehydration or reduced fluid intake or an anal fissure causing pain.

Hirschsprung disease

The abnormal bowel extends from the rectum for a variable distance proximally, ending in a normally innervated, dilated colon. Presentation is usually in the neonatal period with intestinal obstruction. Occasionally, infants present with severe, life-threatening Hirschsprung enterocolitis during the first few weeks of life. Later in childhood, presentation is with chronic constipation. Growth failure may also be present.

Exercise 9
Answer the following questions. Prepare short talks and/or dialogues on these topics

1. Characterize causes of nutrient malabsorption (cholestatic liver disease or biliary atresia, exocrine pancreatic dysfunction, small-intestinal mucosal disease, lymphatic leakage or obstruction, short bowel syndrome, loss of terminal ileal function, chronic non-specific diarrhoea).
2. Describe inflammatory bowel disease.
3. Explain presentation of Crohn's disease in children and adolescents (growth failure, puberty delayed, general ill health, extra intestinal manifestations).
4. What do you know about ulcerative colitis, constipation and Hirschsprung disease?

Translation 5
1. Absent lipase, proteases, and amylase lead to defective digestion on triglyceride, protein, and starch ('pan-nutrient malabsorption'). 2. Small-intestinal mucosal disease means loss of absorptive surface area, specific enzyme defects, and specific transport defects. 3. In short bowel syndrome small-intestinal resection, due to congenital anomalies or necrotizing enterocolitis, leads to nutrient, water and electrolyte malabsorption. 4. Chronic non-specific diarrhoea is the most common cause of persistent loose stools in preschool children. 5. The diarrhoea may result from undiagnosed coeliac disease or excessive ingestion of fruit juice, especially apple juice. 6. Crohn's disease can affect any part of the gastrointestinal tract from mouth to anus, whereas in ulcerative colitis the inflammation is confined to the colon. 7. Inflammatory bowel disease may cause poor general health, restrict growth, and have an adverse effect on psychological well-being.

Exercise 10
Study the following summary and then interpret basic information in English.

1. Lethargy and general ill health without gastrointestinal symptoms can be mistaken for psychological problems.

2. Ulcerative colitis is a recurrent, inflammatory and ulcerating disease involving the mucosa of the colon.
3. Characteristically, the disease presents with rectal bleeding, diarrhoea and colicky pain.
4. Parents may use the term constipation to describe decreased frequency of defecation, the degree of hardness of the stool or painful defecation.
5. The constipation may have been precipitated by dehydration or reduced fluid intake or an anal fissure causing pain.
6. In Hirschsprung disease the abnormal bowel extends from the rectum for a variable distance proximally, ending in a normally innervated, dilated colon.
7. Occasionally, infants present with severe, life-threatening Hirschsprung enterocolitis during the first few weeks of life.

Text 6
Infection and immunity

Features of infection and immunity in children are:

- acute respiratory infections, diarrhoea, neonatal infection, malaria, measles, and HIV infection, often accompanied by undernutrition.
- serious infections still occur, e.g. pneumonia, sepsis and meningitis, and require early recognition and treatment
- some diseases have emerged again, e.g. tuberculosis (TB)
- there has been a rise of methicillin-resistant Staphylococcus aureus
- with air travel, 'tropical diseases' are now encountered in all countries. Epidemics are spreading more rapidly, e.g. severe acute respiratory syndrome (SARS) and H1N1 influenza virus
- immunization has played a major role in reducing morbidity and mortality of infections throughout the world

Worldwide causes of death in children < 5 years
Neonatal (< 4 weeks)

- Neonatal infection
- Congenital anomalies
- Intrapartum related complications including birth asphyxia
- Prematurity

Post neonatal (4 weeks — 5 years)

- Pneumonia
- Diarrhoea
- Malaria
- HIV/AIDS
- Measles

- Injuries
- Congenital anomalies

The febrile child
Most febrile children have a brief, self-limiting viral infection, e.g. otitis media or tonsillitis.

Clinical features
How is fever identified in children?
A fever in children is a temperature over 37.5°C. In general, axillary temperatures underestimate body temperature by 0.5°C.

How old is the child?
- Febrile infants less than 3 months of age can present with non-specific clinical features. During the first few months of life infants are relatively protected against common viral infections because of passive immunity acquired by transplacental transfer of antibodies from their mothers.

Are there risk factors for infection?
These include:
- illness of other family members
- specific illness prevalent in the community
- lack of immunization
- recent travel abroad (consider malaria, typhoid, and viral hepatitis)
- contact with animals (consider brucellosis, Q fever, and haemolytic uremic syndrome)
- increased susceptibility from immunodeficiency

How ill is the child?
- Fever over 38°C if aged less than 3 months, 39°C if 3 months to 6 months of age
- colour — pale, mottled, or cyanosed
- level of consciousness is reduced, neck stiffness, bulging fontanelle, status epilepticus, focal neurological signs, or seizures
- significant respiratory distress
- bile-stained vomiting
- severe dehydration and shock

Is there a rash?
- Rashes often accompany febrile illnesses, e.g. a purpuric rash in meningococcal septicaemia

Is there a focus of infection?
- Identify a focus of infection. However, if no focus is identified, this is often because it is the prodromal phase of a viral illness, but may indicate potentially serious bacterial infection, especially urinary tract infection or septicaemia.

Management

Children who are significantly unwell, particularly if there is no focus of infection, will require investigations and observation or treatment in a paediatric assessment unit. Parenteral antibiotics should be given immediately to seriously unwell children. The use of antipyretic agents should be considered. Either paracetamol or ibuprofen can be used.

Diagnostic clues to evaluating the febrile child
- Upper respiratory tract infection — Very common, may be coincidental with another more serious illness
- Otitis media — Always examine tympanic membranes in febrile children
- Tonsillitis — Erythema or exudate on the tonsils?
- Viral croup?
- Bacterial tracheitis?
- Pneumonia — Fever, cough, raised respiratory rate, chest recession, abnormal auscultation. In infants, auscultation may be normal — diagnosis may require chest X-ray
- Septicaemia — Can be difficult to recognize in absence of rash before shock develops; Early signs of tachycardia, tachypnoea, and poor perfusion
- Need to start antibiotics on clinical suspicion without waiting for culture results
- Meningitis/encephalitis — Lethargy, loss of interest in surrounding, drowsiness or coma, seizures
- Older children — headache, photophobia, neck stiffness, positive Kernig sign (pain on leg straightening)
- Younger children and infants — non-specific symptoms and signs
- Raised intracranial pressure — reduced conscious level, abnormal pupillary responses, abnormal posturing, Cushing triad (bradycardia, hypertension, abnormal pattern of breathing)

- Late signs — papilledema, bulging fontanelle in infants, opisthotonos (hypertension of head and back)
- Seizure — Febrile seizure?
- Meningitis?
- Encephalitis?
- Periorbital cellulitis
- Redness and swelling of the eyelids — May spread to orbit of the eye
- Rash
- Viral exanthem?
- Purpura from meningococcal infection
- Urinary tract infection — Urine sample needed for any seriously ill young child or any febrile illness that does not settle
- Abdominal pain?
- Appendicitis?
- Pyelonephritis?
- Hepatitis?
- Diarrhoea
- Gastroenteritis?
- Fever with blood and mucus in the stool: Shigella, Salmonella, or Campylobacter
- Osteomyelitis or septic arthritis
- Suspect if painful bone or joint or reluctance to move limb
- Prolonged fever

Exercise 11
Study the following summary and then interpret basic information in English.

1. Hirschsprung disease
Absence of myenteric plexuses of rectum and variable distance of colon.
Presentation — usually intestinal obstruction in the newborn period following delay in passing meconium. In later childhood — profound chronic constipation, abdominal distension, and growth failure.
2. The febrile child
Upper respiratory tract infection is a very common cause
Diagnosis — suction rectal biopsy.
Check for otitis media
Serious bacterial infection must be considered, especially urinary tract infection or septicaemia

The younger the child, the lower the threshold for performing a septic screen and starting antibiotics.

Exercise 12
Answer the following questions. Prepare short talks and/or dialogues on these topics

1. What are features of acute respiratory infections, diarrhoea, neonatal infection, malaria, measles, HIV infection, and undernutrition?
2. Describe serious infections (pneumonia, sepsis and meningitis, tuberculosis, methicillin-resistant Staphylococcus aureus, severe acute respiratory syndrome (SARS), and H1N1 influenza virus).
3. Describe worldwide causes of death in children < 5 years.
4. Characterize clinical features of the febrile child.
5. What do you know about the risk factors for infection?
6. Characterize diagnostic clues to evaluating the febrile child (upper respiratory tract infection, otitis media, tonsillitis, viral croup, bacterial tracheitis, pneumonia, septicaemia, meningitis, encephalitis).
7. Speak about other diagnostic clues (photophobia, positive Kernig sign, abnormal pupillary responses, abnormal posturing, Cushing triad, papilledema).
8. What are non-specific symptoms and signs in younger children and infants (abnormal pupillary responses, abnormal posturing, Cushing triad, papilledema, opisthotonos)
9. Characterize febrile seizure, meningitis, encephalitis, periorbital cellulitis, redness and swelling of the eyelids, rash.
10. Explain the terms: viral exanthem, purpura from meningococcal infection, appendicitis, pyelonephritis, hepatitis, gastroenteritis, osteomyelitis and septic arthritis.

Translation 6

1. Features of infection in children are: acute respiratory infections, diarrhoea, neonatal infection, malaria, measles, and HIV infection. 2. Serious infections still occur, e.g. pneumonia, sepsis and meningitis, tuberculosis (TB), methicillin-resistant Staphylococcus aureus, severe acute respiratory syndrome (SARS) and H1N1 influenza virus. 3. Immunization has played a major role in reducing morbidity and mortality of infections throughout the world. 4. Worldwide causes of death in children under 5 years are: neonatal infection, congenital anomalies, intrapartum related

complications, prematurity. 5. Most febrile children have a brief, self-limiting viral infection, e.g. otitis media or tonsillitis. 6. During the first few months of life infants are relatively protected against common viral infections because of passive immunity acquired by transplacental transfer of antibodies from their mothers. 7. The risk factors for infection include: illness of other family members, lack of immunization, recent travel abroad, contact with animals. 8. Children who are significantly unwell, particularly if there is no focus of infection, will require investigations and observation or treatment in a paediatric assessment unit. 9. Parenteral antibiotics should be given immediately to seriously unwell children. 10. The use of antipyretic agents should be considered. 11. Diagnostic clues to evaluating the febrile child are: upper respiratory tract infection, otitis media, tonsillitis, viral croup, bacterial tracheitis, pneumonia, septicaemia, meningitis, encephalitis, drowsiness or coma, and seizures.

Key 1
Exercise 5
1b; 2c; 3a

Exercise 7
1b; 2a; 3d; 4c

VOCABULARY 1

abdominal /æbˈdɒm.ɪ.nəl/
abruption /əˈbrʌp.ʃən/
abscess /ˈæb.ses/
achondroplasia /eɪˌkɒn.drəˈpleɪ.ʒə/
acrodermatitis /ˌækrəʊ.dɜːməˈtaɪtɪs/
acrodermatitis /ˌækrəʊ.dɜːməˈtaɪtɪs/ **chronica** /krɒnɪkə/
act /ækt/ **out** /aʊt/
adenomatoid /ˈædɪ.nɔˈmæ.tɔɪd/
adhere /ədˈhɪər/
aggravate /ˈæg.rə.veɪt/
alcohol /ˈæl.kə.hɒl/ **syndrome** /ˈsɪndrəʊm/
alert /priː.əˈlɜːt/
alkalosis /al.kə.ˈləʊ.səs/
altered /ˈɒl.tərd/
amniotic /ˌæm.niˈɒt.ɪk/ **fluid** /ˈfluː.ɪd/
anal /ˈeɪ.nəl/
anencephaly /æn.en.ˈse.fə.liː/
antepartum /ˈæn.tiˈpɑː.təm/
antibody /ˈæn.tiˌbɒd.i/
antipyretic /ˈæn.tɪpaɪəˈret.ɪk/
anti-thyroid /ˌæn.ti.thaɪ.ˌrɔːid/ **drug** /drʌg/
aorta /eɪˈɔː.tə/
apathetic /ˌæpəˈθetɪk/
apnoea /ˈæp.ni.ə/
appendicectomy /əˌpendɪˈsektəmɪ/
array /əˈreɪ/
artery /ˈɑːtərɪ/
arthralgia /ɑːˈθrældʒə/
assumption /əˈsʌmp.ʃən/
atherosclerosis /ˌæθ.ə.rəʊ.skləˈrəʊ.sɪs/
atrophicans /əˈtrɒfɪkəns/
autosomal /ˌɔː.tə.ˈsəʊ.məl/ **recessive** /rɪˈses.ɪv/ **disorder** /dɪsˈɔːdə/
aware /əˈweər/
axial /ˈæk.si.əl/
barley /ˈbɑː.li/
behave /bɪˈheɪv/
bile /baɪl/ **salts** /sɒlts/
bilious /ˈbɪliəs/
biopsy /ˈbaɪɒpsɪ/
birthweight /bɜːθ.weɪt/
bizarre /bɪˈzɑːr/
bloating /ˈbləʊ.tɪŋ/
blue-veined /bluː ˈveɪnd/ **cheese** /tʃiːz/
bolus /bəʊ.ləs/
bowel /ˈbaʊ.əl/

25

brie /briː/
Brucellosis /ˌbruː.səˈləʊ.səs/
buggery /ˈbʌgərɪ/
burdensome /ˈbɜːdən.səm/
calculus /ˈkæl.kjʊ.ləs/ pl **calculi**
campylobacter /ˌkam.pi.ləʊ.ˈbak.tər/
cardiomyopathy /ˌkɑːr.diə.maɪˈɒp.ə.θi/
catch /kætʃ/ **up** /ʌp/ **with** /wɪð/
cervical /səˈvai.kəl/
childcare /ˈtʃaɪldˌkeə/
chorioamnionitis /ˌkɔːri.əˌæm.ni.əˈnaɪ.tɪs/
chorionic /ˈkɔːr.ɪ.ən.ɪk/
chromosomal /ˌkrəʊ.məˈzəʊ.məl/
chylomicron /ˌkaɪ.ləʊ.ˈmaɪk.rəʊn/
cleft /kleft/ **lip** /lɪp/
coagulation /kəʊˈæg.jʊ.leɪˌʃən/
coarctation /ˌkəʊˈɑːkteɪˌʃən/
coeliac /ˈsiːlɪˌæk/ **disease** /dɪˈziːz/
coercive /kəʊˈɜːsɪv/
colorectal /kəʊ.ləʊˈrek.təl/
comforting /ˈkʌm.fə.tɪŋ/
confirmed /kənˈfɜːmd/
confront /kənˈfrʌnt/
conscious /ˈkɒn.tʃəs/
constellation /ˌkɒnstɪˈleɪʃən/
constipation /ˌkɒnt.stɪˈpeɪˌʃən/
conventional /kənˈventˌʃən.əl/
coronary /ˈkɒr.ən.ər.i/
correction /kəˈrekˌʃən/
craniofacial /ˌkreɪ.ni.əʊˌfeɪ.ʃəl/
crease /kriːs/
cubitus /kjuː.bit.əs/
cyst /sɪst/
dangerous /ˈdeɪn.dʒər.əs/
decompensated /diːˈkɒmpenˌseɪt.əd/
decrease /dɪˈkriːs/
defecation /ˌdef.əˈkeɪˌʃən/
delinquent /dɪˈlɪŋkwənt/
diabetic /ˌdaɪəˈbet.ɪk/ **ketoacidosis** /ˈkiːtəʊˌæs.ɪˈdəʊ.sɪs/
diaphragmatic /ˌdaɪə.frægˈmæt.ɪk/ **hernia** /ˈhɜː.ni.ə/
diligent /ˈdɪl.ɪ.dʒənt/
disabled /dɪˈseɪ.bəld/
discourage /dɪˈskʌr.ɪdʒ/
disease /dɪˈziːz/
dislocation /ˌdɪs.ləˈkeɪˌʃən/
disorder /dɪˈsɔː.dər/
distended /dɪˈstend.ɪd/

distinction /dɪˈstɪŋk.ʃən/
distinguish /dɪˈstɪŋ.gwɪʃ/
distressed /dɪˈstrest/
distressing /dɪˈstresɪŋ/
domestic /dəˈmes.tɪk/
donate /dəʊ ˈneɪt/
duct /dʌkt/
dysgenesis /ˌdis.ˈdʒe.nə.səs/
dysmenorrhoea /ˌdɪs.men.əˈriə/
dyspepsia /dɪˈspep.si.ə/
dysplastic /ˌdɪs.ˈplæs.tɪk/
Edwards /ˈed.wərdz/ **syndrome** /ˈsɪndrəʊm/
egression /iːˈgre.ʃən/
emerge /ɪˈmɜːdʒ/
empty /ˈemp.ti/
encephalocele /ɪn.ˈsef.ə.ləʊ.ˌsiːl/
encompass /ɪnˈkʌm.pəs/
engender /ɪnˈdʒendə/
enteropathy /ˌentərɒpəθɪ/
enticing /ɪnˈtaɪ.sɪŋ/
entirely /ɪnˈtaɪə.li/
enuresis /ˌen.jʊəˈriː.sɪs/
epicanthic /e.pəˈkan.thik/
epigastric /ˌep.ɪˈgæs.trɪk/
eruption /ɪˈrʌp.ʃən/
erythema /ˌer.ɪˈθiː.mə/
escalate /ˈes.kə.leɪt/
evasive /ɪˈveɪ.sɪv/
evert /ɪˈvɜːt/
exanthem /eg.ˈzan.thəm/
exocrine /ˈek.səʊ.kraɪn/
exomphalos /ˈeksˈɒmfəˌlɒs/
expertise /ˌek.spɜːˈtiːz/
exploitation /ˌek.splɔɪˈteɪ.ʃən/
eyelid / ˈaɪ.lɪd/
fabricate /ˈfæbrɪˌkeɪt/
fat-soluble /fæt ˈsɒljʊbəl/
femur /ˈfiː.mər/ pl **femora**
fertilization /ˌfɜːtɪlaɪˈzeɪʃən/
fetoscopy /ˈfiːtə.skə.piː/
fever /ˈfiː.vər/
field /fiːld/
fissure /ˈfɪʃ.ər/
flat /flæt/
flatus /ˈfleɪ.təs/
foetal /ˈfiː.təl/
fold /fəʊld/

forensic /fəˈren.zɪk/
forward /ˈfɔː.wəd/
fraction /ˈfræk.ʃən/
fretful /ˈfretfəl/
galactose /gəˈlak.ˌtəʊs/
gastroschisis /ˌgæs.trəʊˌs.kə.səs/
gene /dʒiːn/
genuinely /ˈdʒen.ju.ɪn.li/
gliadin /ˈglaɪ.ə.dən/
glucose /ˈgluː.kəʊs/
gluten /ˈgluːtən/
goitre /ˈgɔɪ.tər/
Graves disease /ˈgreɪvz dɪˌziːz/
gynecomastia /ˌgaɪ.nɪ.kəʊˈmæst.i.ə/
H1N1 influenza /ˌɪn.fluˈen.zə/ **virus** /ˈvaɪə.rəs/
haemolytic /ˌhiː.məˈlɪt.ɪk/
handwriting /ˈhændˌraɪtɪŋ/
hardness /ˈhɑːdnɪs/
harm /hɑːm/
helplessness /ˈhelplɪsnɪs/
hernial /ˈhɜː.ni.əl/
Hirschsprung /hirʃˈsprɜːng/ **disease** /dɪˈziːz/
hit /hɪt/
hydrolysis /haɪˈdrɒl.ə.sɪs/
hydronephrosis /haɪˈdrɒˈnef.rəʊ.sɪs/
hypercalcaemia /ˌhaɪ.pə.kælˈsiː.mi.ə/
hyperinsulinism/ˌhaɪ.pər.ˈint.sə.lə.ˌni.zəm/
hypertrophic /ˌhaɪ.pərˈtrɒf.ɪk/
hypertrophy /haɪˈpɜː.trə.fi/
hypochloraemia /ˈhaɪpəˈklɔː riːmɪə/
hypogonadism /ˌhaɪ.pəʊ.ˈgəʊ.ˌnad.ˌiz.əm/
hypokalaemia /ˌhaɪ.pəʊ.kæˈliː.mi.ə/
hypospadia /ˌhaɪ.pəʊˈspæ.di.ə/
identify /aɪˈden.tɪ.faɪ/
imbalance /ˌɪmˈbæl.ənt s/
implement /ˈɪm.plɪ.ment/
in vitro /ˌɪnˈviː.trəʊ/
incompatibility /ˌɪn.kəmˌpætəˈbɪlɪtɪ/
incomplete /ˌɪn.kəmˈpliːt/
inconsistency /ˌɪnkənˈsɪstənsɪ/
inconsolable /ˌɪnkənˈsəʊləbəl/
indifference /ɪnˈdɪf.ər.əns/
indifferent /ɪnˈdɪf.ər.ənt/
induced /ɪnˈdjuːst/
infertility /ˌɪn.fəˈtɪl.ɪ.ti/
inflamed /ɪnˈfleɪmd/
inflammatory /ɪnˈflæm.ə.tər.i/

inflict /ɪnˈflɪkt/
inherit /ɪnˈherɪt/
inheritance /ɪnˈherɪtəns/
innervate /ˈɪn.ə.vəɪt/
instability /ˌɪn.stəˈbɪl.ɪ.ti/
instance /ˈɪn.stəns/
insufflation /ˌɪn.səˈfleɪ.ʃən/
intra-abdominal /ɪn.trə.æbˈdɒm.ɪ.nəl/
intrapartum /ɪn.trəˈpɑː.təm/
intrusive /ɪnˈtruː.sɪv/
invagination /in.ˌva.dʒəˈneɪ.ʃən/
invent /ɪnˈvent/
investigation /ɪnˌves.tɪˈgeɪ.ʃən/
ischaemic /ɪˈskiː.mɪk/
jig /dʒɪg/
jitteriness /ˈdʒɪ.tə.rɪː.nəs/
junction /ˈdʒʌŋk.ʃən/
Kernig /ˈker.nig/ **sign** /saɪn/
Klinefelter's /ˈklaɪnˌfeltərz/ **syndrome** /ˈsɪndrəʊm/
lawyer /ˈlɔːjə/
laxity /ˈlæksɪtɪ/
ligature /ˈlɪg.ə.tʃər/
lipase /ˈlaɪ.peɪz/
litter /lɪtə/
lobe /ləʊb/
lymphangiectasia /lɪmfˌædʒɪekˈteɪ.zɪə/
lymphoedema /lɪm.fəˈdiːmə/
macrocephaly /ˌmækrəʊ.ˈsef.ə.li/
macroorchidism /ˈmæk.rəɔː.kɪd.ɪz.əm/
macrosomia /ˌmak.rə.ˈsəʊ.miː.ə/
magnitude /ˈmægnɪˌtjuːd/
mainstay /meɪnˌsteɪ/
maintenance /ˈmeɪntɪnəns/
maltreatment /ˌmælˈtriːt.mənt/
mandible /ˈmæn.dɪ.bəl/
Meckel /ˈmek.əl/ **diverticulum** /ˌdaɪ.vəˌtɪk.jʊ.ləm/ pl **diverticula**
membrane /ˈmem.breɪn/
Mendelian /men.ˈdiː.liː.ən/ **disorder** /dɪˈsɔː.dər/
mercury /ˈmɜː.kjʊ.ri/
methicillin /ˌmɛθ.ɪˈsɪl.ɪn/
methicillin-resistant /ˌmɛθ.ɪˈsɪl.ɪn rɪˈzɪstənt/
meticulous /məˈtɪk.jʊ.ləs/
micro /ˈmaɪ.krəʊ/
micronutrient /maɪˈkrɒ.ˈnjuː.tri.ənt/
microphthalmia /maɪˈkrɒ.ɑːf.ˈthal.miː.ə/
microvascular /ˌmaɪ.krəʊˈvæs.kjə.lər/
minority /maɪˈnɒrɪtɪ/

miscarriage /ˈmɪsˌkær.ɪdʒ/
miserable /ˈmɪzərəbəl/
mode /məʊd/
mole /məʊl/
motility /ˌməʊ.ˈtil.i.ˈtiː/
MRI—magnetic /mægˈnet.ɪk/ **resonance** /ˈrez.ən.əns/ **imaging** /ɪˈmɪdʒ.ɪŋ/
mucosa /mjuːˈkəʊ.sə/
mucous membrane /ˌmjuː.kəsˈmem.breɪn/
mucousy /mjuːˈkəʊ.sə/
mucus /ˈmjuː.kəs/
mutilation /ˌmjuː.tɪˈleɪ.ʃən/
myenteric /ˌmaɪ.ən.ˈter.ik/
nasal /ˈneɪ.zəl/
neural /ˈnjʊə.rəl/
nodose /nəʊ.ˈdəʊ.s/
non-adherence /ədˈhɪə.rənt s/
nonattendance /əˈten.dənts/
non-ulcer stomach /nɒn.ʌl.səˈstʌm.ək/ **pain** /peɪn/
Noonan /nuː.nən/ **syndrome** /ˈsɪndrəʊm/
noxious /ˈnɒk.ʃəs/
nuchal /nuː.kəl/
occiput /ˈɒk.sɪ.pʌt/
oesophageal /iːˌsɒfəˈdʒiːəl/
oligohydramnios /ˌɒlɪgəʊˈhaɪdrˈæmnɪəs/
ongoing /ˈɒŋˌgəʊ.ɪŋ/
oppositional /ˌɒp.əˈzɪʃ.ᵊn.ᵊl/
orbit /ˈɔːbɪt/
orifice /ˈɒr.ɪ.fɪs/
outlet /ˈaʊt.let/
ovarian /əʊˈveə.ri.ən/
overdistended /ˌəʊ.və.dɪˈstend.ɪd/
overlap /ˌəʊ.vəˈlæp/
overlying /ˌəʊ.vəlˈaɪ.ɪŋ/
overstimulation /ˌəʊ.vəˌstɪmjʊˈleɪʃən/
ovum /ˈəʊvəm/ **pl ova**
pallor /ˈpæl.ər/
palmar /pælm.ər/
palpable /ˈpæl.pə.bļ/
palpebral /ˈpæl.pɪ.brəl/
pancreatitis /ˌpæŋ.kri.əˈtaɪ.tɪs/
papilledema /pəˈpɪl.ə.ɪˈdiː.mə/
passage /ˈpæs.ɪdʒ/
Patau-syndrome /pɑːˈtau ˈsɪndrəʊm/
pâté /ˈpæteɪ/
pelvic /ˈpel.vɪk/ **inflammatory** /ɪnˈflæm.ə.tər.i/ **disease** /dɪˈziːz/
pelvi-ureteric /ˈpel.vəˌjʊr.ə.ˈter.ik/
perceive /pəˈsiːv/

performance /pəˈfɔː.məns/
perianal /ˌper.ɪ.ˈeɪ.nəl/
periorbital /ˌper.ɪ.ˈɔːbɪtəl/
periumbilical /ˌper.ɪ.ʌmˈbɪl.ɪ.kəl/
perpetrator /ˈpɜːpɪˌtreɪtə/
pervade /pɜːˈveɪd/
photophobia /ˈfəʊ.təʊˈfəʊ.bi.ə/
plausibility /ˌplɔːzəˈbɪlɪtɪ/
pleural /ˈplʊə.rəl/
plexus /ˈplek.səs/
poisoning /ˈpɔɪ.zən.ɪŋ/
pollutant /pəˈluːtənt/
polycythaemia /ˌpɒl.i.ˌsaɪ.ˈthiː.miː.ə/
polydactyly /ˌpaː.liː.ˈdak.tə.li/
polygenic /ˌpaː.liː.ˈdʒiː.nik/
polyhydramnios /ˈpaː.liː.haɪ.ˈdram.ni.ˌaːs/
positive /ˈpɒ.zɪ.tɪv/
posturing /ˈpɒs.tʃər.ɪŋ/
potassium /pəˈtæs.i.əm/
Prader-Willi /ˈpraː.dər.ˈvi.liː/ syndrome /ˈsɪndrəʊm/
precipitate /prɪˈsɪp.ɪ.teɪt/
pre-eclampsia /ˌpriː.ɪˈklæmp.si.ə/
prodromal /pro.drə.məl/
progression /prəˈgreʃ.ən/
prolapse /ˈprəʊ.læps/
protamine /ˈprəʊ.tə.mən/
protease /ˈprəʊ.tiː.eɪz/
protruding /prəˈtruːd.ɪŋ/
proximal /ˈprɒk.sɪ.məl/
pupillary /pjuː.pɪl.ər.i/
purpura /ˈpər.pjə.rə/
pyloric /paɪ.ˈlɔːr.ik/
Q: cardiac /ˈkaːdɪˌæk/ minute /ˈmɪnɪt/ output /ˈaʊtˌpʊt/
ravenously /ˈrævənəslɪ/
rearrangement / riː ˈəˈreɪndʒ.mənt/
rebound /ˌriːˈbaʊnd/ tenderness /ˈten.dər.nəs/
recessive /rɪˈses.ɪv/
refuse /rɪˈfjuːz/
rehydration /ˌriː.haɪˈdreɪˌʃən/
reluctance /rɪˈlʌktəns/
reproductive /ˌriː.prəˈdʌk.tɪv/
resection /rɪˈsek.ʃ°n/
rocker-bottom /ˈraː.kər ˈbaː.təm/
rush /rʌʃ/
rye /raɪ/
salmonella /ˌsæl.məˈnel.ə/ pl salmonellae
scalp /skælp/

scan /skæn/

Schönlein-Henoch purpura /ˌʃœn.laɪn ˈhen.əḵ ˈpər.pjə.rə/

schooling /ˈskuːlɪŋ/

scream /skriːm/

segment /ˈseg.mənt/

self-harm /ˌself hɑːm/

sensation /senˈseɪ.ʃən/

separation /ˌsepəˈreɪʃən/

septal /ˈsep.tᵊl/

serology /sɪˈrɒl.ə.dʒi/

settle /ˈset.l̩/

severe /sɪˈvɪə/ **acute** /əˈkjuːt/ **respiratory** /rɪˈspɪr.ə.tər.i/ **syndrome** /ˈsɪn.drəʊm/, **SARS**

shake /ʃeɪk/ **(shook, shaken)**

Shigella /ʃɪˈgel.ə/

shin /ʃɪn/

sickle-cell /ˈsɪk.l̩ sel/ **disease** /dɪˈziːz/

sodium /ˈsəʊ.di.əm/ **chloride** /ˈklɔːraɪd/

soil /sɔɪl/

solid /ˈsɒl.ɪd/

solubilization /ˌsɒljʊbəlaɪˈzeɪʃən/

splash /splæʃ/

spoil /spɔɪl/

spoon /spuːn/ **shaped** /ʃeɪpt/

Staphylococcus /ˌstæf.ɪl.əˈkɒk.əs/ *aureus* /ˈɔːriəs/

starch /stɑːtʃ/

stature /ˈstætʃ.ər/

stenosis /steˈnəʊ.sɪs/

stepparent /ˈstepˌpeərənt/

stiffness /ˈstɪf.nəs/

stillbirth /ˈstɪlˌbɜːθ/

stocking /ˈstɒkɪŋ/

straight /streɪt/

strain /streɪn/

stretch /stretʃ/

suffocate /ˈsʌf.ə.keɪt/

sunken /ˈsʌŋ.kən/

supplement /ˈsʌp.lɪ.mənt/

supplementation /ˌsʌpləmenˈteɪʃən/

supravalvular /ˈsuːprə.ˈvælv.jə.lər/

susceptibility /səˌsep.tɪˈbɪl.ɪ.ti/

swab /swɒb/

swordfish /ˈsɔːdˌfɪʃ/

talipes equinovarus /tal.ə.piːz ek.wi.noˈva.rəs/

tearless /ˈtɪə.ləs/

teething /tiːθɪŋ/

testosterone /ˌtesˈtɒs.tər.əʊn/

therapy /ˈθerəpɪ/
thoracic /θɔːˈræs.ɪk/
thrive /θraɪv/
throw /θrəʊ/ (**threw, thrown**)
tonsillitis /ˌtɒn.sɪˈlaɪ.təs/
tracheitis /ˌtreɪkɪˈaɪ.tɪs/
translucency /trænzˈluːsən.si/
transplacental /trænsˈpləˈsen.təl/
treatment /ˈtriːt.mənt/
trident /ˈtraɪ.dᵊnt/
triglyceride /traɪ.glɪs.ə.raɪd/
trunk /trʌŋk/
tube /tjuːb/
turgor /ˈtɜːgə/
Turner /tɜːrˈnər/ **syndrome** /ˈsɪndrəʊm/
typhoid fever/ˌtaɪ.fɔɪd ˈfiː.vərˈ/
ulceration /ˌʌl.sərˈeɪ.ʃən/
ultrasound /ˈʌl.trə.saʊnd/
uncommon /ʌnˈkɒm.ən/
unconcerned /ˌʌnkənˈsɜːnd/
undercooked /ˌʌn.dəˈkʊkt/
undernutrition /ˌʌndəˈnjuːˈtrɪʃ.ᵊn/
undigested /ˌʌndaɪˈdʒestɪd/
unduly /ʌnˈdjuːlɪ/
unrecognized /ʌnˈrek.əg.naɪzd/
uppermost /ˈʌpəˌməʊst/
upslanted /ʌpˈslɑːn.tɪd/
uremic /ˌjʊəˈriː.mɪk/
uterine /ˈjuː.tər.aɪn/
uveitis /ˌju.viˈaɪ.tɪs/
vaginosis /ˌvædʒɪˈnəʊsɪs/
vague /veɪg/
valgus /ˈvæl.gəs/
vicious /ˈvɪʃ.əs/
villus /ˈvɪl.əs/ pl **villi** /ˈvɪl.aɪ/
viral /ˈvaɪə.rəl/
warm /wɔːm/
web /web/
wheat /wiːt/
Williams /wɪljəmz/ **syndrome** /ˈsɪndrəʊm/
wind /wɪnd/
wing /wɪŋ/
withdrawal /wɪðˈdrɔː.əl/
witness /ˈwɪtnəs/
worry /ˈwʌr.i/
yawn /jɔːn/

Serious life-threatening infections; Specific bacterial infections; Common viral infection; Infectious mononucleosis (glandular fever); Prolonged fever; HIV

Text 1
Serious life-threatening infections

Meningitis

Meningitis occurs when there is inflammation of the meninges covering the brain. Viral infections are the most common cause of meningitis, and most are self-resolving. Bacterial meningitis may have severe consequences. Bacterial infection of the meninges usually follows bacteraemia. The release of inflammatory mediators leads to cerebral oedema, raised intracranial pressure, and decreased cerebral blood flow. The classical meningitis symptoms are headache, neck stiffness, and photophobia. Children with meningitis may also have sepsis, signs of shock, such as tachycardia, tachypnoea, prolonged capillary refill time and hypotension. Purpura in a febrile child of any age should be assumed to be due to meningococcal sepsis. It is imperative that there is no delay in the administration of antibiotics and supportive therapy.

Assessment of meningitis/encephalitis

History: fever, headache, photophobia, lethargy, poor feeding/vomiting, irritability, hypotonia, drowsiness, loss of consciousness, seizures.

Examination: Fever, purpuric rash, (meningococcal disease), neck stiffness (not always present in infants), bulging fontanelle in infants, opisthotonos (arching of back), positive Brudzinski/Kernig signs, signs of shock, focal neurological signs, altered conscious level, papilledema (rare)

Signs associated with neck stiffness

Brudzinski sign — flexion of the neck with the child supine causes flexion of the knees and hips

Kernig sign — with the child lying supine and with the hips and knees flexed, there is back pain on extension of the knee

Contraindications to lumbar puncture:
- Cardiorespiratory instability
- Focal neurological signs
- Signs of raised intracranial pressure, e.g. coma, high BP, low heart rate or papilledema
- Coagulopathy
- Thrombocytopenia
- Local infection at the site of LP
- If it causes undue delay in starting antibiotics

Cerebral complications
These include:
- Hearing impairment — inflammatory damage to the cochlear hair cells may lead to deafness. Children with hearing impairment may benefit from hearing amplification or a cochlear implant

- Local vasculitis — this may lead to cranial nerve palsies
- Local cerebral infarction — this may result in seizures, which may result in epilepsy
- Subdural effusion — most result spontaneously, but some require neurosurgical intervention
- Hydrocephalus — may result from impaired resorption of CSF or blockage of the cerebral aqueduct or ventricular outlets by fibrin. A ventricular shunt may be required
- Cerebral abscess — the temperature will continue to fluctuate. Drainage of the abscess is required.

Encephalopathy
In meningitis there is inflammation of the meninges, whereas in encephalitis there is inflammation of the brain substance. Encephalitis may be caused by:
- direct invasion of the brain by a neurotoxic virus
- delayed brain swelling following a response to an antigen, e.g. following chickenpox
- a slow virus infection, such as HIV infection or subacute sclerosing panencephalitis (SSPE) following measles

Toxic shock syndrome
Toxin producing S. Aureus and group A streptococci can cause this rare syndrome, which is characterized by:

- fever over 39°C
- hypotension
- diffuse erythematous, macular rash

The toxin can be released from infection at any site, including small abrasions or burns. It causes organ dysfunction, including:

- mucositis conjunctivae, oral mucosa, genital mucosa
- gastrointestinal dysfunction
- renal impairment
- liver impairment
- clotting abnormalities and thrombocytopenia
- CNS: altered consciousness

About 1 week to 2 weeks after the onset of the illness, there is desquamation of the palms, soles, fingers, and toes.

Exercise 1
Answer the following questions. Prepare short talks and/or dialogues on these topics

1. Characterize meningitis.
2. Describe assessment of meningitis and encephalitis (history, examination).
3. What are signs associated with neck stiffness?
4. Speak about contraindications to lumbar puncture.
5. Describe cerebral complications.
6. What is the difference between meningitis and encephalopathy?
7. Characterize toxic shock syndrome.

Translation 1

1. The septicaemia is usually accompanied by a purpuric rash, which may start anywhere on the body and then spreads. 2. Any febrile child with a purpuric rash should be given intramuscular benzylpenicillin immediately and transferred urgently to hospital. 3. S. pneumoniae may cause pharyngitis, otitis media, conjunctivitis, sinusitis, as well as 'invasive' disease (pneumonia, bacterial sepsis, and meningitis). 4. Impetigo is a localized, highly contagious, staphylococcal or streptococcal skin infection. 5. Lesions are usually on the face, neck, and hands and begin as erythematous macules that may become vesicular/pustular or even bullous. 6. Rupture of the vesicles with exudation of fluid leads to the characteristic confluent honey-coloured crusted lesions. 7. Boils are infections of hair follicles or sweat

glands, usually caused by S. aureus. 8. In periorbital cellulitis there is fever with erythema, tenderness, and oedema of the eyelid. 9. It may spread from a paranasal sinus infection or dental abscess. 10. Staphylococcal scalded skin syndrome is caused by an exfoliative staphylococcal toxin. 11. Infants and young children develop fever and malaise and may have a purulent crusting and localized infection around the eyes, nose, and mouth.

Text 2
Specific bacterial infections
Meningococcal infection

The septicaemia is usually accompanied by a purpuric rash, which may start anywhere on the body and then spreads. Characteristic lesions are non-blanching on palpation, irregular in size and outline, and may have a necrotic centre. Any febrile child with a purpuric rash should be given intramuscular benzylpenicillin immediately and transferred urgently to hospital.

Pneumococcal infections

S. pneumoniae is often carried in the nasopharynx of healthy children. Asymptomatic carriage is particularly prevalent among young children and may be responsible for the transmission of pneumococcal disease to other individuals by respiratory droplets. The organism may cause pharyngitis, otitis media, conjunctivitis, sinusitis, as well as 'invasive' disease (pneumonia, bacterial sepsis, and meningitis).

H. influenzae infection

Hib was an important cause of systemic illness in children including otitis media, pneumonia, epiglottitis, cellulitis, osteomyelitis, and septic arthritis. Immunization has been highly effective and Hib now rarely causes systemic disease.

Exercise 2
Study the following summary and then interpret basic information in English.

1. Meningitis
Predominantly a disease of infants and children.
Incidence has been reduced by immunization.
Clinical features: fever, poor feeding, vomiting, irritability, lethargy, drowsiness, seizures, or reduced consciousness; late signs- bulging fontanelle, neck stiffness, and arched back (opisthotonos)

| Septicaemia can kill in hours; good outcome requires prompt resuscitation and antibiotics. |
| Any febrile child with a purpuric rash should be given intramuscular benzylpenicillin immediately and transferred urgently to hospital. |
| **2. Encephalitis** |
| Onset can be insidious and includes behavioural change. |
| Consider if HSF could be the cause. |
| Treat potential HSV with parenteral high-dose acyclovir until this diagnosis is excluded. |
| **3. Pneumococcal infection** |
| Causes not only minor infections such as otitis media but also severe invasive disease. |
| Susceptibility is increased by hyposplenism (e.g. sickle cell disease) and nephrotic syndrome. |
| **4. H. influenzae infection** |
| Can cause severe invasive infections, including sepsis and meningitis |
| Hib disease is now rare following the introduction of the Hib vaccine |

Staphylococcal and group A streptococcal infections

Staphylococcal and streptococcal infections are usually caused by direct invasion of the organisms. They may also cause disease by releasing toxins.

Impetigo

This is a localized, highly contagious, staphylococcal or streptococcal skin infection. It is more common in children with pre-existing skin disease, e.g. atopic eczema. Lesions are usually on the face, neck, and hands and begin as erythematous macules that may become vesicular/pustular or even bullous. Rupture of the vesicles with exudation of fluid leads to the characteristic confluent honey-coloured crusted lesions. Topical antibiotics are sometimes effective for mild cases. Narrow-spectrum system antibiotics are generally needed for more severe infections. Affected children should not go to nursery or school until the lesions are dry.

Boils

These are infections of hair follicles or sweat glands, usually caused by S. aureus. Treatment is with systemic antibiotics. Recurrent boils are usually from persistent nasal carriage in the child or family acting as a reservoir for reinfection.

Periorbital cellulitis

In periorbital cellulitis there is fever with erythema, tenderness, and oedema of the eyelid. It may follow local trauma to the skin. It may spread from a paranasal sinus infection or dental abscess. In orbital cellulitis, there is proptosis, painful or limited ocular movement with or without reduced visual acuity.

Staphylococcal scalded skin syndrome

This is caused by an exfoliative staphylococcal toxin. It mainly affects infants and young children, who develop fever and malaise and may have a purulent crusting and localized infection around the eyes, nose, and mouth. Areas of epidermis separate on gentle pressure, leaving denuded areas of skin. Management is with intravenous anti-staphylococcal antibiotics, analgesia, and monitoring of hydration and fluid balance.

Text 3
Common viral infection

Many of the common childhood infections present with fever and rash. The infectious period begins a day or two before the rash appears and, for purposes of nursery/school exclusion, is generally considered to last until the rash has resolved or the lesions have dried up.

Enteroviruses

Human enteroviruses are a common cause of childhood infection. Transmission is primary by the faecal-oral and respiratory droplet routes. Following the pharynx and gut, the virus spreads to infect other organs.

Herpes simplex virus infections

HSV usually enters the body through the mucous membranes or skin, and the site of primary infection may be associated with intense local mucosal damage. Treatment is with acyclovir which may be used to treat severe symptomatic skin, ophthalmic, cerebral, and systemic infections.

Gingivostomatitis

This is the most common form of primary HSV illness in children. It usually occurs from 10 months to 3 years of age. There are vesicular lesions on the lips, gums, and anterior surfaces of the tongue and hard palate. There is a high fever and the child is very miserable. Eating and drinking are painful, which may lead to dehydration. Management is symptomatic but severe diseases may necessitate intravenous fluids and acyclovir.

Skin manifestation

- 'Cold sores' are recurrent HSV lesions on the gingival/lip margin.

- Eczema herpeticum — In this serious condition, widespread vesicular lesions develop on eczematous skin.
- Herpetic whitlows — These are painful, erythematous, oedematous white pustules on the site of broken skin, typically on fingers.

Eye disease

It may extend to involve the cornea, producing dendritic ulceration. This can lead to corneal scarring and ultimately loss of vision. Any child with herpetic lesions requires urgent ophthalmic assessment.

Disseminated infection

- Neonatal HSV infection — The infection may be focal, affecting the skin or eyes, or encephalitis, or may be disseminated.
- Infection in the immunocompromised host — infection may be severe. Cutaneous lesions may spread, e.g. oesophagitis and proctitis. Pneumonia and disseminated infections involving multiple organs are serious complications.

Chickenpox (primary varicella zoster infection)
Clinical features

- Lesions start on head and trunk, progress to peripheries. Appear as crops of papules, vesicles with surrounding erythema and pustules at different times for up to one week. Lesions may occur on the palate.
- Itchy and scratching; may result in permanent, depigmented scar formation or secondary infection.
- New lesions appearing beyond 10 days suggest defective cellular immunity.
- Watch for the child with chickenpox whose fever initially settles, but then recurs a few days later — this is likely to be due to secondary bacterial infection.
- Beware of admitting a chickenpox contact to a clinical area with immunocompromised children in whom it can disseminate and cause potentially fatal disease.

Complications

Bacterial superinfection

Staphylococcal; Streptococcal - may lead to toxic shock syndrome or necrotizing fasciitis

Central nervous system
Cerebellitis
Generalized encephalitis
Aseptic meningitis
Immunocompromised
Haemorrhagic lesions
Pneumonitis
Progressive and disseminated infection
Disseminated intravascular coagulation

Shingles (herpes zoster)
Shingles in childhood is more common in those who have primary varicella zoster infection in the 1ˢᵗ year of life. In the immunocompromised individuals reactivated infection can also disseminate to cause severe disease.

Exercise 3
Study the following summary and then interpret basic information in English.

1. Staphylococcal and streptococcal infections
Symptoms are caused by direct invasion of bacteria or by release of toxins.
Can cause a broad range of diseases, including toxic shock syndrome.
Immune-mediated diseases following streptococcal infections include glomerulonephritis and rheumatic fever.
Impetigo is highly contagious.
Periorbital cellulitis should be treated aggressively with intravenous antibiotics to prevent spread to the orbit or brain.
Scalded skin syndrome is a rare but serious disease.
2. Herpes simplex virus infections
Most are asymptomatic
Gingivostomatitis — may necessitate intravenous fluids and acyclovir.
Skin manifestations — mucocutaneous junctions, e.g. lips and damaged skin.
Eczema herpeticum — may result in secondary bacterial infection and septicaemia.
Herpetic whitlows — painful pustules on the fingers.
Eye disease — blepharitis, conjunctivitis, and corneal ulceration.
CNS — aseptic meningitis, encephalitis.
Pneumonia and disseminated infection in the immunocompromised.
3. Chickenpox
Clinical features — fever and itchy, vesicular rash, which crops up to 7 days.

Complications — secondary bacterial infection, encephalitis; disseminated disease in the immunocompromised.
Human varicella zoster immunoglobulin — if immunocompromised or if there is maternal chickenpox shortly before or after delivery.
Treatment is mainly supportive.

Exercise 4
Answer the following questions. Prepare short talks and/or dialogues on these topics

1. Describe common viral infection (herpes simplex virus infections, Shingles, gingivostomatitis, 'cold sores', eye disease, disseminated infection).
2. What are clinical features of chickenpox and its complications?

Translation 2

1. Many of the common childhood infections present with fever and rash. 2. Herpes simplex virus usually enters the body through the mucous membranes or skin, and the site of primary infection may be associated with intense local mucosal damage. 3. Gingivostomatitis is the most common form of primary HSV illness in children. 4. There are vesicular lesions on the lips, gums, and anterior surfaces of the tongue and hard palate. 5. Management is symptomatic but severe diseases may necessitate intravenous fluids and acyclovir. 6. 'Cold sores' are recurrent HSV lesions on the gingival/lip margin. 7. Eye disease may extend to involve the cornea, producing dendritic ulceration. 8. Neonatal HSV infection may be focal, affecting the skin or eyes, or encephalitis, or may be disseminated. 9. Pneumonia and disseminated infections involving multiple organs are serious complications. 10. Clinical features of chickenpox are: lesions starting on head and trunk, progressing to peripheries, itchy and scratching; they may result in permanent, depigmented scar formation or secondary infection. 11. In immunocompromised children it can disseminate and cause potentially fatal disease.

Text 4
Infectious mononucleosis (glandular fever)

Transmission usually occurs by oral contact and the majority of infections are subclinical. Older children, and occasionally young children, may develop a syndrome with:
- fever
- malaise

- tonsillitis/pharyngitis — breathing may be compromised
- lymphadenopathy — prominent cervical lymph nodes, often with diffuse lymphadenopathy elsewhere.

Other possible features include:
- petechiae on the soft palate
- splenomegaly, hepatomegaly
- a maculopapular rash
- jaundice

Diagnosis is supported by:
- atypical lymphocytes
- a positive monospot test
- seroconversion with production of three antibodies

Symptoms may persist for 1 months to 3 months but ultimately resolve. Fatigue is often a prominent feature in adolescents and adults. Treatment is symptomatic.

Cytomegalovirus

CVM is usually transmitted via saliva, genital secretions, or breastmilk, and more rarely via blood products and organ transplants as well as transplacentally. In the immunocompromised host, CMV can cause rhinitis, pneumonitis, bone marrow failure, encephalitis, hepatitis, oesophagitis, and enterocolitis. It is a very important pathogen following bone marrow and organ transplantation

Human parvovirus B 19

Human parvovirus causes erythema infectiosum or fifth disease. Infections can occur at any time of the year, although outbreaks are most common during the spring.

Clinical syndromes:
- asymptomatic infection
- erythema infectiosum — the most common illness with viraemic phase of fever, malaise, headache, and myalgia followed by a characteristic rash on the face, progressing to a maculopapular 'lace'-like rash on the trunk and limbs.
- Aplastic crisis — it occurs in children with chronic haemolytic anaemias.
- Foetal disease — may lead to foetal hydrops and death due to severe anaemia.

Complications
Respiratory
Pneumonia
Secondary bacterial infection and otitis media
Tracheitis

Neurological
Febrile seizures
EEG abnormalities
Encephalitis
Subacute sclerosing panencephalitis (SSPE)

Other
Diarrhoea
Hepatitis
Appendicitis
Corneal ulceration
Myocarditis

Measles
Clinical features and complications of measles

Rash
Spreads downwards, from behind the ears to the whole of the body. Discrete, maculopapular rash initially, becomes blotchy and confluent. May desquamate in the second week.

Koplik spots
White spots on buccal mucosa, seen against bright red background. Pathognomonic, but difficult to see.

Conjunctivitis and coryza
Cough
Mumps
Mumps occur worldwide, but its incidence has declined dramatically because of the mumps component of the MMR vaccine. The virus gains access to the parotid glands before further dissemination to other tissues.

Clinical features
The incubation period is 15 days to 24 days. Onset of the illness is with fever, malaise, and parotitis. Only one side of the face may be swollen

initially, but bilateral parotid involvement may occur over the next few days. Children may complain of earache or pain on eating or drinking. The parotid duct may show redness and swelling. When associated with abdominal pain, there may be evidence of pancreatic involvement. The illness is generally mild and self-limiting.

Orchitis

This is the most feared complication, although it is uncommon in prepubertal males. When it does occur, it is usually unilateral. Although there is some evidence of a reduction in sperm count, infertility is actually very unusual. Rarely, oophoritis, mastitis, and arthritis may occur.

Rubella (German measles)

Rubella is generally a mild disease in childhood. It typically occurs in the winter and spring. It can cause severe damage to the foetus. The incubation period is 15 days to 20 days. It is spread by the respiratory route. The maculopapular rash is often the first sign of infection, appearing initially on the face. It fades in 3 days to 5 days. Lymphadenopathy, particularly the suboccipital and postauricular nodes is prominent. Complications include arthritis, encephalitis, thrombocytopenia, and myocarditis.

Exercise 5
Study the following summary and then interpret basic information in English.

1. Parvovirus
Usually asymptomatic or erythema infectiosum
Can cause aplastic crisis in patients with haemolytic anaemia (e.g. sickle cell disease and thalassemia) or the foetus (foetal hydrops)
2. Enterovirus infection
Mostly asymptomatic or self-limiting illness with rash, which may be petechial.
Can cause hand, foot, and mouth disease; herpangina; meningitis/encephalitis; myocarditis/pericarditis; and neonatal sepsis syndrome.
3. Measles
Incidence has declined dramatically since immunization was introduced; a recent small increase has resulted from the decline in immunization uptake.
Clinical features: fever, cough, runny nose, conjunctivitis, marked malaise, Koplik spots, and maculopapular rash.
Complications: common if malnourished or immunocompromised.
4. Rubella

Generally, a mild illness, but can cause devastating congenital infection.

Exercise 6
Answer the following questions. Prepare short talks and/or dialogues on these topics

1. Characterize infectious mononucleosis (glandular fever).
2. Describe cytomegalovirus, and human parvovirus B 19.
3. What do you know about enteroviruses?
4. Speak about clinical features and complications of measles.
5. Speak about clinical features of mumps and orchitis.
6. Characterize rubella (German measles).

Translation 3

1. Transmission of infectious mononucleosis usually occurs by oral contact and the majority of infections are subclinical. 2. Older children may develop a syndrome with: fever, malaise, tonsillitis/pharyngitis, lymphadenopathy, petechiae on the soft palate, splenomegaly, hepatomegaly, a maculopapular rash, and jaundice. 3. In the immunocompromised host, cytomegalovirus can cause renitis, pneumonitis, bone marrow failure, encephalitis, hepatitis, oesophagitis, and enterocolitis. 4. Human parvovirus causes erythema infectiosum or fifth disease. 5. Clinical syndromes are: asymptomatic infection, erythema infectiosum with fever, malaise, headache, and myalgia, aplastic crisis and foetal disease. 6. Human enteroviruses are a common cause of childhood infection; transmission is primary by the faecal-oral and respiratory droplet routes.

Exercise 7
Fill in the missing words. Choose the correct ones.

1. Clinical features and _____ __ _____are: rash, Koplik spots, _____, _____, and cough.	a conjunctivitis b complications of measles c coryza
2. _____ of mumps ____ _____ dramatically because of the mumps component of the ___ _____.	a MMR vaccine b Incidence c has declined

3. _____ of the illness is with fever, _____, and _____.	a parotitis.
	b malaise
	c Onset
4. Children may complain of _____ or pain on eating or drinking; when _____ ____ abdominal pain, there may be evidence of _____ _____.	a pancreatic involvement
	b associated with
	c earache
5. _____ is the most _____ complication in _____ males.	a prepubertal
	b feared
	c Orchitis
6. Although there is some evidence of a reduction in _____ _____, _____ is actually very _____.	a unusual
	b infertility
	c sperm count
7. _____, particularly the _____ and _____ nodes is prominent.	a suboccipital
	b postauricular
	c Lymphadenopathy
8. Complications include, _____ , _____, thrombocytopenia, and _____.	a myocarditis
	b encephalitis
	c arthritis

Text 5
Prolonged fever

Most childhood infections are acute and resolve in a few days. If not, the child needs to be reassessed for complications of the original illness.

Causes of prolonged fever

Infective	Non-infective
• Localized infection: e.g. osteomyelitis	• Systemic onset juvenile idiopathic arthritis
• Bacterial infections: e.g. typhoid, Bartonella henselae (cat scratch disease), Brucella species	• Systemic lupus erythematosus
• Deep abscesses: e.g. intra-abdominal, retroperitoneal, pelvic	• Vasculitis (including Kawasaki disease)
• Infective endocarditis	• Inflammatory bowel disease (Crohn's disease and ulcerative colitis)
• Tuberculosis	• Sarcoidosis
• Nontuberculous mycobacterial infections: e.g. Mycobacterium avium complex	• Malignancy: e.g. leukaemia, lymphoma, neuroblastoma, Ewing sarcoma
• Viral infections: e.g. Epstein-Barr virus, cytomegalovirus, HIV (human immunodeficiency virus)	• Macrophage activation syndromes: e.g. hemophagocytic lympho-histiocytosis
	• Drug fever
Parasitic infections: e.g. malaria, toxocariasis, Entamoeba histolytica	• Fabricated or induced illness (including Munchausen syndrome by proxy).

Kawasaki disease

Kawasaki disease is a systemic vasculitis. Although uncommon, it is important to establish the diagnosis early, because aneurysms of the coronary arteries are a potentially devastating complication.

Tuberculosis

The decline of the incidence and mortality from TB in developed countries was hailed as an example of how public health measures and antimicrobial therapy can dramatically modify a disease. However, TB is again becoming a public health problem. Spread of TB is almost invariably by the respiratory route. Children usually acquire TB from an infected adult in the same household. The clinical features of active TB are often nonspecific, such as prolonged fever, malaise, anorexia, weight loss, or focal signs of infection.

Tropical infections

A febrile child returning from the tropics — most common causes are non — tropical infections, but consider malaria, typhoid fever, and other tropical infections.

An approach to the febrile child returning from the tropics
History

All places visited and duration of stay. Immunization, malaria prophylaxis. History of food, drink (infected water), accommodation (exposure to insect vectors), infectious contacts e.g. TB, swimming (infested rivers and lakes).

⇓

Examination

Particular reference to: fever, jaundice, anaemia, enlarged liver or spleen

⇓

Non-tropical causes of fever

Consider non-tropical causes of fever in childhood — upper and lower respiratory tract infections, gastroenteritis, urinary tract infection, septicaemia, meningitis, osteomyelitis, hepatitis, etc.

⇓

Tropical infections
Malaria

The clinical features include fever, diarrhoea, vomiting, flulike symptoms, jaundice, anaemia, and thrombocytopenia. Whilst typically the onset is 7-10 days after inoculation, infections can present months later. Children are particularly susceptible to severe anaemia and cerebral malaria. Diagnosis is by examination of thick blood films. Rapid diagnostic tests (RDTs) can also be used to establish the diagnosis.

Typhoid

A child with worsening fever, headaches, cough, abdominal pain, anorexia, malaise, and myalgia may be suffering from infection with Salmonella typhi or paratyphi. Gastrointestinal symptoms (diarrhoea or constipation) may not appear until the second week. Splenomegaly, bradycardia, and rose-coloured spots on the trunk may be present. The serious complications of this disease include gastrointestinal perforation, myocarditis, hepatitis, and nephritis.

Viral infections transmitted by mosquitoes

Dengue fever is wide spread in the tropics. The primary infection is characterized by a fine erythematous rash, myalgia, arthralgia, and high fever. After resolution of the fever, a secondary rash with desquamation may occur. Dengue haemorrhagic fever, (dengue shock syndrome), occurs when a previously infected child has a subsequent infection with a different strain of the virus. The partially effective host immune response augments the severity of infection causing severe capillary leak syndrome leading to hypotension as well as haemorrhagic manifestations. With fluid resuscitation, most children recover fully.

Gastroenteritis and dysentery

Gastroenteritis frequently accompanies foreign travel. 'Traveller's diarrhoea' is commonly caused by a change in gut flora, viruses including rotavirus and by E. Colli. It rarely needs more than attention to rehydration. Fever accompanied by loose stools with blood or mucus suggests dysentery caused by Shigella, Salmonella, Campylobacter, or Entamoeba histolytica. Blood cultures and stool cultures should be taken and appropriate antibiotics started if indicated.

Viral haemorrhagic fevers

These rare infections are imported, are highly contagious, and have a high mortality. If suspected, strict isolation procedures should be initiated for any symptomatic patient who has returned from an endemic area within 21-day incubation period of these infections. Specialist advice should be sought.

Exercise 8
Answer the following questions. Prepare short talks and/or dialogues on these topics

1. Describe infective and non-infective causes of prolonged fever.
2. Explain the term Kawasaki disease.
3. Characterize tuberculosis.
4. What is meant by tropical infections (malaria, typhoid)?
5. Speak about viral infections transmitted by mosquitoes.
6. What do you know about gastroenteritis and dysentery and viral haemorrhagic fevers?

Translation 4
1. Infective causes of prolonged fever are: localized infection, bacterial infections, infective endocarditis, nontuberculous mycobacterial infections, viral infections, parasitic infections. 2. Non-infective causes of prolonged fever are: systemic juvenile idiopathic arthritis, systemic lupus erythematosus, vasculitis, sarcoidosis, inflammatory bowel disease, malignancy, macrophage activation syndromes, drug fever, fabricated or induced illness. 3. Kawasaki disease is a systemic vasculitis; aneurysms of the coronary arteries are a potentially devastating complication. 4. The clinical features of active TB are often nonspecific, such as prolonged fever, malaise, anorexia, weight loss, or focal signs of infection. 5. In a febrile child returning from the tropics consider malaria, typhoid fever, and other tropical infections.

Exercise 9
Match the column A with the column B. Try to learn the expressions and/or sentences by heart.

A
1. The clinical features of malaria include …
2. A child with worsening fever, headaches, cough, abdominal pain, anorexia, malaise, and myalgia …
3. The serious complications of this disease include …
4. Dengue fever is wide spread in the tropics; …
5. 'Traveller's diarrhoea' is commonly caused by …
6. Blood cultures and stool cultures should be taken …
7. Viral haemorrhagic fevers …

B
a. … *the primary infection is characterized by a fine erythematous rash, myalgia, arthralgia, and high fever.*
b. … *and appropriate antibiotics started if indicated.*
c. … *fever, diarrhoea, vomiting, flulike symptoms, jaundice, anaemia, and thrombocytopenia.*
d. … *may be suffering from infection with Salmonella typhi or paratyphi.*
e. … *are highly contagious, and have a high mortality.*
f. … *a change in gut flora, viruses including rotavirus and by E. Colli.*
g. … *gastrointestinal perforation, myocarditis, hepatitis, and nephritis.*

Text 6
HIV

All infants born to HIV-infected mothers should be tested for HIV infection, whether or not they are symptomatic. A proportion of HIV-infected infants progress rapidly to symptomatic disease and onset of acquired immune deficiency syndrome (AIDS) in the 1st year of life; however, other infected children remind asymptomatic for months or years.

Children with mild immunocompromise may only have lymphadenopathy or parotid enlargement; if moderate, they may have recurrent bacterial infections, candidiasis, chronic diarrhoea, and lymphocytic interstitial pneumonitis. Severe AIDS diagnoses include opportunistic infections. Children with persistent lymphadenopathy, hepatosplenomegaly, recurrent fever, parotid swelling, thrombocytopenia, or any suggestion of serious, persistent, unusual, recurrent infections should be tested for HIV.

Aspects of management include:
- Immunization
- Multidisciplinary management of children if possible, in a family clinic
- Regular follow-up

Mothers who are most likely to transmit HIV to their infants are those with a high HIV viral load and more advanced disease. Avoidance of breastfeeding reduces the rate of transmission. In high-income countries, perinatal transmission of HIV has been reduced to less than 1% by using a combination of interventions:
- use of effective ART during pregnancy and intrapartum.
- postexposure prophylaxis given to the infant after birth
- avoidance of breastfeeding
- active management of labour and delivery
- prelabour caesarean section

Exercise 10
Study the following summary and then interpret basic information in English.

1. Kawasaki disease
Mainly affects infants and young children.
The diagnosis is made on clinical features — fever over 5 days, nonpurulent conjunctivitis, red mucous membranes, cervical lymphadenopathy, rash, red and oedematous palms and soles or peeling of fingers and toes.
Complications — coronary artery aneurysm and sudden death.

Treatment — intravenous immunoglobulin and aspirin.
2. Tuberculosis
TB affects millions of children worldwide; low but increasing incidence in many high-income countries.
Clinical features follow a sequence — primary infection, then latency, which may be followed by conversion to active TB months to years later.
Diagnosis is often difficult, so the decision to treat is then based on contact history, tuberculin skin test and interferon-gamma release assay results, X-ray findings, and clinical features.
Adherence to drug therapy is essential for successful treatment.
Contact tracing and identification of children with latent TB are important.
TB is more likely to disseminate in immunocompromised individuals.
3. HIV
Affects over 3 million children (<15 years) worldwide
Treatment includes combination ART and prophylaxis against Pneumocystis jirovecii pneumonia
The majority of perinatally infected children are surviving into adulthood if ART is available and adhered to.
Raises complex psychosocial issues for the family and healthcare providers, including when and what to tell the HIV-infected child (and siblings), confidentiality, and adherence support.
Antenatal antiretroviral treatment, active management of labour and delivery, and avoidance of breastfeeding can reduce the vertical transmission rate of HIV to less than 1%.

Lyme disease

Infections occur most commonly in the summer months in rural settings.

Clinical features

An erythematous macule at the site of the tick bite enlarges to cause the classical skin lesion, a painless red expanding lesion with a bright red outer spreading edge. During early disease, the skin lesion if often accompanied by fever, headache, malaise, myalgia, arthralgia, and lymphadenopathy. These features fluctuate over several weeks and then resolve. Dissemination of infection may lead to cranial nerve palsies, meningitis, arthritis, or carditis. The late stage of Lyme disease occurs after weeks to months with neurological, cardiac, and joint manifestations. Neurological disease includes meningoencephalitis and cranial (particularly facial nerve) and peripheral neuropathies. Recurrent attacks of arthritis are common.

Immunization

Immunization is one of the most effective and economic public health measures to improve the health of both children and adults. The most notable success has been the worldwide eradication of smallpox.

Immunization schedule

- BCG is given to newborn infants at high risk of TB infection
- the '5 in 1' vaccine is given, against diphtheria, tetanus, pertussis, Hib and inactivated (killed) polio – at 2 months, 3 months and 4 months of age
- pneumococcal conjugate vaccine (PCV 13) is given at 2 months, 4 months, and 12 months, and 12 months of age.
- Rotavirus vaccine is given orally at 2 months and 3 months of age.
- Booster Hib and MenC, a conjugate vaccine against group C meningococcus is given at 1 year.
- MMR against measles, mumps, and rubella is given at 1 year and 3 years 4 months.
- HPV, human papilloma virus vaccine, is given to girls at 12 years to 13 years of age.
- Meningococcal ACWY conjugate vaccine is given at 14 years.

Complications and contraindications

Following vaccination, there may be swelling and discomfort at the injection site and a mild fever and malaise. More serious reactions, including anaphylaxis, can occur but are very rare. Vaccination should be postponed if the child has an acute illness; however, a minor infection without fever of systemic features is not a contraindication. The controversy regarding a possible association between MMR vaccination and autism and inflammatory bowel disease has been discredited by a large number of well-conducted studies.

Immunodeficiency

Immunodeficiency may be Primary (uncommon) a genetically determined defect in the immune system, or Secondary (more common), such as malignancy/chemotherapy, malnutrition, HIV infection, immunosuppressive therapy, splenectomy, or nephrotic syndrome.

Presentation of immunodeficiency
- Recurrent (proven) bacterial infections
- Severe infections (e.g. meningitis, osteomyelitis, pneumonia)
- Infections that present atypically, are unusually severe or chronic or fail to respond to regular treatment
- Infections caused by an unexpected or opportunistic pathogen or a pathogen the child has been immunized against
- Severe or long-lasting warts, generalized molluscum contagiosum
- Extensive candidiasis
- Complications following live vaccinations
- Abscesses of internal organs; recurrent skin abscesses
- Prolonged or recurrent diarrhoea (often combined with faltering growth)

Management
Management options include:
- Antimicrobial prophylaxis
- Antibiotic treatment
- Prompt treatment of infections
- Appropriate choice of antibiotics to cover likely organisms
- Generally longer courses
- Screening for end-organ disease e.g. CT scan in children with antibody deficiency
- Immunoglobulin replacement therapy for children with antibody deficiency can be given intravenously, which may require central venous line insertion, or subcutaneously
- Bone marrow transplantation e.g. for severe combined immunodeficiency, chronic granulomatous disease can be matched sibling donor, matched unrelated donor, or parental transplant
- Gene therapy — currently an evolving area and not widely available

Exercise 11
Answer the following questions. Prepare short talks and/or dialogues on these topics

1. Speak about infants born to HIV-infected mothers.
2. What does management include?
3. What do you know about postexposure prophylaxis?
4. What are clinical features of Lyme disease?
5. Explain the principle of immunization and its complications and contraindications.

6.   What is meant by immunodeficiency and its management?

Translation 6
1. All infants born to HIV-infected mothers should be tested for HIV infection, whether or not they are symptomatic. 2. Children with mild immunocompromise may only have lymphadenopathy or parotid enlargement; if moderate, they may have recurrent bacterial infections, candidiasis, chronic diarrhoea, and lymphocytic interstitial pneumonitis. 3. Children with persistent lymphadenopathy, hepatosplenomegaly, recurrent fever, parotid swelling, thrombocytopenia, or any suggestion of serious, persistent, unusual, recurrent infections should be tested for HIV. 4. Aspects of management include: active management of labour and delivery, prelabour caesarean section, immunization, multidisciplinary management, regular follow-up. 5. Clinical features of Lyme disease are: an erythematous macule at the site of the tick bite enlarges to cause the classical skin lesion, a painless red expanding lesion with a bright red outer spreading edge. 6. The skin lesion if often accompanied by fever, headache, malaise, myalgia, arthralgia, and lymphadenopathy.

Exercise 12
Match the column A with the column B. Try to learn the expressions and/or sentences by heart.

A
1.   Dissemination of infection may lead to...
2.   Neurological disease includes...
3.   The most notable success has been ...
4.   Following vaccination, there may be swelling and discomfort ...
5.   The controversy regarding a possible association between MMR vaccination ...
6.   Presentation of immunodeficiency includes: ...
7.   Management options include: ...

B
a.   ... *meningoencephalitis and cranial (particularly facial nerve) and peripheral neuropathies.*
b.   ... *antimicrobial prophylaxis, antibiotic treatment, prompt treatment of infections, screening for end-organ disease, immunoglobulin replacement therapy, bone marrow transplantation, and gene therapy.*
c.   ... *cranial nerve palsies, meningitis, arthritis, or carditis.*

d. … *and autism and inflammatory bowel disease has been discredited by new studies.*

e. … *recurrent bacterial infections, severe infections, infections that present atypically, severe or long-lasting warts, extensive candidiasis, complications following live vaccinations, abscesses of internal organs, prolonged or recurrent diarrhoea.*

f. … *at the injection site and a mild fever and malaise.*

g. … *the worldwide eradication of smallpox.*

Key 2
Exercise 7
1 b, a, c; 2 b, c, a; 3 c, b, a; 4 c, b, a; 5 c, b, a; 6 c, b, a; 7 c, a, b; 8 c, b, a

Exercise 9
1c; 2 d; 3 g; 4 a; 5 f; 6 b; 7 e

Exercise 12
1c; 2 a; 3 g; 4 f; 5 d; 6 e; 7 b

VOCABULARY 2

acyclovir /əˈsaɪkləʊvɪr/
adherence /ədˈhɪə.rənt s/
adulthood /ˈæd.ʌlt.hʊd/
anaphylaxis /ˌæn.ə.fɪˈlæk.sɪs/
aneurysm /ˈæn.jʊə.rɪ.zəm/
anterior /ænˈtɪə.ri.ər/
antigen /ˈæn.tɪ.dʒən/
antiretroviral /æn.tiˌret.rəʊˈvaɪə.rəl/
aplastic /əˈplæs.tɪk/
aqueduct /ˈækwɪˌdʌkt/
arch /ɑːtʃ/
arthralgia /aːˈθræl.dʒɪ.ə/
aspect /ˈæs.pekt/
assay /əˈseɪ/
atopic /əˈtɒp.ɪk/ eczema /ˈek.sɪ.mə/
augmentation /ˌɔːgmenˈteɪʃən/
Bartonella henselae /bahr,təʊ.nelˈæ henˈse.liː/
bartonellosis /ˈbɑːtᵊn.eəʊ.sɪs/
benzylpenicillin /ben.zɪlˌpen.əˈsɪl.ɪn/
beware /bɪˈweə/
blepharitis /ˌblef.əˈraɪ.təs/
blotchy /blɒtʃ.i/
booster /ˈbuː.stər/
Brucella /bruːsɪˈllə/
Brudzinski sign /bruːˌdʒinˈskiː saɪn/
buccal /ˈbʌk.əl/
bullous /ˈbʊ.ləs/
burn /bɜːn/
candidiasis /ˈkændɪ.daɪə.sɪs/
carditis /kɑːˈdaɪ.tɪs/
carriage /ˈkær.ɪdʒ/
cellular /ˈsel.jʊ.lər/
central /ˈsen.trəl/ venous /ˈviː.nəs/ line /laɪn/
chickenpox /ˈtʃɪk.ɪn.pɒks/
cling film /ˈklɪŋ ˌfɪlm/
confluent /kənˈfluː.ənt/
conjunctiva /ˌkɒn.dʒʌŋkˈtaɪ.və/ pl conjunctivae
conjunctivitis /kənˌdʒʌŋk.tɪˈvaɪ.tɪs/
contraindication /ˌkɒn.trəˌɪn.dɪˈkeɪ.ʃən/
controversy /ˈkɒntrəˌvɜːsɪ/
conversion /kənˈvɔː.ʃən/
cornea /ˈkɔːnɪə/ pl corneae
coryza /kəˈraɪ.zə/
crop /krɒp/
crust /krʌst/

crusted /ˈkrʌs.tɪd/
cutaneous /kjuːˈteɪ.ni.əs/
deafness /ˈdef.nəs/
decline /dɪˈklaɪn/
defective /dɪˈfek.tɪv/
delivery /dɪˈlɪv.ər.i/
dendritic /denˈdrɪ.tɪk/
dengue /ˈdeŋɡɪ/ **fever** /ˈfiː.və/
denude /dɪˈnjuːd/
depigmented /deˈpɪɡ.mənt.ɪd/
desquamate /ˈdeskwəˈmeɪt/
desquamation /ˌdeskwəˈmeɪ.ʃən/
devastating /ˈdev.ə.steɪ.tɪŋ/
diphtheria /dɪfˈθɜɪr.i.ə/
discredit /dɪsˈkredɪt/
discrete /dɪsˈkriːt/
disseminate /dɪˈsem.ɪ.neɪt/
donor /ˈdəʊ.nər/
drainage /ˈdreɪ.nɪdʒ/
droplet /ˈdrɒp.lət/
duct /dʌkt/
dysentery /ˈdɪs.ənˌter.i/
dysfunction /dɪsˈfʌŋk.ʃən/
earache /ˈɪə.reɪk/
eczema /ˈek.sɪ .mə/
eczematous /ekˈsem.ə.təs/
endemic /enˈdem.ɪk/
enlarge /ɪnˈlɑːdʒ/
Entamoeba /ˌentəˈmiːbə/ **histolytica** /ˌhɪs.təˈlɪ.tɪ.kə/
enterovirus /ˌɛn.tə.roʊˈvaɪ.rəs/
epidermis /ˌep.ɪˈdɜː.mɪs/
epiglottitis /ˌep.ɪ.gləˈtaɪ.tɪs/
Epstein-Barr /ˈep.ˌstaɪn bɑː/ **virus** /ˈvaɪrəs/
eradication /ɪˌrædiˈkeɪ.ʃən/
erythema /ˌer.ɪˈθiː.mə/
erythematous /ˌer.ɪ.ˈθiː.mə.təs/
Ewing /juˈing/ **sarcoma** /sɑːˈkəʊ.mə/
exfoliative /eksˈfəʊlɪˌeɪ.tɪv/
exudation /ˌek.sjuːˈdəɪ.ʃən/
fade /feɪd/
faecal-oral /ˈfiː.kəl ˈɔː.rəl/
fasciitis /ˈfeɪʃ.ɪaɪ.tɪs/
fatal /ˈfeɪ.təl/
fatigue /fəˈtiːg/
flection /ˈflek.ʃən/
flulike /ˈfluː.laɪk/
foetal /ˈfiː.təl/

gingival /dʒɪnˈdʒaɪ.vəl/
gingivostomatitis /ˈdʒɪn.dʒɪ.vəˈstəʊməˈtaɪ.tɪs/
glandular /ˈɡlæn.djʊ.lər/
glomerulonephritis /ɡlɒˌmer.jʊ.ləʊ.nɪˈfraɪ.tɪs/
granulomatous /ˌɡrænjʊˈlɒm.ə.təs/
hemophagocytosis /ˈhiːməˌfæɡə.saɪˈtəʊ.sɪs/
hailed /heɪld/
hard /hɑːd/ **palate** /ˈpæl.ət/
herpangina /ˈhɜːpænˈdʒaɪ.nə/
herpetic /həːpetɪk/
herpetic /hɜːˈpetɪk/ **whitlow** /ˈwɪtləʊ/
Hib, /ˈhib/ *Haemophilus* /ˌhiːmˈhiːməʊˌfɪləs/ *influenzae* /ˌinˌflʊ.ˈen.zə/
human /ˈhjuː.mən/ **papilloma virus** /ˌpa.pə.ˈləʊ.məˈvaɪə.rəs/
hydrops /haɪdrɒps/
hyposplenism /ˈhaɪ.pəʊ ˈspliː.nɪzm/
immuno-suppressive /ˌimjʊnəʊ.səˈpresiv/
imperative /ɪmˈper.ə.tɪv/
infective /ɪnˈfek.tɪv/
infested /ɪnˈfest.ɪd/
inoculation /ɪˌnɒk.jʊˈleɪ.ʃən/
insect /ˈɪn.sekt/
insidious /ɪnˈsɪdɪəs/
interferon-gamma /ˌɪn.təˈfɪə.rɒnˈɡæm.ə/
interstitial /ˌɪn.təˈstɪʃ.əl/
intravascular /ˌɪn.trəˈvæs.kjʊ.lər/
intravenously /ˌɪn.trəˈviː.nəs.li/
invariably /ɪnˈveə.ri.ə.bli/
involvement /ɪnˈvɒlv.mənt/
itchy /ˈɪtʃ.i/
junction /ˈdʒʌŋk.ʃən/
Kawasaki disease /kɑːwəˈsɑːki dɪˌziːz/
Koplik spots /kopˈlik spots/
labour /ˈleɪ.bər/
lace /leɪs/
latency /ˈleɪ.tən.si/
load /ləʊd/
localized /ˈləʊ.kəl.aɪzd/
lupus /ˈluː.pəs/
Lyme disease /ˈlaɪm dɪˌziːz/
lymphocyte /ˈlim.fə.saɪt/
lymphocytic /ˌlɪɪmfəʊˈsɪtɪk/
lympho-histiocytosis /ˌlɪmfəʊˈhɪstɪəˌsaɪtəʊsis/
maculovesicular /ˌmæk.jʊ.lə veˈsɪkjʊlə/
malaise /mælˈeɪz/
marrow /ˈmær.əʊ/
mastitis /mæˈstaɪ.tɪs/
mediator /ˈmiː.di.eɪ.tər/

molluscum /mɒˈlʌskəm/ **contagiosum** /kənˈteɪdʒɪəs.əm/

monospot /ˈmɒnəʊ.spɒt/

mucocutaneous /mjuːkəʊ.kjuːˈteɪn.ɪəs/

mucositis /mjuːˈkəʊ.saɪ.tɪs/

mucous membrane /ˌmjuː.kəsˈmem.breɪn/

myalgia /maɪˈæl.dʒi.ə/

mycobacterium /ˌmaɪkəʊ bækˈtɪərɪəm/

myocarditis /ˌmaɪ.əʊ.kɑːdˈaɪ.tɪs/

necessitate /nəˈses.ɪ.teɪt/

nephritis /nɪˈfraɪ.tɪs/ pl **nephritides**

nephrotic /nɪˈfrɒt.ɪk/

neurotoxic /ˌnjʊə.rəʊˈtɒk.sɪk/

non-blanching /nɒn.blɑːntʃ.ɪŋ/

nontuberculous /ˌnɒn.tjʊˌbɜːkjʊˈləs/

notable /ˈnəʊ.tə.bl̩/

oophoritis /ˌəʊvə.fəˈraɪ.tɪs/

opisthotonos /ˌɒpɪsθɒtənəs/

orchitis /ˈɔː.kaɪ.tɪs/

outbreak /ˈaʊtˌbreɪk/

outline /ˈaʊt.laɪn/

palm /pɑːm/

palsy /ˈpɔːl.zi/

pancreatic /ˌpæŋ.krɪˈæ.tɪk/

panencephalitis /pænˌen.kef.əˈlaɪ.tɪs/

parotid /pəˈrɒt.ɪd/ **gland** /glænd/

pathogen /ˈpæθ.ə.dʒən/

pathognomonic /ˌpath.əg.ˈnɒm.ɒ.nik/

peel /piːl/

pericarditis /ˌper.ɪ.kɑːdˈaɪ.tɪs/

pharyngitis /ˌfær.ɪnˈdʒaɪ.tɪs/

Pneumocystis /njuːməʊˈsɪstɪs/ **jirovecii** /dʒaɪ.rəʊ.viːˈsaɪ/ (**carinii**) /kæ.raɪ.niːaɪ/

polio /ˈpəʊ.li.əʊ/

porosis /ˈpɔːrəsɪs/

postauricular /ˈpəʊst ɔːˈrɪkjʊlə/

postexposure /ˈpəʊst.ɪkˈspəʊ.ʒəʳ/

postpone /pəʊstˈpəʊn/

prelabour /ˌpriːˈleɪ.bəʳ/

prominent /ˈprɒm.ɪ.nənt/

proptosis / prɒpˈtoʊ sɪs /

purulent /ˈpjʊə.rʊ.lənt/

pustular /ˈpʌs.tjuːl.əʳ/

pustule /ˈpʌstjuːl/

recur /rɪˈkɜːr/

recurrent /rɪˈkʌrənt/

reference /ˈref.ər.ənt s/

regular /ˈreg.jʊ.lər/

release /rɪˈliːs/

replacement / rɪˈpleɪs.mənt/

resorption /ˌriː.ˈsɔːrp.ʃən/

retroperitoneal /ˌretrəʊˌperɪˈniːəl /

rheumatic /ruːˈmætɪk/

rhinitis /raɪˈnaɪ.tɪs/

rotavirus /ˈrəʊtəˌvaɪrəs/

sarcoidosis /ˌsɑr.kɔɪˈdoʊ.sɪs/

scarring /skɑːr.ɪŋ/

scratch /skrætʃ/

seek /siːk/ **(sought, sought)**

self-limiting /selfˈlɪm.ɪ.tɪŋ/

self-resolving /ˌself rɪˈzɒlv.ɪŋ/

separate /ˈsep.ər.ət/

seroconversion /sɪˈrɒ.kənˈvɜː.ʃ°n/

sinusitis /ˌsaɪˌnəˈsaɪ.tɪs/

smallpox /ˈsmɔːl.pɒks/

soft /sɒft/ **palate** /ˈpæl.ət/

sole /səʊl/

species /ˈspiː.ʃiːz/

splenectomy /spləˈnek.tə.mi/

spread /spred/

subclinical /sʌbˈklɪn.ɪ.kəl/

subcutaneously /ˌsʌb.kjʊˈteɪ.ni.əs.li/

suboccipital /ˌsʌb.ɒkˈsɪp.ɪ.təl/

supportive /səˈpɔː.tɪv/

survive /səˈvaɪv/

tetanus /ˈtet.ən.əs/

thick /θɪk/

tick /tɪk/

toxocariasis /ˌtɒksəkəˈraɪəsɪs /

trace /treɪs/

tuberculin /tjuːˈbɔː.kjə.lɪn/

ulcerative /ˈʌl.sər.ə.tɪv/ **colitis** /kəʊˈlaɪ.təs/

ultimately /ˈʌl.tɪ.mət.li/

undue /ʌnˈdjuː/

unexpected /ˌʌn.ɪkˈspek.tɪd/

unusually /ʌnˈjuːʒʊəl.i/

uptake /ˈʌp.teɪk/

vector /ˈvek.tər/

viraemic /vaɪˈri.mik/

Allergy; Food allergy and food intolerance; Respiratory disorders; Tonsillectomy and adenoidectomy; Basic management of acute upper airways obstruction; Asthma

Text 1
Allergy
Features of allergic disorders in children are:
- allergic rhinitis, eczema or asthma, food allergy
- they have increased in prevalence in many countries
- they are the most common chronic diseases of childhood and the most common cause of school absence and acute hospital admissions
- they cause significant morbidity and can be fatal

An abnormal immune system may result in:
- allergic diseases
- immune deficiencies
- autoimmune disorders — either organ specific (e.g. type 1 diabetes mellitus) or systemic (systemic lupus erythematosus).

Mechanisms of allergic disease

Allergic diseases occur when individuals make an abnormal immune response to harmless environmental stimuli, usually proteins. The developing immune system must be 'sensitized' to an allergen. Sensitization can be 'occult'.

Only a few stimuli account for most allergic diseases:
- Inhalant allergens, e.g. house-dust mite, plant pollens, pet dander and moulds.
- Ingestant allergens, e.g. cow's milk, nuts, soya, egg, wheat, seeds, legumes, seafood and fruits
- Insect stings/bites, drugs, and natural rubber latex.

Allergy definitions
- Hypersensitivity — reproducible symptoms or signs following exposure to a defined stimulus (e.g. food, drug, pollen) at a dose that is usually tolerated by most people.

- Allergy — a hypersensitivity reaction initiated by specific immunological mechanisms
- Atopy — a personal and/or familial tendency to produce IgE antibodies in response to ordinary exposures to potential allergens, usually proteins. Strongly associated with asthma, allergic rhinitis and conjunctivitis, eczema and food allergy.
- Anaphylaxis — a serious allergic reaction with bronchial, laryngeal, or cardiovascular involvement that is rapid in onset and may cause death.

Hygiene hypothesis
Developed urban environment $\Rightarrow$ Allergy and autoimmune disease
Family size — small
Exposure to parasites — low
Infections — few
Antibiotic exposure —high
Farming exposure — low
Microbial exposure — low

Developing rural environment $\Rightarrow$ No allergy or autoimmune disease
Family size — large
Exposure to parasites — high
Infections — many
Antibiotic exposure — low
Farming exposure — high
Microbial exposure — high

The allergic march
Allergic children develop individual allergic disorders at different ages:
- Eczema and food allergy usually develop in infancy.
- Allergic rhinitis, conjunctivitis and asthma begin most often in preschool and primary school years.
- Rhinitis and conjunctivitis may precede the development of asthma.

Prevention of allergic diseases
Many interventions have been tried to prevent allergic disease. Those with some evidence base include avoiding the use of formula milk from cow's milk, using probiotics during late pregnancy and lactation for preventing eczema and early introduction of peanut or egg to the infant diet to prevent peanut or egg allergy.

History and examination

As allergic diseases are multisystem, examination may reveal:

- mouth breathing. Children may have obstructed nasal airway from rhinitis, and there may also be history of snoring or obstructive sleep apnoea
- an allergic salute, from rubbing an itchy nose
- pale and swollen inferior nasal turbinates
- hyperinflated chest from undertreated asthma
- atopic eczema affecting the limb flexures
- allergic conjunctivitis and blue-grey discoloration below the lower eyelids

Growth needs to be checked, especially in those with food allergy and in those treated with high-dose inhaled/nasal/topical corticosteroids.

Management

Allergic diseases co-exist and it is therefore helpful to consider allergy as a systemic disease. In addition, specific allergen immunotherapy can be used for treating allergic rhinitis and conjunctivitis, insect stings, anaphylaxis, and asthma. Immunotherapy must be carried out under specialist supervision due to the risk of inducing severe allergic reactions (anaphylaxis).

Exercise 1
Answer the following questions. Prepare short talks and/or dialogues on these topics

1. Describe features of allergic disorders in children.
2. Describe mechanisms of allergic disease.
3. Explain allergy definitions.
4. What are the differences between developed urban environment and developing rural environment?
5. Characterize prevention of allergic diseases.
6. Describe history, examination and management of paediatric allergy.

Translation 1

1. Features of allergic disorders in children are: allergic rhinitis, eczema or asthma, and food allergy. 2. An abnormal immune system may result in: allergic diseases, immune deficiencies, and autoimmune disorders. 3. Allergic diseases occur when individuals make an abnormal immune response to harmless environmental stimuli, usually proteins. 4. Only a few stimuli

account for most allergic diseases: inhalant allergens, ingestant allergens, insect stings/bites, and drugs. 5. Hypersensitivity means reproducible symptoms or signs following exposure to a defined stimulus (e.g. food, drug, pollen). 6. Allergy is a hypersensitivity reaction initiated by specific immunological mechanisms. 7. Atopy is a personal and/or familial tendency to produce IgE antibodies in response to ordinary exposures to potential allergens, usually proteins. 8. Anaphylaxis is a serious allergic reaction with bronchial, laryngeal, or cardiovascular involvement that is rapid in onset and may cause death. 9. Interventions to prevent allergic disease include avoiding the use of formula milk from cow's milk, using probiotics during late pregnancy and lactation. 10. As allergic diseases are multisystem, examination may reveal: mouth breathing, rubbing an itchy nose, atopic eczema, or allergic conjunctivitis. 11. Specific allergen immunotherapy can be used for treating allergic rhinitis, conjunctivitis, insect stings, anaphylaxis, and asthma.

Text 2
Food allergy and food intolerance

A food allergy occurs when a pathological immune response is mounted against a specific food protein. A non-immunological hypersensitivity reaction to a specific food is called food intolerance.

Presentation varies with the agent and the child's age:

*   in infants — the most common causes are milk, egg and peanut
*   in older children — peanut, tree nut, fish and shellfish.

Food allergy can also be secondary, which is usually due to cross-reactivity between proteins present in fresh fruits/vegetables/nuts and those present in pollens. This common condition is termed the 'pollen food allergy syndrome'.

Non-IgE food allergy typically occurs hours after ingestion and usually involves the gastrointestinal tract. Food allergy and intolerance are different from food aversion, where the person refuses the food for psychological or behavioural reasons.

Diagnosis

For IgE mediated food allergy, the most helpful confirmatory tests are skin-prick tests and measurement of specific IgE antibodies in blood. Non-IgE mediated food allergies are harder to diagnose. If indicated, endoscopy and intestinal biopsy may be obtained. The test should be performed in hospital with full resuscitation facilities available, and close monitoring for signs of an allergic reaction. Clinical features of an acute allergic reaction:

Mild reaction
- Urticaria and itchy skin
- Facial swelling

Severe reaction
- Wheeze
- Stridor
- Abdominal pain, vomiting, diarrhoea
- Shock, collapse

Management
The child and family must be able to manage an allergic attack. Written self-management plans and adequate training are essential. If the child has a severe reaction (i.e. with cardiovascular laryngeal or bronchial involvement), treatment is with epinephrine (adrenaline) given intramuscularly by autoinjector (e.g. EpiPen), which the child or parent should carry with them at all times. The diagnosis of food allergy should not be made lightly — dietary restrictions and fear of accidental reactions make a major impact on family life.

Eczema
Atopic eczema is classified as an allergic disease as many affected children have a family history of allergy.

Allergic rhinitis and conjunctivitis
Rhino-conjunctivitis is classified according to the pattern and severity of symptoms experienced. Therefore, it may be intermittent or persistent and mild, moderate or severe. In temperate climates it is often classified as seasonal (related to seasonal grass, weed or tree pollens) and perennial (related to perennial allergens such as house dust mite or pets. It can also present as 'cough-variant rhinitis' due to a post-nasal drip or as a chronically blocked nose causing sleep disturbance with impaired daytime behaviour and concentration, or with predominant eye symptoms. It is associated with eczema, sinusitis, and adenoid hypertrophy.

Asthma
Allergy is an important component of asthma. Affected children often have IgE antibodies to aero-allergens (house dust mite, tree, grass and weed pollens; moulds; animal danders).

Classification of urticaria/angioedema

Acute — resolves within 6 weeks; infection, food allergy and drug reactions are common triggers

Chronic idiopathic — intermittent for at least 6 weeks

Physical urticarias

- cold, delayed pressure, heat contact, solar, and vibratory urticaria

Other causes

- water (aquagenic), sweating (cholinergic), exercise induced
- aspirin and other nonsteroidal anti-inflammatory agents
- C1 esterase inhibitor deficiency (angioedema, but no urticaria or pruritus)

Insect sting hypersensitivity

This arises from bee and wasp stings and some ant species. The severity of the allergic reaction may be:

- mild — local swelling
- moderate — generalized urticaria
- severe — systemic symptoms with wheeze or shock.

Exercise 2
Answer the following questions. Prepare short talks and/or dialogues on these topics

1. Characterize food allergy and food intolerance.
2. Describe clinical features of an acute allergic reaction (urticaria and itchy skin, facial swelling, wheeze, stridor, abdominal pain, vomiting, diarrhoea, shock, collapse).
3. What is the treatment if the child has a severe reaction (i.e. with cardiovascular laryngeal or bronchial involvement)?
4. What are the signs of eczema, allergic rhinitis and conjunctivitis, asthma?
5. What can you say about classification of urticaria/angioedema?
6. What do you know about insect sting hypersensitivity?

Translation 2

1. A food allergy occurs when a pathological immune response is mounted against a specific food protein. 2. A non-immunological

hypersensitivity reaction to a specific food is called food intolerance. 3. Food allergy can also be secondary, which is usually due to cross-reactivity between proteins present in fresh fruits/vegetables/nuts and those present in pollens. 4. Food allergy and intolerance are different from food aversion, where the person refuses the food for psychological or behavioural reasons. 5. The child and family must be able to manage an allergic attack. 6. If the child has a severe reaction (i.e. with cardiovascular laryngeal or bronchial involvement), treatment is with epinephrine (adrenaline) given intramuscularly by autoinjector (e.g. EpiPen). 7. Atopic eczema is classified as an allergic disease as many affected children have a family history of allergy. 8. Rhino-conjunctivitis is classified according to the pattern and severity of symptoms experienced. 9. It can also present as 'cough-variant rhinitis' due to a post-nasal drip or as a chronically blocked nose. 10. It is associated with eczema, sinusitis, and adenoid hypertrophy. 11. Allergy is an important component of asthma. 12. Insect sting hypersensitivity arises from bee and wasp stings and some ant species.

Text 3
Respiratory disorders
Presentation of respiratory disorders in children with:
- upper respiratory tract symptoms of coryza, sore throat, earache, sinusitis or stridor
- lower respiratory tract symptoms of cough, wheeze and respiratory distress.

Children are particularly susceptible to respiratory failure, and early detection and prevention are the cornerstone of management.

Signs of respiratory distress are:
- moderate — tachypnoea, tachycardia, nasal flaring, use of accessory respiratory muscles, intercostal and subcostal recession, head retraction and inability to feed
- severe — cyanosis, tiring because of increased work of breathing, reduced conscious level, oxygen saturation < 92% despite oxygen therapy.

Oxygen saturation monitoring is helpful to detect hypoxaemia and to titrate the amount of additional oxygen required. Narrowing of the airway due to inflammation is a feature of many respiratory pathologies. Upper airway narrowing results in increased effort and added respiratory noises during inspiration — stridor is harsh but musical whilst snoring (stertor) is rough and lacks a single note! Lower airway narrowing results in increased effort and added respiratory noises during expiration, such as crepitations and wheeze.

Upper respiratory tract infection

The term URTI embraces a number of different conditions:

- common cold (coryza)
- sore throat (pharyngitis, including tonsillitis)
- acute otitis media
- sinusitis

The most common presentation is a child with a combination of these conditions.

URTIs may cause:

- difficulty in feeding in infants as their noses are blocked and this obstructs breathing
- febrile seizures
- acute exacerbations of asthma

The common cold (coryza)

This is the common infection of childhood. Classical features include a clear or mucopurulent nasal discharge and nasal blockage. Colds are self-limiting and have no specific curative treatment. Pain is best treated with paracetamol or ibuprofen. Antibiotics are of no benefit as the common cold is viral in origin.

Sore throat (pharyngitis and tonsillitis)

In pharyngitis, the pharynx and soft palate are inflamed and local lymph nodes are enlarged and tender. Tonsillitis is a form of pharyngitis, where there is intense inflammation of the tonsils. It is not possible to distinguish clinically between viral and bacterial causes. Headache, apathy and abdominal pain, white tonsillar exudate and cervical lymphadenopathy is more common with bacterial infection. Antibiotics are often prescribed for severe pharyngitis and tonsillitis. They may hasten recovery from streptococcal infection. Rarely, in severe cases, children may require hospital admission for intravenous fluid administration and analgesia if they are unable to swallow solids or liquids. Occasionally, group A streptococcal infection results in scarlet fever. A typical appearance will include a 'sandpaper-like' maculopapular rash with flushed cheeks and perioral sparing. The tongue is often white and coated and may be sore or swollen. It is not possible to distinguish clinically between viral and bacterial tonsillitis.

Acute otitis media

Most children will have at least one episode of acute otitis media. Eustachian tubes are short, horizontal, and function poorly. There is pain in the ear and fever. Every child with a fever must have his/her tympanic membranes examined. The tympanic membrane is seen to be bright red and bulging with loss of the normal light reflection. Occasionally, there is acute perforation of the eardrum with pus visible in the external canal. Serious complications are mastoiditis and meningitis. Pain should be treated with an analgesic such as paracetamol or ibuprofen. Antibiotics marginally shorten the duration of pain but have not be shown to reduce the risk of hearing loss. Recurrent ear infections can lead to otitis media with effusion (also called glue ear). The eardrum is seen to be dull and retracted with a fluid level visible. It usually resolves spontaneously, but may cause conductive hearing loss. Hearing loss in children can interfere with normal speech development and result in learning difficulties in school. Insertion of ventilation tubes (grommets) is often performed. If problems recur after grommet extrusion, then reinsertion of grommets with adjuvant adenoidectomy is often advocated.

Exercise 3
Answer the following questions. Prepare short talks and/or dialogues on these topics

1. Characterize respiratory disorders.
2. Speak about upper respiratory tract infection.
3. Describe the common cold (coryza), sore throat (pharyngitis and tonsillitis) and acute otitis media.

Translation 3

1. Upper respiratory tract symptoms include coryza, sore throat, earache, sinusitis or stridor. 2. Lower respiratory tract symptoms include cough, wheeze and respiratory distress. 3. Signs of respiratory distress are: moderate (tachypnoea, tachycardia, nasal flaring, use of accessory respiratory muscles, intercostal and subcostal recession, head retraction and inability to feed) or severe (cyanosis, tiring because of increased work of breathing, reduced conscious level, oxygen saturation < 92% despite oxygen therapy). 4. The term URTI embraces a number of different conditions: common cold (coryza) sore throat (pharyngitis, including tonsillitis) acute otitis media, sinusitis. 5. URTIs may cause: difficulty in feeding in infants, febrile seizures, and acute exacerbations of asthma. 6. Classical features of the

common cold (coryza) include a clear or mucopurulent nasal discharge and nasal blockage.

Exercise 4
Match the column A with the column B. Try to learn the expressions and/or sentences by heart.

A

1. In pharyngitis, the pharynx and soft palate are...
2. Tonsillitis is a form of pharyngitis, ...
3. Headache, apathy and abdominal pain, white tonsillar exudate and cervical lymphadenopathy ...
4. Occasionally, group A streptococcal infection ...
5. In acute otitis media the tympanic membrane ...
6. Occasionally, there is acute perforation of the eardrum ...
7. Recurrent ear infections can lead ...
8. Hearing loss in children can interfere with ...

B

a. *... is more common with bacterial infection.*
b. *... normal speech development and result in learning difficulties in school.*
c. *... inflamed and local lymph nodes are enlarged and tender.*
d. *... is seen to be bright red and bulging with loss of the normal light reflection.*
e. *... where there is intense inflammation of the tonsils.*
f. *... to otitis media with effusion (also called glue ear).*
g. *... results in scarlet fever.*
h. *... with pus visible in the external canal; serious complications are mastoiditis and meningitis.*

Text 4
Tonsillectomy and adenoidectomy
Children with recurrent tonsillitis are often referred for removal of their tonsils. The indications for tonsillectomy include:

*   recurrent severe tonsillitis
*   a peritonsillar abscess (quinsy)
*   obstructive sleep apnoea (the adenoids will also often be removed)

Like tonsils, adenoids increase in size until about the age of 8 years and then gradually regress. The airway may narrow the posterior nasal space sufficiently to justify adenoidectomy. Indications include:

- recurrent otitis media with effusion with hearing loss
- obstructive sleep apnoea
- stridor

Stridor is a harsh, musical sound due to partial obstruction of the lower portion of the upper airway including the upper trachea and the larynx. Most common cause is laryngeal and tracheal infection, where mucosal inflammation and swelling can rapidly cause life-threatening obstruction of the airway in young children. The severity is best assessed clinically by characteristics of the stridor (none, only on crying, at rest, or biphasic), and the degree of chest retraction (none, only on crying, at rest). Severe obstruction also leads to increasing respiratory rate, heart rate, and agitation. Central cyanosis, drooling or reduced level of consciousness suggest impending complete airway obstruction. The most reliable objective measure of hypoxaemia is measuring the oxygen saturation by pulse oximetry. Total obstruction of the upper airway may be precipitated by examination of the throat using a spatula.

Differential diagnosis of acute stridor (upper airway obstruction)
Common causes
- Viral laryngotracheobronchitis ('croup')
- Rare causes
- Epiglottitis
- Bacterial tracheitis
- Laryngeal or oesophageal foreign body
- Allergic laryngeal angioedema (seen in anaphylaxis and recurrent croup)
- Inhalation of smoke and hot fumes in fires
- Trauma to the throat
- Retropharyngeal abscess
- Hypocalcaemia
- Severe lymph node swelling (tuberculosis, infectious mononucleosis, malignancy)
- Measles
- Diphtheria
- Psychological — vocal cord dysfunction

Croup

Croup typically occurs from 6 months to 6 years of age. It is most common in the autumn. Hoarseness due to inflammation of the vocal cords, a barking cough, due to tracheal oedema and collapse, harsh stridor, variable degree of difficulty breathing with chest retraction, the symptoms often start, and are worse, at night. When the upper airway obstruction is mild, the stridor and chest recession disappear when the child is at rest and the child can usually be managed at home. Inhalation of warm moist air is a traditional and widely used therapy but it has not been shown to be beneficial. In severe upper airways obstruction, nebulized epinephrine (adrenaline) with oxygen by face mask provides rapid but transient improvement

Acute epiglottitis

In acute epiglottitis there is intense swelling of the epiglottis and surrounding tissues associated with septicaemia. It is a life-threatening emergency. It is important to distinguish clinically between epiglottitis and croup as they require quite different treatment. The onset of epiglottitis is usually very acute, with:

- high fever in a very ill, toxic-looking child
- an intensely painful throat that prevents the child from speaking or swallowing; saliva drools down the chin
- soft inspiratory stridor and rapidly increasing respiratory difficulty
- the child sitting immobile, upright, with an open mouth

In contrast to viral croup, cough is minimal or absent. If the diagnosis of epiglottitis is suspected, urgent hospital admission and treatment are required. A senior anaesthetist, paediatrician, and ear, nose and throat (ENT) surgeon should be summoned and treatment initiated without delay. The child should be transferred directly to the intensive care unit. The child should be intubated. Rarely, this is impossible, and urgent tracheostomy is life-saving. Only after the airway is secured should blood be taken and intravenous antibiotics started. With appropriate treatment, most children recover completely within 2-3 days.

Clinical features of croup (viral laryngotracheobronchitis) and epiglottitis

	Croup	Epiglottitis
Onset	Over days	Over hours
Preceding coryza	Yes	No

Cough	Severe, barking	Absent or slight
Able to drink	Yes	No
Drooling saliva	No	Yes
Appearance	Unwell	Toxic, very ill
Fever	<38.5°C	>38.5°C
Stridor	Harsh, rasping	Soft, whispering
Voice, cry	Hoarse	Muffled, reluctant to speak

Exercise 5
Answer the following questions. Prepare short talks and/or dialogues on these topics

1. Describe tonsillectomy and adenoidectomy.
2. What are common causes of acute stridor?
3. What is meant by the term croup?
4. Characterize acute epiglottitis.
5. Characterize clinical features of croup and epiglottitis.

Translation 4

1. The indications for tonsillectomy include: recurrent severe tonsillitis, a peritonsillar abscess (quinsy), obstructive sleep apnoea (the adenoids will also often be removed). 2. Indications of adenoidectomy include: recurrent otitis, obstructive sleep apnoea, stridor. 3. Stridor is a harsh, musical sound due to partial obstruction of the lower portion of the upper airway including the upper trachea and the larynx. 4. Mucosal inflammation and swelling can rapidly cause life-threatening obstruction of the airway in young children. 5. Severe obstruction also leads to increasing respiratory rate, heart rate, and agitation. 6. Central cyanosis, drooling or reduced level of consciousness suggest impending complete airway obstruction. 7. Common causes of acute stridor are: viral laryngotracheobronchitis, epiglottitis, bacterial tracheitis, laryngeal or oesophageal foreign body, allergic laryngeal angioedema, inhalation of smoke and hot fumes, trauma to the throat, abscess, hypocalcaemia, lymph node swelling, measles, diphtheria. 8. The symptoms of croup often start, and are worse, at night.

Exercise 6
Match the column A with the column B. Try to learn the expressions and/or sentences by heart.

A

1. In severe upper airways obstruction, ...
2. In acute epiglottitis there is intense swelling ...
3. It is important to distinguish clinically between ...
4. The onset of epiglottitis is usually very acute, ...
5. If the diagnosis of epiglottitis is suspected, ...
6. Only after the airway is secured ...
7. Features of croup are: ...
8. Clinical features of epiglottitis are: ...

B

a. *... urgent hospital admission and treatment are required.*
b. *... onset over hours, drooling saliva, toxic, very ill appearance, stridor muffled, reluctant to speak*
c. *... nebulized epinephrine (adrenaline) with oxygen by face mask provides rapid but transient improvement*
d. *... should blood be taken and intravenous antibiotics started.*
e. *... onset over days, preceding coryza, severe, barking cough, unwell appearance, harsh stridor.*
f. *... of the epiglottis and surrounding tissues associated with septicaemia.*
g. *... with high fever, an intensely painful throat, and respiratory difficulty.*
h. *... epiglottitis and croup as they require quite different treatment.*

Text 5
Basic management of acute upper airways obstruction is:
- Reduce anxiety by being calm, confident, and well organized
- Observe carefully for signs of hypoxia or deterioration — agitation or fatigue or drowsiness or cyanosis. Provide oxygen if required and tolerated.
- Do not examine the throat with a spatula! It may precipitate upper airway obstruction
- Oral, nebulized or intravenous steroids are beneficial in croup and have similar speed of onset (90-120 min)
- If severe, administer nebulized epinephrine (adrenaline) and contact an anaesthetist

- If respiratory failure develops from increasing airways obstruction, exhaustion or secretions blocking the airway, urgent tracheal intubation is required.

Clinical conditions
Croup:
- Mostly viral
- 6 months to 6 years of age
- Coryza and mild fever, hoarse voice, barking cough

Epiglottitis:
- Caused by H. influenzae type b, rare since Hib immunization
- Mostly aged 1-6 years
- Acute, life-threatening illness
- High fever, ill, toxic looking
- Painful throat, unable to swallow saliva, which drools down the chin

Bacterial tracheitis:
- High fever, toxic
- Loud, harsh stridor

Inhaled foreign body:
- Choking on peanut or toy or object in mouth
- Sudden onset of cough or respiratory distress

Chronic stridor:
- Recurrent or continuous stridor since birth or early infancy from laryngomalacia, congenital airway abnormality, or external compression, e.g. vascular ring.

Wheeze
Acute wheeze is due to a partial obstruction of the intrathoracic airways.

Bronchiolitis
Bronchiolitis is the most common serious respiratory infection of infancy. There is evidence that co-infection with more than one virus may lead to a more severe illness. Recurrent apnoea is a serious complication especially in young infants. Hospital admission is indicated if any of the following are present:

- apnoea
- persistent oxygen saturation of < 90% when breathing air
- inadequate oral fluid intake
- severe respiratory distress — grunting, marked chest recession, or a respiratory rate over 70 breaths/minute

Humidified oxygen is either delivered via nasal canulae or using a head box. Most infants recover from the acute infection within 2 weeks. However, as many as half will have recurrent episodes of cough and wheeze.

Clinical features of severe bronchiolitis in an infant:
Dry, wheezy cough
Cyanosis or pallor

Hyperinflation of the chest:
- sternum prominent
- liver displaced downwards

Subcostal and intercostal recession

Auscultation:
- fine end-inspiratory crackles (crepitations)
- prolonged expiration/wheeze

Treatment
O_2 therapy via nose
Intravenous infusion

Causes of acute respiratory distress in an infant:
- Bronchiolitis
- Viral episodic wheeze
- Pneumonia
- Heart failure
- Foreign body
- Anaphylaxis
- Pneumothorax or pleural effusion
- Metabolic acidosis
- Severe anaemia

Viral episodic wheeze

Most wheezy preschool children have viral episodic wheeze. This is thought to result from small airways being more likely to narrow and obstruct. Some children have recurrent wheeze triggered by many stimuli, cold air, dust, animal danger and exercise. Evidence of allergy may be accompanied by positive skin-prick testing. Atopic asthma is strongly associated with other atopic diseases, such as eczema, rhinoconjunctivitis and blood allergy.

Causes of recurrent or persistent childhood wheeze
- Viral episodic wheeze
- Multiple trigger wheeze
- Asthma
- Recurrent anaphylaxis (e.g. in food allergy)
- Chronic aspiration
- Cystic fibrosis
- Bronchopulmonary dysplasia
- Bronchiolitis obliterans
- Tracheobronchomalacia

Exercise 7
Answer the following questions. Prepare short talks and/or dialogues on these topics

1. Describe basic management of acute upper airways obstruction.
2. Describe clinical features and treatment of severe bronchiolitis in an infant.
3. What are causes of acute respiratory distress in an infant?
4. What do you know about viral episodic wheeze?
5. What are causes of recurrent or persistent childhood wheeze?

Translation 5

1. In acute upper airways obstruction observe carefully for signs of hypoxia or deterioration — agitation or fatigue and drowsiness or cyanosis. 2. Do not examine the throat with a spatula because it may precipitate upper airway obstruction. 3. If respiratory failure develops from increasing airways obstruction, exhaustion or secretions blocking the airway, urgent tracheal intubation is required. 4. In the child with stridor clinical features to assess are: fever, hoarse, barking cough, level of consciousness and chest recession. 5. Clinical conditions of croup are: mostly viral, coryza and mild fever, hoarse voice, and barking cough. 6. Epiglottitis is acute, life-threatening

illness with high fever, ill, toxic looking and painful throat, and the child is unable to swallow saliva. 7. Inhaled foreign body causes sudden onset of cough or respiratory distress. 8. Chronic stridor is caused by congenital airway abnormality, or external compression, e.g. vascular ring. 9. Acute wheeze is due to a partial obstruction of the intrathoracic airways. 10. Bronchiolitis is the most common serious respiratory infection of infancy.

Exercise 8
Match the column A with the column B. Try to learn the expressions and/or sentences by heart.

A

1. Hospital admission is indicated if any of the following are present: …
2. Humidified oxygen is either delivered via …
3. Clinical features of severe bronchiolitis in an infant are: …
4. Causes of acute respiratory distress in an infant are: …
5. Some children have recurrent wheeze …
6. Atopic asthma is strongly associated with …
7. Causes of recurrent or persistent childhood wheeze are: …

B

a. … *bronchiolitis, viral episodic wheeze, pneumonia, heart failure, foreign body, anaphylaxis, pneumothorax, metabolic acidosis, severe anaemia.*
b. … *asthma, recurrent anaphylaxis, chronic aspiration, cystic fibrosis, bronchopulmonary dysplasia, bronchiolitis obliterans, tracheobronchomalacia.*
c. … *apnoea, inadequate oral fluid intake, or severe respiratory distress.*
d. … *dry, wheezy cough, cyanosis or pallor, hyperinflation of the chest, subcostal and intercostal recession.*
e. … *nasal canulae or using a head box.*
f. … *other atopic diseases, such as eczema, rhino-conjunctivitis and blood allergy.*
g. … *triggered by many stimuli, cold air, dust, animal danger and exercise.*

Text 6
Asthma
Asthma is the most common chronic respiratory disorder in childhood. It is an important cause of absence from school, restricted activity, and

anxiety for the child and family. Diagnosing asthma in preschool children is often difficult. In general, these are three patterns of wheezing:
- viral episodic wheezing – wheeze only in response to viral infections
- multiple trigger wheeze – in response to multiple triggers
- asthma

Pathophysiology of asthma
- Genetic predisposition
- Atopy
- Environmental triggers:

Upper respiratory tract infections
- Allergens (e.g. house-dust mite, grass pollens, pets)
- Smoking (active or passive)
- Cold air
- Exercise
- Emotional upset or anxiety
- Chemical irritants (e.g. paint, aerosols)

Bronchial inflammation	Oedema Excessive mucus production Infiltration with cells (eosinophils, mast cells, neutrophils, lymphocytes)
Bronchial hyperresponsiveness	Exaggerated 'twitchiness' to inhaled stimuli
Airway narrowing	Reversible airflow obstruction (e.g. peak flow variability)
Symptoms	Wheeze Cough Breathlessness Chest tightness

Clinical features
Ideally, the presence of wheeze is confirmed on auscultation by health professionals to distinguish it from transmitted upper respiratory noises. Asthmatic wheeze is a polyphonic (multiple pitch) noise coming from the airways.

Key features associated with a high probability of a child having asthma include:
- Symptoms worse at night and in the early morning
- Symptoms that have non-viral triggers
- Interval symptoms, i.e. symptoms between acute exacerbations

- Personal or family history of an atopic disease
- Positive response to asthma therapy.

Once suspected, the pattern should be further explored by asking
- How frequent are the symptoms?
- What triggers the symptoms?
- How often is sleep disturbed by asthma?
- How severe are the interval symptoms between exacerbations?
- How much school has been missed due to asthma?

The presence of a wet cough or sputum production, finger clubbing or poor growth suggests a condition characterized by chronic infection such as cystic fibrosis or bronchiectasis. Always monitor the growth of children with asthma, especially if taking regular inhaled or oral corticosteroids.

Acute asthma

With each acute attack, the duration of symptoms, the treatment already given, and the course of previous attacks should be noted. Children require hospital admission if, after high-dose inhaled bronchodilator therapy, they:
- have not responded adequately clinically, i.e. there is persisting breathlessness or tachypnoea
- are becoming exhausted

Causes of acute breathlessness in the older child:
- Asthma
- Pneumonia or lower respiratory tract infection
- Foreign body
- Anaphylaxis
- Pneumothorax or pleural effusion
- Metabolic acidosis — diabetic ketoacidosis, inborn error of metabolism, lactic acidosis
- Severe anaemia
- Heart failure
- Panic attacks (hyperventilation)

Assessment of the child with acute asthma

Determine the severity of the attack:	• Mild • Moderate • Severe • Life-threatening • This is determined by clinical features

Too breathless to talk	• Severe
Increased work of breathing Check respiratory rate: Chest recession: Auscultation:	• Tachypnoea — varies with age • Moderate — some intercostal recession • Severe — use of accessory neck muscles • Life-threatening — poor respiratory effort • Wheeze • Silent chest — poor air entry from poor expiratory effort or exhaustion in life-threatening
Cardiovascular	• Tachycardia — varies with age; better guide to severity than respiratory rate but affected by Beta 2-agonists • Arrythmia, hypotension — life-threatening
Altered consciousness	• Agitation or confusion — life-threatening • Exhaustion — life-threatening
Tongue	• Cyanosis
Peak flow (1% predicted or best or unusual measurement):	• Moderate >50% • Severe — 33-50% • Life-threatening <33%
O_2 saturation	• Moderate ≥ 92% • Severe or life-threatening <92%
Is there a trigger for the attack?	• URTI or other viral illness • Allergen, e.g. animal dander • Exercise • Cold air

Periodic assessment of the child with asthma

Clinical features to check
Growth and nutrition
Peak flow/spirometry

Check for:
• Hyperinflation
• Harrison's sulcus
• Wheeze

Are there other allergic disorders?
• Allergic rhinitis
• Eczema
• Food allergy

If atypical features present:

- Sputum
- Finger clubbing
- Growth failure
- then seek another diagnosis

Monitor:
- Peak flow diary
- Severity and frequency of symptoms
- Exercise tolerance
- interference with life, time off school
- Is sleep disturbed?
- Use of preventer and reliever medication – are they appropriate?
- Inhaler technique
- Lung function test

Consider triggers:
- Untreated allergic rhinitis
- Allergen or cigarette smoke
- Stress

Check:
- Child has an up to date personalized asthma management action plan
- Family have necessary medication/equipment to manage an acute exacerbation

Exercise 9
Answer the following questions. Prepare short talks and/or dialogues on these topics

1. What can you say about diagnosing asthma in preschool children?
2. What are causes of upper respiratory tract infections?
3. Describe clinical features of wheeze.
4. Which are key features associated with a high probability of a child having asthma?
5. Which condition is suggested by the presence of a wet cough or sputum production, finger clubbing or poor growth?
6. Which conditions should be noted (the duration of symptoms, the treatment already given, and the course of previous attacks)?
7. What are causes of acute breathlessness in the older child?
8. Characterize assessment of the child with acute asthma.

9.   Describe clinical features to check in the child with asthma.

Exercise 10
Study the following summary and then interpret basic information in English.

1. Food allergy
Affects up to 6% of children.
The most common causes are milk, egg, nuts, seafood, wheat, legumes, seeds and fruits.
Diagnosis of IgE-mediated food allergy is based on a suggestive history supported by skin-prick tests or specific IgE antibodies in blood.
Supervised food challenge is sometimes necessary to clarify the diagnosis.
Those at risk of a severe reaction, e.g. with previous anaphylaxis or coexistent asthma, should carry an epinephrine (adrenaline) autoinjector.
2. Paediatric allergy
Includes food allergy, eczema, allergic rhinitis and conjunctivitis, asthma, urticaria, insect sting hypersensitivity and anaphylaxis.
Occurs when a genetically susceptible person reacts abnormally to an environmental antigen.
There is an 'allergic march' of disorders.
Different allergic diseases often co-exist – if a child has one, look for others.
3. Insect sting hypersensitivity
Mainly to bee and wasp stings
Following a severe reaction, an epinephrine (adrenaline) autoinjector should be carried.
Immunotherapy is effective for preventing further reactions.
4. Acute otitis media
Is diagnosed by examining the tympanic membrane.
Antibiotics marginally shorten the duration of pain but do not reduce hearing loss.
If recurrent, may result in otitis media with effusion, which may cause speech and learning difficulties from hearing loss

Translation 6

1. Asthma is the most common chronic respiratory disorder in childhood. 2. Upper respiratory tract infections are caused by allergens (e.g. house-dust mite, grass pollens, pets), smoking, cold air, exercise, emotional upset or anxiety, or chemical irritants (e.g. paint, aerosols). 3. Asthmatic wheeze is a noise coming from the airways. 4. Key features include: symptoms worse at night and in the early morning, symptoms between acute exacerbations, history of an atopic disease. 5. The presence of a wet cough or sputum production, finger clubbing or poor growth suggests a condition characterized by chronic infection such as cystic fibrosis or bronchiectasis.

6. With each acute attack, the duration of symptoms, the treatment already given, and the course of previous attacks should be noted. 7. Causes of acute breathlessness in the older child are: asthma, pneumonia, foreign body, anaphylaxis, pneumothorax, metabolic acidosis, severe anaemia, heart failure, and panic attacks. 8. Periodic assessment of the child with asthma include: growth and nutrition, and peak flow/spirometry. 9. Check for these clinical features: hyperinflation, Harrison's sulcus, wheeze, allergic rhinitis, eczema, food allergy, sputum, finger clubbing, and growth failure. 10. Monitor severity and frequency of symptoms, inhaler technique, lung function test, and consider triggers.

Key 3
Exercise 4
1c; 2e; 3a; 4g; 5d; 6h; 7f; 8b

Exercise 6
1c; 2f; 3h; 4g; 5a; 6d; 7e; 8b

Exercise 8
1c; 2e; 3d; 4a; 5g; 6f; 7b

VOCABULARY 3

added /ˈædɪd/
adenoid /ˈædɪˌnɔɪd/
adenoidectomy /ˈædɪˌnɔɪd.ek.tə.mi/
adjuvant /ˈædʒəvənt/
admission /ədˈmɪʃ.ən/
adrenaline /əˈdren.əl.ɪn/
advocated /ˈæd.vəˌkeɪt.ɪd/
agitation /ˌædʒ.ɪˈteɪ.ʃən/
aquagenic /ˈækwədʒənɪk/
autoinjector /ˌɔːtəʊ.ɪnˈɪndʒektᵊr/
aversion /əˈvɜːʃən/
bark /bɑːk/
biphasic /baɪˈfeɪz.ɪk/
breathlessness /ˈbreθlɪs.nɪs/
bronchiectasis /ˌbrɒŋ.kɪˈɛktə.sɪs/
carry /ˈkær.i/ out /aʊt/
cell /sel/
challenge /ˈtʃæl.ɪndʒ/
cholinergic /ˌkəʊlɪˈnɜːdʒɪk/
co-exist /ˌkəʊɪgˈzɪst/
coexistent /ˌkəʊɪgˈzɪstənt/
conductive /kənˈdʌk.tɪv/
confident /ˈkɒn.fɪ.dənt/
confirmatory /kənˈfɜː.mə.tər.i/
crepitation /ˌkrep.ɪˈteɪ.ʃən/
curative /ˈkjʊərətɪv/
drip /drɪp/
eardrum /ˈɪə.drʌm/
embrace /ɪmˈbreɪs/
endoscopy /enˈdɒskəpɪ/
environmental /ɪnˌvaɪə.rənˈmen.təl/
eosinophil /ˌiːəʊˈsɪnə.fɪl/
epinephrine /ˌepɪˈnef.riːn/
esterase /es.təˌreɪs/
Eustachian /juːˈsteɪ.ki.ən/ tube /tjuːb/
exaggerated /ɪgˈzædʒ.ə.reɪ.tɪd/
exhaustion /ɪgˈzɔːs.tʃən/
expiration /ˌek.spəˈreɪ.ʃən/
extrusion /ɪkˈstrʊ.ʒən/
exudate /ɪgˈzjuːdəɪt/
farming /ˈfɑːmɪŋ/
flexure /ˈflek.ʃər/
flushed /flʌʃt/
fume /fjuːm/
harmless /ˈhɑːm.ləs/

hasten /ˈheɪ.sən/
humidified /hjuːˈmɪd.ɪ.faɪd/
hyperinflation /ˌhaɪpəɪnˈfleɪʃən/
immunotherapy /ˌɪm.jə.nəʊˈθe.rə.pi/
improvement /ɪmˈpruː.v.mənt/
inferior /ɪnˈfɪə.ri.ər/
ingestion /ɪnˈdʒest.ʃən/
interfere /ˌɪn.təˈfɪər/
lactation /lækˈteɪ.ʃən/
legume /ˈlegjuːm/
marginal /ˈmɑːdʒɪnᵊl/
mast /mɑːst/ **cell** /sel/
mastocyte /mæst.ə.saɪt/
mastoiditis /ˌmæstɔɪˈdaɪ.tɪs/
mediated /ˈmiː.di.eɪt.ɪd/
microbial /ˈmaɪ.krəʊ.baɪ.əl/
mite /maɪt/
mould /məʊld/
mounted /ˈmaʊn.tɪd/
mucopurulent /mjuːˈkəʊ ˈpjʊə.rʊ.lənt/
muffled /ˈmʌf.ļd/
narrowing /ˈnær.əʊ.ɪŋ/
nebulized /ˈneb.jə.laɪzd/
obliterans /əˈblɪtəˌrəns/
obliterate /əˈblɪtəˌreɪt/
occult /əˈkʌlt/
origin /ˈɒr.ɪ.dʒɪn/
peak /piːk/ **flow** /fləʊ/
perennial /pəˈrenɪəl/
peritonsillar /ˌperɪˈtɒns.ələ/
pitch /pɪtʃ/
pollen /ˈpɒl.ən/
polyphonic /ˈpɒlɪˈfɒnɪk/
precede /prɪˈsiːd/
predisposition /ˌpriːdɪs.pəˈzɪʃ.ən/
prevalence /ˈprevələns/
prevent /prɪˈvent/
pruritus /prʊəˈraɪ.təs/
pus /pʌs/
quinsy /ˈkwɪnzɪ/
rasping /ˈrɑːspɪŋ/
recovery /rɪˈkʌv.ər.i/
refer /rɪˈfɜːr/
reliable /rɪˈlaɪə.bļ/
relieve /rɪˈliːv/
reluctant /rɪˈlʌktənt/
reproducible /ˌriː.prə.djuːsɪ.bļ/

retract /rɪˈtrækt/
retraction /rɪˈtrækˌʃən/
retropharyngeal /ˌretrəʊˌfærɪnˈdʒiːəl/
reveal /rɪˈviːl/
rhinitis /raɪˈnaɪtɪs/
rough /rʌf/
salute /səˈluːt/
sandpaper /ˈsændˌpeɪpə/
scarlet /ˈskɑːlɪt/ **fever** /ˈfiːvə/
seafood /ˈsiːˌfuːd/
seed /siːd/
sensitization /ˌsen.sɪ.taɪˈzeɪ.ʃən/
sensitize /ˈsen.sɪ.taɪz/
shellfish /ˈʃel.fɪʃ/
skin-prick /skɪn prɪk/
sparing /ˈspeə.rɪŋ/
species /ˈspiː.ʃiːz/
sputum /ˈspjuː.təm/ pl **sputa**
sternal /ˈstɜː.nəl/
sternum /ˈstɜː.nəm/
stertor /ˈstɜr.tər/
stimulus /ˈstɪm.jʊ.ləs/ pl **stimuli**
sting /stɪŋ/
suggestive /səˈdʒes.tɪv/
summon /ˈsʌm.ən/
temperate /ˈtempərɪt/
tightness /ˈtaɪt.nəs/
titrate /ˈtɑɪ.treɪt/
tonsillar /ˈtɒnt .səl.ər/
tonsillectomy /ˌtɒn.səˈl.ek.tə.mi/
tonsillitis /ˌtɒnsɪ laɪ.tɪs/
tracheobronchomalacia /ˈtreɪkɪəʊˈbrɒnkə məˈleɪ.ʃɪə/
treat /triːt/
tree /triː/ **nut** /nʌt/
trigger /ˈtrɪg.ər/
turbinate bone /ˈtəːbɪnɪt ˈbone/
twitching /ˈtwɪtʃ.iŋ/
under /ˈʌn.dər/
upset /ʌpˈset/
urban /ˈɜːbən/
vibratory /ˈvaɪ.brə.tɜː.ri:/
wasp /wɒsp/
weed /wiːd/
whispering /ˈwɪs.pər.ɪŋ/

Other causes of acute wheezing; Cystic fibrosis; Cardiac disorders; Kidney and urinary tract disorder; Incomplete bladder emptying; Enuresis; Haematuria; Dialysis

Text 1
Other causes of acute wheezing:

- Atypical pneumonia
- Foreign body inhalation — abrupt onset of cough followed by wheeze in a previously well child
- Anaphylaxis — suspect if acute urticaria, facial swelling, stridor, or previous reaction to an allergen

Acute cough

Cough is the most common symptom of respiratory disease. Identifying if the cough is dry or moist can be helpful diagnostically. A dry cough suggests that there is some narrowing of airways. A barking cough suggests that a degree of tracheal inflammation. A moist cough suggests that there is either increased mucus secretion or infection in the lower airway. The cough reflex functions to expel unwanted material from the airway below the glottis.

Whooping cough (pertussis)

This is a highly contagious respiratory infection caused by Bordetella pertussis. After a week of coryza, the child develops a characteristic paroxysmal or spasmodic cough followed by a characteristic inspiratory whoop. The spasms of cough are often worse at night and may culminate in vomiting. The child goes red or blue in the face, and mucus flows from the nose and mouth. The symptoms gradually decrease (convalescent phase), but may persist for many months. Siblings, parents and school contacts may develop a similar cough and close contacts should receive macrolide prophylaxis.

Persistent or recurrent cough

A cough that lasts more than 8 weeks or one that has not improved after 3-4 weeks should be considered persistent in the absence of recurrent URTI. Most children will swallow rather than expectorate sputum. In any child with a severe, persistent cough, tuberculosis should be considered. Asthma is another common cause of recurrent cough.

Causes of persistent or recurrent cough
- Recurrent respiratory infections
- Following specific respiratory infections (e.g. pertussis, respiratory syncytial virus, Mycoplasma)
- Asthma
- Persistent lobar collapse following pneumonia
- Suppurative lung diseases (e.g. cystic fibrosis, ciliary dyskinesia or immune deficiency)
- Recurrent aspiration (±gastro-oesophageal reflux)
- Persistent bacterial bronchitis
- Inhaled foreign body
- Cigarette smoking (active or passive)
- Tuberculosis
- Habit cough
- Airway anomalies (e.g. tracheobronchomalacia, tracheooesophageal fistula)

Pneumonia

It is a major cause of childhood mortality in low and middle-income countries. Viruses are the most common cause in younger children, whereas bacteria are more common in older children. Fever, cough and rapid breathing are the most common presenting symptoms. Other symptoms include lethargy, poor feeding, and 'unwell' child. Localized chest, abdominal, or neck pain is a feature of pleural irritation. Examination reveals tachypnoea, nasal flaring and chest indrawing. There may be end-inspiratory coarse crackles over the affected area. Oxygen saturation may be decreased. General supportive care should include oxygen for hypoxia and analgesia if there is pain. Intravenous fluids should be given if necessary, to correct dehydration and maintain adequate hydration and sodium balance. Consider pneumonia in children with neck stiffness or acute abdominal pain.

Chronic lung infection

Any child with a persistent cough that sounds 'wet' (i.e. sounds like there is excess sputum in the chest) or is productive requires further investigations. Referral to a specialist in paediatric respiratory disorders is indicated.

Exercise 1
Answer the following questions. Prepare short talks and/or dialogues on these topics

1. Which are causes of acute wheezing (acute cough, whooping cough, persistent or recurrent cough).
2. Characterize causes of persistent or recurrent cough.
3. What do you know about pneumonia and chronic lung infection?

Translation 1

1. Causes of acute wheezing are: atypical pneumonia, foreign body inhalation, and anaphylaxis. 2. Cough is the most common symptom of respiratory disease. 3. Identifying if the cough is dry or moist can be helpful diagnostically. 4. Whooping cough (pertussis) is a highly contagious respiratory infection. 5. After a week of coryza, the child develops a characteristic paroxysmal or spasmodic cough followed by a characteristic inspiratory whoop. 6. The child goes red or blue in the face, and mucus flows from the nose and mouth. 7. The symptoms gradually decrease (convalescent phase), but may persist for many months. 8. In any child with a severe, persistent cough, tuberculosis should be considered. 9. Causes of persistent or recurrent cough are: pertussis, respiratory syncytial virus, lobar collapse, mycoplasma, suppurative lung diseases, persistent bacterial bronchitis, inhaled foreign body, cigarette smoking, tuberculosis, airway anomalies. 10. Pneumonia is a major cause of childhood mortality in low and middle-income countries. 11. Fever, cough and rapid breathing are the most common presenting symptoms. 12. Examination reveals tachypnoea, nasal flaring and chest indrawing. 13. General supportive care should include oxygen for hypoxia and analgesia if there is pain.

Text 2
Cystic fibrosis

CF is the most common life-limiting autosomal recessive condition in Caucasians. It is well recognized but less common in other ethnic groups. Average life expectancy has increased for current newborns into the 40s.

Clinical features of cystic fibrosis
Newborn

- Diagnosed through newborn screening
- Meconium ileus

Infancy
- Prolonged neonatal jaundice
- Growth faltering
- Recurrent chest infections
- Malabsorption, steatorrhea

Young child
- Bronchiectasis
- Rectal prolapse
- Nasal polyp
- Sinusitis

Older child and adolescent
- Allergic bronchopulmonary aspergillosis
- Diabetes mellitus
- Cirrhosis and portal hypertension
- Distal intestinal obstruction (meconium ileus equivalent)
- Pneumothorax or recurrent haemoptysis
- Sterility in males

Diagnosis

The essential diagnostic procedure is the sweat test, to confirm that the concentration of chloride in sweat is markedly elevated. Cystic fibrosis should be considered in any child with recurrent infections, loose stools or faltering growth.

Management

The effective management of CF requires a multidisciplinary team approach. With regular treatment, many infants and children will have no respiratory symptoms, and often have no abnormal signs. From diagnosis, children should have physiotherapy at least twice a day, aiming to clear the airways of secretions. In younger children, parents are taught to perform airway clearance at home using chest percussion and postural drainage. Physical exercise is beneficial and is encouraged.

Periodic review of the child with cystic fibrosis

Siblings	May be affected, too	Monitor for potential complications:	• Nasal polyps, sinusitis, rectal prolapse • Allergic bronchopulmonary aspergillosis (ABPA) • Diabetes mellitus (often insulin dependent) • Cirrhosis and portal hypertension • Distal intestinal obstruction syndrome (DIOS), meconium ileus equivalent) • Pneumothorax or recurrent haemoptysis Concern about sterility in males
Sweat	salty, may lead to dehydration in hot weather	Sputum	Acute or chronic colonisation with Pseudomonas aeruginosa or Burkholderia cepacian
Central venous line, e.g. Portacath	for intravenous antibiotics to aggressively treat infection	Growth	Aim for normal growth
Chest — determine if:	• Hyper-expansion due to air trapping • Harrison's sulcus • Coarse inspiratory crepitations and/or expiratory wheeze Chest infection	Nutrition	• Gastrostomy for overnight feeding for extra calories? • Pancreatic exocrine insufficiency • Taking sufficient pancreatic replacement therapy? • Taking fat-soluble vitamins?
Clubbing of fingers?		Review of chest problems	• Spirometry to identify deterioration • Regular breathing exercises? • Physiotherapy and exercise? • Bronchodilator therapy – is it optimal? • Chest infection — acute or chronic and its treatment? • Nebulised antipseudomonal antibiotics and DNAse? • Avoidance of direct contact with other affected patients other than family members?
Scar from operation for meconium ileus as neonate (10-20%)		General overview	• School attendance and performance • Specific problems with managing their disease • Psychological needs

Immunodeficiency

Children with immunodeficiency may develop severe, unusual, or recurrent chest infections.

Tuberculosis

Tuberculosis remains an important cause of chronic lung infection. All children with a persistent productive cough should have a chest X-ray and either a tuberculin skin test or Tuberculosis blood test.

Sleep-disordered breathing

Sleep-disordered breathing occurs either due to airway obstruction, central hypoventilation or a combination of these. Key aspects of the history include loud snoring, witnessed pauses in breathing (apnoeas), restlessness, and disturbed sleep. Obstructive sleep apnoea leads to excessive daytime sleepiness, or hyperactivity, learning and behaviour problems, faltering growth, and in severe cases, pulmonary hyperextension. In most basic assessment is overnight pulse oximetry, which can be performed in the child's home.

Tracheostomy

If a child with a tracheostomy develops sudden and severe breathing difficulties, it may be that the tracheostomy tube is blocked with secretions and needs urgent suction or needs changing immediately. All children with a tracheostomy should have a spare tracheostomy tube with them at all times, and a carer competent to change it.

Long term ventilation

An increasing number of children are receiving long-term respiratory support. Preterm infants with severe bronchopulmonary dysplasia may require additional oxygen for many months. Children who have more severe respiratory failure may need 24-hour respiratory support via a tracheostomy.

Some indications for tracheostomy in children

Narrow upper airways	Subglottic stenosis Laryngeal anomalies (e.g. atresia, haemangiomas, webs) Pierre Robin sequence (small jaw and cleft palate) Other craniofacial anomalies (e.g. Crouzon disease)
Lower airway anomalies	Severe tracheobronchomalacia
Long-term ventilation	Muscle weakness Head or spinal injury
Wean from ventilation	Any prolonged period of ventilation

Airway protection	To facilitate clearance of secretions

Exercise 2
Answer the following questions. Prepare short talks and/or dialogues on these topics

1. What are clinical features of cystic fibrosis?
2. Describe diagnosis, management and periodic review of the child with cystic fibrosis.
3. Speak about immunodeficiency, tuberculosis and sleep-disordered breathing.
4. What are indications for tracheostomy in children?

Translation 2

1. Cystic fibrosis is the most common life-limiting autosomal recessive condition in Caucasians. 2. Clinical features of cystic fibrosis are: prolonged neonatal jaundice, growth faltering, recurrent chest infections, malabsorption, steatorrhea, bronchiectasis, rectal prolapse, sinusitis, cirrhosis and portal hypertension, intestinal obstruction, pneumothorax or recurrent haemoptysis. 3. The essential diagnostic procedure is the sweat test, to confirm that the concentration of chloride in sweat is markedly elevated. 4. Cystic fibrosis should be considered in any child with recurrent infections, loose stools or faltering growth. 5. Children should have physiotherapy at least twice a day, aiming to clear the airways of secretions. 6. Children with immunodeficiency may develop severe, unusual, or recurrent chest infections. 7. All children with a persistent productive cough should have a chest X-ray and either a tuberculin skin test or Tuberculosis blood test. 8. Key aspects of the sleep-disordered breathing include: loud snoring, witnessed pauses in breathing (apnoeas), restlessness, and disturbed sleep. 9. If a child with a tracheostomy develops sudden and severe breathing difficulties, it may be that the tracheostomy tube is blocked with secretions and needs urgent suction or needs changing immediately. 10. Children who have more severe respiratory failure may need 24-hour respiratory support via a tracheostomy. 11. Some indications for tracheostomy in children are: narrow upper airways, lower airway anomalies, long-term ventilation, wean from ventilation, airway protection.

Text 3
Cardiac disorders
Heart disease in children is mostly congenital.

The most common congenital heart lesions
Left-to-right shunts (breathless)
- Ventricular septal defect
- Persistent arterial duct
- Atrial septal defect

Right-to-left shunts (blue)
- Tetralogy of Fallot
- Transposition of the great arteries

Common mixing (breathless and blue)
- Atrioventricular septal defect (complete)

Outflow obstruction in a well child (asymptomatic with a murmur)
- Pulmonary stenosis
- Aortic stenosis

Outflow obstruction in a sick neonate (collapsed with shock)
- Coarctation of the aorta

Heart murmurs
The most common presentation of congenital heart disease is with a heart murmur. Even so, the vast majority of children with murmurs have a normal heart. They have an 'innocent murmur'. The features of an innocent murmur can be remembered as the five Ss: Innocent murmur = Soft, Systolic, asymptomatic, left sternal edge.

Heart failure
Symptoms:
- Breathlessness (particularly on feeding or exertion)
- Sweating
- Poor feeding
- Recurrent chest infections

Signs:
- Poor weight gain or faltering growth
- Tachypnoea
- Tachycardia
- Heart murmur, gallop rhythm
- Enlarged heart
- Hepatomegaly

- Cool peripheries.

Causes of heart failure
- Neonates — obstructed (duct-dependent) systemic circulation
- Hypoplastic left heart syndrome
- Critical aortic valve stenosis
- Severe coarctation of the aorta
- Interruption of the aortic arch
- Infants (high pulmonary blood flow)
- Ventricular septal defect
- Atrioventricular septal defect
- Large persistent ductus arteriosus
- Older children and adolescents (right or left heart failure)
- Eisenmenger syndrome (right heart failure only)
- Rheumatic heart disease
- Cardiomyopathy.

Cyanosis
- Peripheral cyanosis (blueness of the hands and feet) may occur when a child is cold or unwell
- Central cyanosis, seen on the tongue as a slate blue colour, is associated with a fall in arterial blood oxygen tension
- Persistent cyanosis in an otherwise well infant is nearly always a sign of structural heart disease.

Cyanosis in a newborn infant with respiratory distress may be due to:
- cardiac disorders
- respiratory disorders
- persistent pulmonary hypertension
- infections
- metabolic acidosis and shock

Exercise 3
Study the following summary and then interpret basic information in English.

1. Pertussis
Caused by Bordetella pertussis
Paroxysmal cough followed by inspiratory whoop and vomiting; in infants, apnoea rather than whoop, which is potentially dangerous.
Diagnosis: culture of organism on pernasal swab, marked lymphocytosis.

2. Sleep disordered breathing
The majority are due to adenotonsillar hypertrophy, and surgical removal usually dramatically improves symptoms.
3. Presentation of congenital heart disease
Antenatal ultrasound screening
Detection of a heart murmur — need to differentiate innocent from pathological
Cyanosis — if duct dependent, prostaglandin to maintain ductal patency is vital to initial survival
Heart failure —usually from left-to-right shunt when pulmonary vascular resistance falls
Shock — when duct closes in severe left heart obstruction.

Exercise 4
Study the following summary and then interpret basic information in English.

Cyanotic congenital heart disease

Lesion	Clinical features	Management
Tetralogy of Fallot	Loud murmur at upper left sternal edge Clubbing of fingers and toes (older) Hyper-cyanotic spells	Surgery at 6 – 9 months of age
Transposition of the great arteries	Neonatal cyanosis No murmur	Prostaglandin infusion
Eisenmenger syndrome	No murmur	Balloon atrial septostomy Arterial switch operation in neonatal period

Common mixing

Lesion	Clinical features	Management
Atrioventricular septal defect (complete)	Down syndrome Cyanosis at birth Breathless at 2 – 3 weeks	Treat heart failure medically Surgical repair at 3 months
Complex diseases (e.g. tricuspid atresia)	Cyanosis Breathless	Shunt or pulmonary artery banding, then surgery

Outflow obstruction in the well child

Lesion	Signs	Management
Aortic stenosis	Murmur, upper right sternal edge; carotid thrill	Balloon dilatation
Pulmonary stenosis	Murmur, upper left sternal edge; carotid thrill	Balloon dilatation
Coarctation (adult type)	Systemic hypertension Radio-femoral artery	Stent insertion or surgery

Left heart outflow obstruction in the sick infant – duct-dependent lesions

Lesion	Clinical features	Management
Coarctation of the aorta	Circulatory collapse Absent femoral pulses	Maintain ABC Prostaglandin infusion
Interruption of the aortic arch	Circulatory collapse Absent femoral pulses and absent left brachial pulse	Maintain ABC Prostaglandin infusion
Hypoplastic left heart syndrome	Circulatory collapse All peripheral pulses absent	Maintain ABC Prostaglandin infusion

Jones criteria for diagnosis of rheumatic fever
Major manifestations

Carditis (50%)
Endocarditis
- significant murmur
- valvular dysfunction

Myocarditis
- may lead to heart failure and death

Pericarditis
- pericardial friction rub
- pericardial effusion
- tamponade

Migratory arthritis (80%)
Ankles, knees, and wrists
Exquisite tenderness, moderate redness and swelling
'Flitting', lasting <1 week in a joint, but migrating to other joints over 1 – 2 months

Sydenham chorea (10%)

2 – 6 months after the streptococcal infection

Involuntary movements and emotional lability for 3 – 6 months

Erythema marginatum (<5%)

Uncommon, early manifestation

Rash on trunk and limbs

Pink macules spread outwards, causing pink border with fading centre.
Borders may unite to give a map like outline

Subcutaneous nodules (rare)

Painless, pea-sized, hard

Mainly on extensor surfaces

Causes of pulmonary hypertension

•   Pulmonary arterial hypertension

Idiopathic: sporadic or familial

Post-tricuspid shunts

HIV infection

Persistent pulmonary hypertension of the newborn

•   Pulmonary venous hypertension

Left-sided heart disease

Pulmonary vein stenosis or compression

•   Pulmonary hypertension with respiratory disease

Chronic obstructive lung disease or bronchopulmonary dysplasia in
preterm infants

Interstitial lung disease

Obstructive sleep apnoea or upper airway obstruction

•   Pulmonary thromboembolic disease

•   Pulmonary inflammatory or capillary disease.

Exercise 5
**Answer the following questions. Prepare short talks and/or dialogues
on these topics**

1.   Which are the most common congenital heart lesions?
2.   Describe heart murmurs.
3.   Characterize symptoms, signs and causes of heart failure.

4. What can you say about cyanosis?
5. What do you know about cyanotic congenital heart disease?
6. Characterize Jones criteria for diagnosis of rheumatic fever.
7. Describe major manifestations of carditis, endocarditis, myocarditis, pericarditis, migratory arthritis, Sydenham chorea, erythema marginatum, subcutaneous nodules).
8. What are causes of pulmonary hypertension?

Translation 3

1. The most common congenital heart lesions are: left-to-right shunts, ventricular septal defect, persistent arterial duct, atrial septal defect, right-to-left shunts, tetralogy of Fallot, transposition of the great arteries, atrioventricular septal defect, common mixing, outflow obstruction, pulmonary stenosis, and coarctation of the aorta. 2. The most common presentation of congenital heart disease is with a heart murmur. 3. Symptoms of heart failure are: breathlessness, sweating, poor feeding, recurrent chest infections. 4. Signs of heart failure are: poor weight gain or faltering growth, tachypnoea, tachycardia, heart murmur, enlarged heart, hepatomegaly, cool peripheries. 5. Peripheral cyanosis (blueness of the hands and feet) may occur when a child is cold or unwell. 6. Central cyanosis, seen on the tongue as a slate blue colour, is associated with a fall in arterial blood oxygen tension. 7. Cyanosis in a newborn infant with respiratory distress may be due to: cardiac disorders, respiratory disorders, persistent pulmonary hypertension, infections, metabolic acidosis and shock.

Text 4
Kidney and urinary tract disorder
Assessment of renal function in children

Plasma creatinine concentration	Main test of renal function. Rises progressively throughout childhood according to height and muscle bulk. May not be outside laboratory 'normal range' until renal function has fallen to less than half normal
Estimated glomerular filtration	Better measure of renal function than creatinine and useful to monitor renal function serially in children with renal impairment
Inulin or EDTA (ethylene diamine tetra acetic acid) glomerular filtration rate	More accurate as clearance from the plasma of substances freely filtered at the glomerulus, and is not secreted or reabsorbed by the tubules. Need for repeated blood sampling over several hours limits use in children.

Creatinine clearance	Requires time for urine collection and blood tests. Rarely done in children as inconvenient and often becomes inaccurate
Plasma urea concentration	Increased in renal failure, often before creatinine starts rising, and raised levels may be symptomatic. Urea levels also increased by high protein diet, in catabolic states, or due to gastrointestinal bleeding.

Some congenital abnormalities of the kidneys and urinary tract

Bilateral renal agenesis or bilateral multicystic dysplastic kidneys
⇓
Reduced foetal urine excretion
⇓
Oligohydramnios causing foetal compression

Potter syndrome

Intrauterine compression of the foetus from oligohydramnios caused by lack of foetal urine causes characteristic facies, lung hypoplasia, and postural deformities including severe talipes. The infant may be stillborn or die soon after birth from respiratory failure.

- Potter facies
- Low-set ears
- Beaked nose
- Prominent epicanthic folds and downward slant to eyes
- Pulmonary hypoplasia causing respiratory failure
- Limb deformities

Urinary tract infection

UTI in childhood is important because:

- up to half of patients have a structural abnormality of their urinary tract.
- Pyelonephritis may damage the growing kidney by forming a scar, predisposing to hypertension and to progressive chronic kidneys if the scarring is bilateral

Presentation of urinary tract infection in infants and children

Infants	Children
Fever	Dysuria, frequency and urgency
Vomiting	Abdominal pain or loin tenderness
Poor feeding/ faltering growth	Fever with or without rigors (exaggerated shivering)
Jaundice	Lethargy and anorexia
Septicaemia	Vomiting, diarrhoea
Offensive urine	Haematuria
Febrile seizure (<6 months)	Offensive/cloudy urine
	Febrile seizure
	Recurrence of enuresis

Methods and interpretation of dipstick testing in children
Methods of dipstick testing

Nitrile stick testing	Positive result useful as very likely to indicate a true urinary tract infection (UTI) But some children with a UTI are nitrite negative
Leucocyte esterase stick testing (for white blood cells)	May be present in children with UTI but may also be negative Present in children with febrile illness, without UTIs Positive in balanitis and vulvovaginitis

Interpretation of results

Leucocyte esterase and nitrite positive	Regard as UTI
Leucocyte esterase negative and nitrite positive	Start antibiotic treatment if clinical evidence of UTI Diagnosis depends on urine culture
Leucocyte esterase positive and nitrite negative	Only start antibiotic treatment if clinical evidence of UTI Diagnosis depends on urine culture

Leucocyte esterase and nitrite negative	UTI unlikely. Repeat or send urine for culture if clinical history suggests UTI
Blood, protein, and glucose present on stick testing	Useful in any unwell child to identify other diseases, e.g. nephritis, diabetes mellitus, but will not discriminate between children with and without UTIs.

Collection of samples

For the child in nappies, urine can be collected by:

- A 'clean catch' sample into a waiting clean pot when the nappy is removed
- an adhesive plastic bag applied to the perineum after careful washing, although there may be contamination from the skin
- a urethral catheter
- suprapubic aspiration, when a fine needle attached to a syringe is inserted directly into the bladder just above the symphysis pubis under ultrasound guidance

In the older child, urine can be obtained by collecting a midstream sample. Ideally, the urine sample should be observed under a microscope to identify organisms and cultured straight away. Dipstick can be used as a screening test. A urine sample should be tested in all infants with an unexplained fever >38°C

Exercise 6

Answer the following questions. Prepare short talks and/or dialogues on these topics

1. How to assess renal function in children?
2. Speak about some congenital abnormalities of the kidneys and urinary tract.
3. What is Potter syndrome?
4. Describe presentation of urinary tract infection in infants and children.
5. Describe methods and interpretation of dipstick testing in children.
6. How to collect samples and interpret results?

Translation 4

1. Assessment of renal function in children includes: plasma creatinine concentration, estimated glomerular filtration, Inulin or EDTA (ethylene diamine tetracetic acid), glomerular filtration rate, creatinine clearance,

plasma urea concentration. 2. These are some congenital abnormalities of the kidneys and urinary tract: bilateral renal agenesis, reduced foetal urine excretion, oligohydramnios. 3. In Potter syndrome intrauterine compression of the foetus from oligohydramnios caused by lack of foetal urine causes characteristic facies, lung hypoplasia, and postural deformities including severe talipes. 4. In urinary tract infection patients have a structural abnormality of their urinary tract. 5. Urinary tract infection in infants includes: fever, vomiting, poor feeding/ faltering growth, jaundice, septicaemia, offensive urine, febrile seizures. 6. Urinary tract infection in children includes: dysuria, frequency and urgency, abdominal pain or loin tenderness, fever with or without rigors, exaggerated shivering, lethargy and anorexia, vomiting, diarrhoea, haematuria, offensive/cloudy urine, febrile seizure, recurrence of enuresis. 7. For the child in nappies, urine can be collected by: a 'clean catch' sample, an adhesive plastic bag, a urethral catheter, or suprapubic aspiration. 8. In the older child, urine can be obtained by collecting a midstream sample. 9. Ideally, the urine sample should be observed under a microscope to identify organisms and cultured straight away.

Text 5
Incomplete bladder emptying
Contributing factors in some children are:
* infrequent voiding, resulting in bladder enlargement
* vulvitis
* incomplete micturition with residual postmicturition bladder volumes
* obstruction by a loaded rectum from constipation
* neuropathic bladder
* vesicoureteral reflux

Vesicoureteral reflux
VUR - associated ureteric dilatation is important as:
* urine returning to the bladder from the ureters after voiding results in incomplete bladder emptying which encourages infection
* the kidneys may become infected (pyelonephritis)
* bladder voiding pressure is transmitted to the renal papillae which may contribute to renal damage.

Infection may destroy renal tissue, leaving a scar, resulting in a shrunken, poorly functioning segment of kidney (reflux nephropathy). Progressive chronic kidney disease may develop.

Reflux is due to a developmental anomaly of the vesicoureteric junction:
- familial
- secondary to bladder pathology
- can occur with UTI (temporary)

Mild reflux
- reflux into ureter only

Severe reflux
- Gross dilatation of ureter, renal pelvis and calyces
- Predisposes to intrarenal reflux and renal scarring with UTI

Investigation
Atypical UTI includes:
- seriously ill or septicaemia
- poor urine flow
- abdominal or bladder mass
- raised creatinine
- failure to respond to suitable antibiotics
- infection with atypical organisms

An initial ultrasound will identify:
- serious structural abnormalities and urinary obstruction
- renal defects

Management
All infants under 3 months of age with suspicion of a UTI or if seriously ill should be referred immediately to hospital. They require intravenous antibiotic therapy. Infants aged over 3 months and children with acute pyelonephritis/upper UTI and fever or bacteruria and loin pain/tenderness are usually treated with oral antibiotics. Children with cystitis/lower UTI can also be treated with oral antibiotics.

Medical measures for the prevention of UTI
The aim is to ensure washout of organisms that ascend into the bladder from the perineum; and to reduce the presence of aggressive organisms in the stool, perineum, and under the foreskin:

- high fluid intake
- regular voiding
- complete bladder emptying

- prevention of constipation
- good perineal hygiene
- Lactobacillus acidophilus, a probiotic to encourage colonization of the gut by this organism
- antibiotic prophylaxis

Follow-up of children with recurrent UTIs, renal scarring, or reflux

In these children:

- urine should be dipsticked with any non-specific illness in case it is caused by a UTI
- long-term, low-dose antibiotic prophylaxis can be used
- circumcision in boys may sometimes be considered
- anti-VUR surgery may be indicated
- blood pressure should be checked annually
- and urinalysis is to check for proteinuria
- regular assessment of renal growth and function if there are bilateral defects because of the risk of progressive chronic kidney disease.

A child with a first urinary tract infection

Why important?	Up to half have a structural abnormality of their urinary tract
	Pyelonephritis may damage the growing kidney by forming a renal scar, which may result in hypertension and chronic renal failure
Predisposing factors	Incomplete bladder emptying
	Constipation
	Vesicoureteral reflux
Diagnosis secure?	Suggestive clinical features?
	Upper or lower urinary tract infection?
	Urine sample properly collected and processed?
	Culture of single organism
Why investigate?	To identify serious structural abnormalities, urinary obstruction, renal scars, vesicoureteral reflux

Management

Treat infection with antibiotics

Advice about medical preventive measures to consider:
- High fluid intake
- Regular voiding, double micturition
- Prevent or treat constipation
- Good perineal hygiene
- Lactobacillus acidophilus

Advise to check urine culture if develops clinical features suggestive of non-specific illness

If renal scarring or reflux on investigation, or develops recurrent UTIs:
- Consider low-dose antibiotic prophylaxis
- Monitor blood pressure, renal growth and function

Exercise 7
Answer the following questions. Prepare short talks and/or dialogues on these topics

1. What are contributing factors of incomplete bladder emptying?
2. Why is vesicoureteral reflux important?
3. What does atypical urinary tract infection (UTI) include?
4. Speak about management of UTI and medical measures for the prevention.
5. Characterize follow-up of children with recurrent UTIs, renal scarring, or reflux.
6. What can you say about a child with a first urinary tract infection and its management?
7. What are medical preventive measures to consider?

Translation 5
1. Contributing factors of incomplete bladder emptying may be: infrequent voiding, vulvitis, incomplete micturition, obstruction from constipation, neuropathic bladder, and vesicoureteral reflux. 2. Vesicoureteral reflux is important as: urine returning to the bladder encourages infection, the kidneys may become infected, or bladder voiding pressure may contribute to renal damage. 3. Infection may destroy renal tissue, leaving a scar, resulting in a shrunken, poorly functioning segment of kidney. 4. Reflux is due to a developmental anomaly of the vesicoureteric junction. 5. Atypical UTI includes: seriously ill or septicaemia, poor urine flow, abdominal or bladder mass, raised creatinine, failure to respond to suitable antibiotics, infection with atypical organisms. 6. An initial ultrasound will identify: serious structural abnormalities, urinary

obstruction, and renal defects. 7. The aim of medical measures for the prevention of UTI is to ensure washout of organisms that ascend into the bladder from the perineum and to reduce the presence of aggressive organisms in the stool, perineum, and under the foreskin. 8. In children with recurrent UTIs, renal scarring, or reflux, urine should be dipsticked; with any non-specific illness, long-term, low-dose antibiotic prophylaxis can be used, circumcision in boys may be considered, anti-VUR surgery may be indicated, blood pressure should be checked, urinalysis to check for proteinuria, and regular assessment of renal growth and function. 9. Advice about medical preventive measures to consider is: high fluid intake, regular voiding, double micturition, prevent or treat constipation, good perineal hygiene, lactobacillus acidophilus. 10. Consider low-dose antibiotic prophylaxis, and monitor blood pressure, renal growth and function.

Text 6
Enuresis
Daytime enuresis
This is a lack of bladder control during the day in a child over the age of 3-5 years. Nocturnal enuresis is also usually present. It may be caused by:
- lack of attention to bladder sensation
- detrusor instability (sudden, urgent urge to void induced by sudden bladder contractions)
- bladder neck weakness
- a neuropathic bladder (bladder is enlarged and fails to empty properly associated with spina bifida and other neurological conditions)
- a UTI (rarely in the absence of other symptoms)
- constipation
- an ectopic ureter, causes constant dribbling and child is always damp

An ultrasound may show bladder pathology, with incomplete bladder emptying or thickening of the bladder wall.

Secondary (onset) enuresis
The loss of previously achieved urinary continence may be due to:
- emotional upset
- UTI
- polyuria in diabetes mellitus, sickle cell disease or chronic kidney disease

Investigation should include:
- testing a urine sample for infection, glycosuria, and proteinuria using a dipstick
- assessment of urinary concentrating ability
- ultrasound of the renal tract

Proteinuria

Persistent proteinuria is significant and should be quantified by measuring the urine protein to creatinine ratio in an early morning sample.

Causes of proteinuria

- Orthostatic proteinuria
- Glomerular abnormalities
- Minimal change disease
- Glomerulonephritis
- Abnormal glomerular basement membrane (familial nephritides)
- Increased glomerular filtration pressure
- Reduced renal mass in chronic kidney disease
- Hypertension
- Tubular proteinuria

Nephrotic syndrome

Clinical signs of the nephrotic syndrome are:

- periorbital oedema (particularly on waking)
- scrotal or vulvar, leg, and ankle oedema
- breathlessness due to pleural effusions and abdominal distension
- infection such as peritonitis, septic arthritis or sepsis

Investigations performed at presentation of nephrotic syndrome

- Urine protein — on test strips (dipstick)
- Full blood count and erythrocyte sedimentation rate
- Urea, electrolytes, creatinine, albumin
- Complement levels — C3, C4
- Anti-streptolysin O or anti DNAse B titres and throat swab
- Urine microscopy and culture
- Urinary sodium concentration
- Hepatitis B and hepatitis C screen
- Malarial screen if travel abroad

Steroid-resistant nephrotic syndrome

Cause	Specific features	Prognosis
Focal segmental glomerulosclerosis	Most common Familial or idiopathic	30% progress to end-stage renal failure in 5 years; Recurrence post-transplant is common
Mesangiocapillary glomerulonephritis (membranoproliferative glomerulonephritis)	More common in older children Haematuria and low complement level present	Decline in renal function over many years
Membranous nephropathy	Associated with hepatitis B May precede SLE (systemic lupus erythematosus)	Most remit spontaneously within 5 years

Exercise 8
Study the following summary and then interpret basic information in English.

1. Enuresis
Daytime enuresis
Consider possible causes: developmental or psychogenic, bladder instability or neuropathy, UTI, constipation, ectopic ureter.
2. Secondary (onset) enuresis
Consider: emotional upset, UTI, polyuria from an osmotic diuresis in diabetes mellitus or a renal concentrating disorder.
3. Nephrotic syndrome
Clinical signs: oedema (periorbital, scrotal, or vulvar, leg and ankle oedema; ascites, pleural effusions.
Diagnosis: heavy proteinuria and low plasma albumin
4. Steroid-sensitive nephrotic syndrome
Characteristic features: 1-10 years-old; no macroscopic haematuria; and normal blood pressure, complement levels, and renal function.
Management: oral corticosteroids, renal biopsy
Complications: hypovolaemia, thrombosis, infection (pneumococcal), hypercholesterolaemia.
Prognosis: may resolve or else there may be infrequent of frequent relapses.

Exercise 9
Answer the following questions. Prepare short talks and/or dialogues on these topics

1. What does the term enuresis mean?
2. What are causes of proteinuria?
3. What investigations are performed at presentation of nephrotic syndrome?
4. What is meant by steroid-resistant nephrotic syndrome?

Translation 6

1. Daytime enuresis is a lack of bladder control during the day in a child over the age of 3-5 years. 2. Nocturnal enuresis may be caused by: lack of attention to bladder sensation, detrusor instability, urgent urge to void, a neuropathic bladder, a UTI, constipation, and an ectopic ureter. 3. The loss of previously achieved urinary continence may be due to: emotional upset, UTI, polyuria in diabetes mellitus, sickle cell disease or chronic kidney disease. 4. Investigation should include: testing a urine sample for infection, glycosuria, and proteinuria and ultrasound of the renal tract. 5. Persistent proteinuria is significant and should be quantified by measuring the urine protein to creatinine ratio in an early morning sample. 6. Causes of proteinuria are: orthostatic proteinuria, glomerular abnormalities, glomerulonephritis, increased glomerular filtration pressure, reduced renal mass, hypertension, tubular proteinuria. 7. Clinical signs of the nephrotic syndrome are: periorbital oedema, scrotal or vulvar, leg, and ankle oedema, breathlessness, infection such as peritonitis, septic arthritis or sepsis. 8. Investigations performed at presentation of nephrotic syndrome are: urine protein – on test strips, full blood count and erythrocyte sedimentation rate, urine microscopy and culture, urinary sodium concentration, hepatitis B and hepatitis C screen, malarial screen if travel abroad. 9. Causes of steroid-resistant nephrotic syndrome are: focal segmental glomerulosclerosis, mesangiocapillary glomerulonephritis, and membranous nephropathy.

Text 7
Haematuria

Urine that is red in colour or tests positive for haemoglobin on urine sticks should be examined under the microscope to confirm haematuria. UTI is the most common cause of haematuria.

Hypertension

Presentation includes vomiting, headaches, facial palsy, hypertensive retinopathy, convulsions, or proteinuria. Faltering growth and cardiac failure are the most common features in infants. Early detection of hypertension is important. All children with a renal tract abnormality should have their blood pressure checked annually throughout life.

Causes of hypertension

- Renal
- Renal parenchymal disease
- Renovascular, e.g. renal artery stenosis
- Polycystic kidney disease (autosomal recessive polycystic kidney disease and autosomal dominant polycystic kidney disease)
- Renal tumours
- Coarctation of the aorta
- Catecholamine excess
- Pheochromocytoma
- Neuroblastoma
- Endocrine
- Congenital adrenal hyperplasia
- Cushing syndrome or corticosteroid therapy
- Hyperthyroidism
- Essential hypertension
- A diagnosis of exclusion

Renal masses

An abdominal mass identified on palpating the abdomen should be investigated promptly by ultrasound scan

Causes of palpable kidneys
Unilateral

- Multicystic kidney
- Compensatory hypertrophy
- Obstructed hydronephrosis
- Renal tumour (Wilms tumour)
- Renal vein thrombosis

Bilateral

- Autosomal recessive polycystic kidneys
- Autosomal dominant polycystic kidneys
- Tuberous sclerosis

- Renal vein thrombosis

Renal calculi

Renal stones are uncommon in childhood. Presentation may be with haematuria, loin or abdominal pain, UTI, or passage of a stone. Stones that are not passed spontaneously should be removed. A high fluid intake is recommended in all affected children

Renal tubular disorders

Proximal tubule cells are especially vulnerable to cellular damage. Fanconi syndrome should be considered in a child presenting with:
- polydipsia and polyuria
- salt depletion and dehydration
- hyperchloremic metabolic acidosis
- rickets
- faltering or poor growth

Causes of Fanconi syndrome
Idiopathic

Secondary to inborn errors of metabolism
- Cystinosis (an autosomal recessive disorder causing intracellular accumulation of cystine)
- Glycogen storage disorders
- Lowe syndrome (oculocerebrorenal dystrophy)
- Galactosemia
- Fructose intolerance
- Tyrosinemia
- Wilson disease

Acquired
- Heavy metals
- Drugs and toxins
- Vitamin D deficiency

Acute kidney injury

Acute kidney injury can be classified as:
- prerenal: the most common cause in children
- renal: there is salt and water retention; blood, protein, and casts in the urine
- postrenal: from urinary obstruction.

Management

Investigation by ultrasound scan will identify obstruction of the urinary tract, the small kidneys of chronic kidney disease, or large, bright kidneys with loss or cortical medullary differentiation typical of an acute process.

Causes of acute kidney injury

Prerenal	Renal	Postrenal
Hypovolaemia: • gastroenteritis • burns • sepsis • haemorrhage • nephrotic syndrome **Circulatory failure**	**Vascular:** • haemolytic uremic syndrome • vasculitis • embolus • renal vein thrombosis **Tubular:** • acute tubular necrosis • ischaemic • toxic • obstructive **Glomerular:** • glomerulonephritis • Interstitial: • interstitial nephritis • pyelonephritis	**Obstruction:** • congenital, e.g. posterior urethral valves • acquired, e.g. blocked urinary catheter

Exercise 10
Answer the following questions. Prepare short talks and/or dialogues on these topics

1. What is the most common cause of haematuria?
2. Why is early detection of hypertension important?
3. What are causes of hypertension?
4. What are causes of palpable kidneys?
5. Characterize renal calculi and renal tubular disorders.
6. What are idiopathic and acquired causes of Fanconi syndrome?
7. How can acute kidney injury be classified?
8. What are causes of acute kidney injury (prerenal, renal, postrenal)?
9. What can be identified by ultrasound scan?

Translation 7

1. Urine that is red in colour or tests positive for haemoglobin on urine sticks should be examined under the microscope to confirm haematuria. 2. Presentation of hypertension includes vomiting, headaches, facial palsy, hypertensive retinopathy, convulsions, or proteinuria. 3. All children with a renal tract abnormality should have their blood pressure checked annually throughout life. 4. Causes of hypertension are: renal, renovascular,

polycystic kidney disease, renal tumours, neuroblastoma, congenital adrenal hyperplasia, Cushing syndrome, hyperthyroidism, and essential hypertension. 5. Causes of palpable kidneys are: multicystic kidney, compensatory hypertrophy, obstructed hydronephrosis, renal tumour, renal vein thrombosis, autosomal recessive polycystic kidneys, autosomal dominant polycystic kidneys, tuberous sclerosis, or renal vein thrombosis. 6. A high fluid intake is recommended in all children affected by renal calculi. 7. Fanconi syndrome should be considered in a child presenting with: polydipsia and polyuria, salt depletion and dehydration, hyperchloremic metabolic acidosis, rickets, faltering or poor growth. 8. Acute kidney injury can be classified as: prerenal, renal and postrenal. 9. Causes of prerenal acute kidney injury are: hypovolaemia and circulatory failure. 10. Causes of renal acute kidney injury are: vascular, tubular, glomerular, and interstitial. 11. Obstruction is the cause of postrenal acute kidney injury.

Text 8
Dialysis
   Dialysis in acute kidney injury is indicated when there is:
   * failure of conservative management
   * hyperkalaemia
   * severe hyponatraemia or hypernatremia
   * pulmonary oedema or severe hypertension due to volume overload
   * severe metabolic acidosis
   * multisystem failure.

If plasma exchange is part of the treatment (e.g. in vasculitis), haemodialysis is used. Continuous arteriovenous or venovenous hemofiltration provides gentle, continuous dialysis and fluid removal. Acute kidney injury in childhood generally carries a good prognosis for renal recovery

Haemolytic uremic syndrome
   HUS is a triad of acute renal failure, microangiopathic haemolytic anaemia, and thrombocytopenia. Typical HUS is secondary to gastrointestinal infection. It follows a prodrome of bloody diarrhoea. The toxin from these organisms enters the gastrointestinal mucosa and localizes to the endothelial cells of the kidney. Other organs such as the brain, pancreas, and heart may also be involved.
   With early supportive therapy, including dialysis, the typical diarrhoea-associated HUS usually has a good prognosis. By contrast, atypical HUS has no diarrhoeal prodrome, may be familial, and frequently relapses. It has a high risk of hypertension and progressive chronic kidney disease.

Haemolytic uremic syndrome — the triad of:
- acute kidney injury
- haemolytic anaemia
- thrombocytopenia

Chronic kidney disease
Chronic kidney disease is progressive loss of renal function due to numerous conditions.

Clinical features
- anorexia and lethargy
- polydipsia and polyuria
- faltering growth/growth failure
- bony deformities from renal osteodystrophy
- hypertension
- acute-on-chronic renal failure (precipitated by infection or dehydration)
- incidental finding of proteinuria
- unexplained normochromic, normocytic anaemia.

Dialysis and transplantation
The optimum management is by renal transplantation. Technically this is difficult in very small children and a minimum weight, e.g. 10 kg, needs to be reached before transplantation. Kidneys obtained from living related donors have a higher success rate than deceased donor kidneys. Ideally, a child is transplanted before dialysis if required, but if this is not possible, a period of dialysis may be necessary.

Exercise 11
Study the following summary and then interpret basic information in English.

1. Acute nephritis
Cause: usually post-infectious or follows a streptococcal infection, but also vasculitis, IgA nephropathy, and familial nephritis.
Clinical features: oedema (around the eyes), hypertension, decreased urine output, haematuria and proteinuria.
Management: fluid and electrolyte balance, diuretics, monitor for rapid deterioration in renal function.
2. Acute kidney injury
Prerenal: from hypovolaemia and circulatory failure

| Renal: most often haemolytic uremic syndrome |
| Management: treat underlying cause, metabolic abnormalities, dialysis if necessary. |
| **3. Chronic kidney disease** |
| Causes: congenital (structural malformations and hereditary nephropathies) most common. |
| Presentation: abnormal antenatal ultrasound, anorexia and lethargy, polydipsia and polyuria, faltering growth/growth failure, renal rickets (osteodystrophy), hypertension, proteinuria, anaemia. |
| Management: diet and nasogastric or gastrostomy feeding, phosphate restriction and activated vitamin D to prevent renal osteodystrophy, salt supplements and free access to water to control salt and water balance, bicarbonate supplements to prevent acidosis, erythropoietin to prevent anaemia, growth hormone, and dialysis and transplantation. |

Exercise 12
Answer the following questions. Prepare short talks and/or dialogues on these topics

1. When is dialysis in acute kidney injury indicated?
2. What can you say about haemolytic uremic syndrome?
3. What are clinical features of chronic kidney disease?
4. Speak about dialysis and transplantation.

Translation 8

1. Dialysis in acute kidney injury is indicated when there is: failure of conservative management, hyperkalaemia, severe hyponatraemia or hypernatremia, pulmonary oedema, metabolic acidosis, or multisystem failure. 2. Continuous arteriovenous or venovenous hemofiltration provides gentle, continuous dialysis and fluid removal. 3. Haemolytic uremic syndrome is a triad of acute renal failure, microangiopathic haemolytic anaemia, and thrombocytopenia. 4. Typical HUS is secondary to gastrointestinal infection. 5. The toxin from these organisms enters the gastrointestinal mucosa and localizes to the endothelial cells of the kidney. 6. Other organs such as the brain, pancreas, and heart may also be involved. 7. Haemolytic uremic syndrome is the triad of: acute kidney injury, haemolytic anaemia and thrombocytopenia. 8. Chronic kidney disease is progressive loss of renal function due to numerous conditions. 9. Clinical features are: anorexia and lethargy, polydipsia and polyuria, faltering growth/growth failure, bony deformities, hypertension, renal failure, proteinuria, anaemia. 10. The optimum management is by renal transplantation. 11. Kidneys obtained from living related donors have a higher success rate than deceased donor kidneys.

VOCABULARY 4

abrupt /ə'brʌpt/
accumulation /əˌkjuːmjʊ'leɪˌʃən/
acetic /ə'siːtɪk/ **acid** /'æsɪd/
acidophil /'æsɪdəʊˌfɪl/
adenotonsillar /ˌædɪnəʊ.tɒn.sələ/
adhesive /əd'hiː.sɪv/
agenesis /eɪ'dʒenɪs.ɪs/
aim /eɪm/ **at** /æt/
angiocapillary /ˌæn.dʒi'ə kə'pɪl.ər.i/
annually /'ænjʊəlɪ/
anomaly /ə'nɒm.ə.li/
anti /'æntɪ/
antipseudomonal /ˌæntɪˌsuː'də.məʊ'nəl/
antistreptolysin /ˌæntɪˌstreptə'laɪ.sɪn/
aortic /eɪ'ɔː.tɪk/ **valve** /vælv/
arterial /ɑː'tɪə.ri.əl/
ascend /ə'send/
aspergillosis /æˌspɔː.dʒɪ'ləʊ.sɪs/
atrial /'eɪ.tri.əl/
atrioventricular /ˌɑː.trɪ.ə.ven'trɪk.jə.lər/
balanitis /ˌbal.ə.'naɪ.təs/
balloon /bə'luːn/
band /bænd/
beak /biːk/
border /bɔː.dər/
Bordetella /bəʊ.də.tel.æ/ *pertussis* /pə'tʌs.ɪs/
breathless /'breθ.lɪs/
Burkholderia cepacia /burk.hol.der'iː.æ siːpeɪ'ʃiː.æ/
calyx /'keɪ.lɪks/
cast /kɑːst/
catabolic /ˌkætə'bɒl.ɪk/
catheter /'kæθ.ɪ.tər/
Caucasian /kɔː'keɪ.ʒən/
chorea /ko'rɪə/
ciliary /'sɪ.lɪː.ˌər.i:/
circumcision /ˌsɜː.kəm'sɪ.ʒən/
cloudy /'klaʊ.di/
coarse /kɔːs/
complement /'kɒm.plɪ.ment/
contagious /kən'teɪ.dʒəs/
continuous /kən'tɪn.ju.əs/
convalescent /ˌkɒnvə'les.ənt/
convulsion /kən'vʌl.ʃən/
culminate /'kʌl.mɪ.neɪt/
cystine /sɪs.tɪn/

cystinosis /ˈsɪstɪ.nəʊ.sɪs/
damp /dæmp/
depletion /dɪˈpliː.ʃən/
detrusor /dɪˈtruːzə/
diamine /ˌdɪˈeɪ.miːn/
differentiation /ˌdɪf.ər.en.ʃiˈeɪ.ʃən/
disturb /dɪˈstɜːb/
diuretic /ˌdaɪ.jʊˈret.ɪk/
DNAse B, deoxyribonuclease / diːˌɒksɪˌraɪbəʊˈnjuːklɪeɪz/
ductus arteriosus /ˈdəktəs ɑːr.ˌtir.iːˈəʊ.səs/
dyskinesia /ˌdɪs.kaɪˈniː.zɪ.ə/
ectopic /ekˌtɒp.ɪk/
Eisenmenger syndrome /aɪˈzen.menˈger ˈsɪn.drəʊm/
embolus /ˈem.bə.ləs/ pl **emboli**
endothelial /ˌendəʊˈθiːlɪəl/
erythema /ˌer.ɪˈθiː.mə/
erythrocyte /ɪˈrɪθ.rəʊ.saɪt/
erythropoietin /eˌrɪθ.rəˈpɒɪ.ə.tɪn/
estimated /ˈes.tɪ.meɪt.ɪd/
ethylene /ˈeθ.ɪ.liːn/
exclusion /ɪkˈskluː.ʒən/
exertion /ɪgˈzɜː.ʃən/
expectorate /ɪkˈspek.tər.eɪt/
exquisite /ɪkˈskwɪzɪt/
Fanconi syndrome /faːn.kəʊˈniː ˈsɪn.drəʊm/
femoral /ˈfemə.rəl/
fistula /ˈfɪs.tʃə.lə/ pl **fistulae**
flit /flɪt/
foreskin /ˈfɔːˌskɪn/
friction /ˈfrɪk.ʃən/
Galactosemia /gəˌlæktəˈsiː.mɪə/
gastrostomy /gæsˈtrə.stə.mi/
gentle /ˈdʒen.tl̩/
glomerular /glɒˈmərʊlə/
glycosuria /ˌglaɪkəʊˈsjʊərɪə/
guidance /ˈgaɪ.dəns/
habit /ˈhæb.ɪt/
haemodialysis /ˌhiː.məʊ.daɪˈæl.ə.sɪs/
hemofiltration /ˈhiː.mə.fɪlˈtreɪ.ʃən/
hyperchloremia /ˈhaɪ.pər.klɔːriː.miː.ə/
hypercyanotic /ˌhaɪ.pə.ˌsaɪəˈn ɒtik/
hyperkalaemia /ˈhaɪ.pər.kæˈliː.mɪ.ə/
hypertrophy /haɪˈpɜː.trə.fi/
hypoplastic /ˌhaɪ.pəʊˈpla.stik/
hypovolaemia /ˌhaɪ.pəʊ.vəˈliː.mɪ.ə/
inaccurate /ɪnˈækjʊrɪt/
incidental /ˌɪnsɪˈdentəl/

inconvenient /ˌɪnkən'viːnjənt/
indrawing /ɪn'drɔːɪŋ/
innocent /'ɪnəs.ənt/
interruption /ˌɪn.tə'rʌp.ʃən/
intracellular /ˌɪn.trə'sel.jə.lər/
inulin /in'ju.lɪn/
lability /leɪ.'bɪ.lə.tiː/
Lactobacillus /ˌlæktəʊ.bə'sɪləs/
life /laɪf/ **expectancy** /ɪk'spek.tən.si/
lobar /'ləʊ.bəʳ/
loin /lɔɪn/
Lowe syndrome / ləʊ 'sɪn.drəʊm/
lymphocytosis /ˌlɪmfəʊs.aɪ'təʊ.sɪs/
macrolide /'maɪkrəʊl.aɪd/
malarial /mə'leərɪəl/
marginal /'mɑː.dʒɪn.əl/
medullary /meˌdʌl.ə.ri/
microangiopathy /ˌmaɪkrəʊ'ændʒɪ'ɒpəθɪ/
micturition /ˌmɪktjʊ'rɪ.ʃən/
midstream /ˌmɪd'striːm/
migratory /'maɪ.grə.tər.i/
mucosa /mjuː'kəʊ.sə/
mycoplasma /ˌmaɪ.kəʊ.'plæz.mə/
nephritis /nɪ'fraɪ.tɪs/ pl **nephritides**
Nitrile /'naɪ.trɪl/
normochromic /ˌnɔː.məʊ'krəm.ɪk/
normocytic /ˌnɔː.məʊ'sɪtɪk/
oculocerebrorenal /ˌɒkjʊləˌserɪbrəʊ'riː.nəl/
oculocerebrorenal syndrome /ˌɒkjʊləˌserɪbrəʊ'riː.nəl 'sɪn.drəʊm/
offensive /ə'fent.sɪv/
orthostatic /ˌɔː.θə'stæt.ɪk/
osteodystrophy /ˌɒstɪəʊ.dɪ'strəʊ.fɪ/
overload /ˌəʊ.və'ləʊd/
overnight /ˌəʊ.və'naɪt/
papilla /pə'pɪlə/ pl **papillae**
pernasal /'pər.'neɪ.zəl/
pheochromocytoma /fiːəʊ.krəʊ.məʊs.aɪ'təʊ.mə/
polydipsia /ˌpɒl.ɪ'dɪp.sɪ.ə/
polyp /'pɒlɪp/
polyuria /ˌpɒl.ɪ'jʊə.rɪ.ə/
portacath /'pɔː.tə'kæθ/
post /'pəʊst/
postrenal /'pəʊst.'riː.nəl/
prerenal /prɪ.'riː.nəl/
preventive /prɪ.ventiv/
prodrome /'prəʊ.drəʊm/
productive /prə'dʌk.tɪv/

prolyferative /prəˈlɪfərətɪv/
prostaglandins /ˌprɒstəˈglændɪnz/
proteinuria /ˈprəʊ.tiːn.jʊəˈriː.ə/
pseudomonas aeruginosa /suː.dəʊ.məʊnæz e.rɜːdʒi.nəʊsæ/
pubis /ˈpjuː.bɪs/
radial /ˈreɪ.dɪəl/
ratio /ˈreɪ.ʃi.əʊ/
recurrence /rɪˈkʌ.rəns/
recurrent /rɪˈkʌ.rənt/
referred /rɪˈfɜːd/
relapse /rɪˈlæps/
remit /rɪˈmɪt/
renal /ˈriː.nəl/ **tubule** /ˈtjuː.bjuːl/
residual /rɪˈzɪd.ju.əl/
restlessness /ˈrest.ləs.nəs/
rickets /ˈrɪk.ɪts/
rigor /ˌrɪg.əˈ/
sample /saːmpl/
scrotal /ˈskrəʊ.təl/
sedimentation /ˌsedɪmenˈteɪ.ʃən/ **rate** /reɪt/
septostomy /sepˈtɒstəmɪ/
serially /ˈsɪə.ri.ə.li/
shivering /ˈʃɪv.ər.ɪŋ/
shrink /ʃrɪŋk/
slant /slaːnt/
slate /sleɪt/
sleepiness /ˈsliː.pɪ.nəs/
sodium /ˈsəʊ.di.əm/ **chloride** /ˈklɔːraɪd/
spasmodic /spæzˈmɒd.ɪk/
spell /spel/
steatorrhea /ˌstɪətəˈrɪə/
stent /stent/
stillborn /ˈstɪl.bɔːn/
sulcus /sʌl.kəs/ pl **sulci**
suppurative /ˈsʌpjʊrə.tɪv/
suprapubic /ˌsuː.prəˈpjuː.bɪk/
suspicion /səˈspɪ.ʃən/
swab /swɒb/
switch /swɪtʃ/
Sydenham /sid'en.ham/ **chorea** /kɒˈrɪə/
symphysis /ˈsɪm.fɪ.sɪs/ **pubis** /ˈpjuː.bɪs/
syringe /sɪˈrɪndʒ/
talipes /tal.ə.piːz/
tamponade /tæm.pəˈneɪd/
temporary /ˈtem.pər.ər.i/
tension /ˈten.ʃən/
tetralogy /teˈtræ.lə.dʒɪ/ **of Fallot**

throat /θrəʊt/ **swab** /swɒb/

thromboembolism /ˌθrɒmbəʊˈembəˌlɪzəm/

titre /ˈtaɪ.tə/

tracheostomy /ˌtræk.iˈɒst.ə.mi/

transposition /ˌtrænspəˈzɪ.ʃən/

tricuspid /traɪˈkʌs.pɪd/

tube /tjuːb/

tyrosinemia /ˌtaɪ.rəʊ.sɪˈniːmɪə/

unite /juːˈnaɪt/

ureter /jʊəˈriː.tər/

urge /ɜːdʒ/

urgency /ˈɜː.dʒən.si/

valvular /ˈvælv.jə.lər/

vasculitis /væskjʊˈlaɪ.tɪs/

vesicoureteric /vesɪ.kəʊ.jʊˈriː.tər.ɪk/

void /vɔɪd/

vulvar /vʌlˈvəl/

vulvitis /vʌlˈvaɪ.tɪs/

wake /weɪk/

washout /ˈwɒʃˌaʊt/

wean /wiːn/

web /web/

whoop /wuːp/

Wilson /wilˈsɒn/ **disease** /dɪˈziːz/

Genital disorders; Other acute inguinoscrotal conditions; Liver disorders; Cystic fibrosis; Cirrhosis and portal hypertension

Text 1
Features of genital disorders in children are:
- hydroceles, inguinal hernias and undescended testes, usually arise from abnormal embryological development
- the acute scrotum is a surgical emergency
- foreskin conditions and hypospadias are common in boys
- vulvovaginitis and labial adhesions are common in girls

Inguinoscrotal conditions
Embryology

Development of a testis from an early indeterminate gonad is determined by genes associated with a Y chromosome. For a testis to descend from its origin on the posterior abdominal wall, it must produce testosterone. The testis migrates down into the inguinal canal. The structures that are found in the scrotum in a boy (testis, vas and blood vessels) or labium in a girl pass through the abdominal wall and pick up layers corresponding to those of the abdominal wall. If it remains patent and in continuity with the abdomen fluid or abdominal contents can become a hydrocele or hernia, respectively.

Inguinal hernia

A hernia presents as a lump in the groin which may extend into the scrotum or labium. They may be intermittent, visible during straining. The contents of the hernia may become irreducible (incarcerated), causing pain or damage to the testis (strangulation). The lump is tender and the infant may be irritable and may vomit. Most hernias can be successfully reduced by 'taxis' (gentle compression in the line of the inguinal canal). If reduction is impossible, emergency surgery is required. Prompt surgical repair is indicated for inguinal hernias in infants to lower the risk of incarceration.

Hydrocele

A hydrocele has the same underlying anatomy as a hernia. Hydroceles are usually asymptomatic and sometimes appear blue. Hydroceles usually resolve spontaneously. Surgery may be considered if it persists beyond the first two years of life.

Varicocele

This is a scrotal swelling comprising dilated (varicose) testicular veins and usually occurs at puberty. Its cause is multifactorial; valvular incompetence plays a role. It is usually asymptomatic, but may cause a dull ache. On examination it may have a bluish colour. Sometimes the testis is smaller or softer than normal. Occlusion of the gonadal veins can be achieved by surgical ligation.

Undescended testis

Most undescended testes become arrested along their normal pathway of descent. The diagnosis should ideally be made at the routine examination of the newborn. Examination of the testes in babies must be made in a warm environment and with warm hands. An undescended testis may be palpable or impalpable. A palpable undescended testis is usually seen or felt in the groin, but cannot be manipulated into the scrotum. Occasionally it can be palpated outside the scrotum — the so-called 'ectopic' testis. If the testis is impalpable, it may be in the inguinal canal but cannot be identified or it may be intra-abdominal or absent. If there are bilateral impalpable testes, the karyotype must be established to exclude disorders of sex development. This should be regarded as a medical emergency. The crucial difference between a retractile and undescended testis is that a retractile testis can be manipulated into the scrotum. Action of the cremaster muscle (as seen in eliciting the cremasteric reflex by light touch on the abdominal wall) pulls up the testis. Undescended testis should be referred to a paediatric surgeon when detected. If surgery is required, the optimum time is within the first year of life.

Investigation and management

Orchidopexy, the surgical placement of the testis in the scrotum, is performed for the following reasons:

- Cosmetic — symmetrical appearance as other boys
- Reduced risk of torsion and trauma
- Fertility — the testis needs to be in the scrotum, below body temperature, in order to allow spermatogenesis. Delaying orchidopexy beyond the first two years of life adversely affects testicular development.

- Malignancy — placing the testis in the scrotum facilitates self-examination

Torsion of the testis

This is commonest in post-prepubertal boys. It is usually very painful, with redness and oedema of the scrotal skin. However, the pain may be localised to the groin or lower abdomen highlighting the need to always examine the testes in a boy presenting with sudden-onset pain in the groin, abdomen, or scrotum. Surgical exploration in any acute scrotal presentation is mandatory.

Torsion of appendix testis

Torsion of appendix testis tends to affect prepubertal boys and is more common than torsion of the testis.

Scrotal exploration of the appendage is often necessary.

Exercise 1
Answer the following questions. Prepare short talks and/or dialogues on these topics

1. What are features of genital disorders in children?
2. Speak about embryology, inguinal hernia, hydrocele, varicocele, and undescended testis.
3. Speak about investigation and management.
4. What do you know about torsion of the testis and torsion of appendix testis?

Translation 1

1. Features of genital disorders in children are: hydroceles, inguinal hernias and undescended testes, the acute scrotum, foreskin conditions and hypospadias and vulvovaginitis and labial adhesions. 2. Development of a testis from an early indeterminate gonad is determined by genes associated with a Y chromosome. 3. The testis migrates down into the inguinal canal. 4. The structures that are found in the scrotum in a boy (testis, vas and blood vessels) or labium in a girl pass through the abdominal wall and pick up layers corresponding to those of the abdominal wall. 5. A hernia presents as a lump in the groin which may extend into the scrotum or labium. 6. Most hernias can be successfully reduced by 'taxis' (gentle compression in the line of the inguinal canal). 7. Prompt surgical repair is indicated for inguinal hernias in infants to lower the risk of incarceration. 8. A hydrocele has the same underlying anatomy as a hernia. 9. Surgery may be considered

if it persists beyond the first two years of life. 10. Varicocele is a scrotal swelling comprising dilated (varicose) testicular veins and occurs usually at puberty. 11. It is usually asymptomatic, but may cause a dull ache. 12. Occlusion of the gonadal veins can be achieved by surgical ligation.

Exercise 2
Match the column A with the column B. Try to learn the expressions and/or sentences by heart.

A

1. Most undescended testes become arrested ...
2. Examination of the testes in babies must be made ...
3. A palpable undescended testis is usually seen or felt ...
4. Occasionally it can be palpated ...
5. If the testis is impalpable, it may be in the inguinal canal ...
6. If there are bilateral impalpable testes, ...
7. Action of the cremaster muscle ...
8. Orchidopexy, the surgical placement of the testis in the scrotum, ...
9. Torsion of the testis is commonest ...
10. It is usually very painful, ...
11. Surgical exploration in any acute ...
12. Torsion of appendix testis tends to affect ...

B

a. ... *is performed for the following reasons: cosmetic, reduced risk of torsion, fertility, malignancy.*
b. ... *prepubertal boys and is more common than torsion of the testis.*
c. ... *along their normal pathway of descent.*
d. ... *but cannot be identified or it may be intra-abdominal or absent.*
e. ... *with redness and oedema of the scrotal skin.*
f. ... *in a warm environment and with warm hands.*
g. ... *the karyotype must be established to exclude disorders of sex development.*
h. ... *scrotal presentation is mandatory.*
i. ... *(as seen in eliciting the cremasteric reflex by light touch on the abdominal wall) pulls up the testis*
j. ... *outside the scrotum – the so-called 'ectopic' testis.*
k. ... *in post-prepubertal boys.*
l. ... *in the groin, but cannot be manipulated into the scrotum.*

Text 2
Other acute inguinoscrotal conditions

Infection may cause an acute scrotum. A urine sample should be obtained to identify an associated urinary tract infection. Pus should be sent at operation for microbiology to characterize the nature of the infection. Trauma to the scrotum is an uncommon cause of testicular damage, but may need exploration, debridement and surgical repair. Sexual abuse needs to be considered in all genital injuries. Torsion of the testis must be excluded (by emergency exploration if necessary) in boys with an 'acute scrotum'. Delay leads to testicular loss.

Abnormalities of the penis
The foreskin

A normal foreskin does not retract in infancy, and retraction should not be attempted. At 1 year of age, about half of uncircumcised boys have a non-retractile (normal) foreskin. Ballooning of the foreskin on urination is a common cause of parental concern. It has no functional consequence, does not represent obstruction, and does not need intervention.

Non-retractile foreskin and phimosis

A foreskin that is pathologically non-retractile will truly render the glans 'muzzled', (Greek word 'phimosis'). The commonest condition that gives rise to a true phimosis is balanitis xerotica obliterans, or BXO, which gives rise to progressive scarring which can extend onto the glans, into the meatus and ultimately into the urethra. BXO is the index indication for circumcision.

Paraphimosis

This is a condition, usually in post-pubertal boys, of as retracted foreskin that cannot be reduced easily. There is a ring of narrower skin and the glans swells. It may result in compromise of the blood supply to the glans.

Circumcision

Circumcision remains a tradition in Jewish and Muslim religions. Medical reasons for circumcision include:
- BXO causing a true phimosis
- recurrent balanoposthitis causing refractory symptoms
- prophylaxis of recurrent urinary infection
- if access to the urethra is required reliably for intermittent catheterization, e.g. spina bifida

There is some evidence that circumcision affords protection against transmission of HIV and HPV (human papillomavirus). Up to one boy in fifty has post-operative bleeding requiring a return to the operating theatre, infection, or ulceration. A non-retractile foreskin is normal in preschool children.

Undescended testis
- Common — up to 5% of term boys
- If testis palpable, requires orchidopexy
- If impalpable, may require laparoscopy to establish presence of a testis
- If bilateral impalpable, urgent karyotype is essential
- Retractile testes usually do not require surgery

Acute scrotal conditions
- May occur at any age but torsion of testis must be considered not only for acute pain of the scrotum but also for acute abdominal and groin pain
- scrotal surgical exploration is required unless torsion of the testis can be reliably excluded

Non-retractile foreskin
- Is normal in preschool children
- Is pathological if associated with BXO
- Circumcision is not recommended routinely but is still traditional in some communities worldwide

Hypospadias
- Common — 1 in 200 boys
- Variable ventral urethral meatus and penile curvature
- Surgery may be required in first two years of life
- Infants with hypospadias must not be circumcised

Genital disorders in girls
Vulvovaginitis/vaginal discharge
The commonest problem is redness of the vulva. In infants, this is often due to a nappy rash. Less often, the vulvovaginitis is infective, occasionally with Candida infection. Vaginal discharge is common. If it is green or offensive it may indicate infection.

Labial adhesions

Fusion of the labia minora can be a cause of local irritation in the prepubertal girl. There is usually an adequate orifice for the passage of urine. Unless the labial adhesion causes significant symptoms, no specific treatment is required.

Other conditions

If there is a bulging introitus that appears blue, the diagnosis is imperforate hymen — and the treatment is hymenotomy under anaesthesia. In contrast to problems with the testes in boys, ovarian problems tend to be more difficult to diagnose because they are intra-abdominal. An ovarian cause for symptoms should be considered in a girl who presents with acute abdominal pain (from ovarian cyst or torsion) or a mass (cyst or tumour). Blood stained vaginal discharge must be investigated.

Exercise 3
Answer the following questions. Prepare short talks and/or dialogues on these topics

1. Describe other acute inguinoscrotal conditions.
2. Describe abnormalities of the penis.
3. What can you say about circumcision?
4. Characterize genital disorders in girls.

Translation 2

1. A urine sample should be obtained to identify an associated urinary tract infection. 2. Pus should be sent at operation for microbiology to characterize the nature of the infection. 3. Sexual abuse needs to be considered in all genital injuries. 4. A normal foreskin does not retract in infancy, and retraction should not be attempted. 5. The commonest condition that gives rise to a true phimosis is balanitis xerotica obliterans, (BXO), which gives rise to progressive scarring which can extend onto the glans, into the meatus and ultimately into the urethra. 6. Paraphimosis is a condition, usually in post-pubertal boys, of as retracted foreskin that cannot be reduced easily. 7. Circumcision remains a tradition in Jewish and Muslim religions.

Exercise 4

Match the column A with the column B. Try to learn the expressions and/or sentences by heart.

A

1. Medical reasons for circumcision include: …
2. There is some evidence that circum affords protection …
3. A non-retractile foreskin …
4. In genital disorders in girls …
5. Less often, the vulvovaginitis is infective, …
6. Fusion of the labia minora can be a cause …
7. There is usually an adequate orifice …
8. If there is a bulging introitus that appears blue, …
9. An ovarian cause for symptoms should be considered …

B

a. … *is normal in preschool children.*
b. … *of local irritation in the prepubertal girl.*
c. … *BXO, recurrent balanoposthitis, prophylaxis of recurrent urinary infection, and if access to the urethra is required for intermittent catheterization.*
d. … *in a girl who presents with acute abdominal pain (from ovarian cyst or torsion) or a mass (cyst or tumour).*
e. … *for the passage of urine.*
f. … *against transmission of HIV and HPV (human papillomavirus).*
g. … *the diagnosis is imperforate hymen – and the treatment is hymenotomy under anaesthesia.*
h. … *occasionally with Candida infection.*
i. … *the commonest problem is redness of the vulva.*

Text 3
Liver disorders
Features of liver disorders in children are:
- Prolonged neonatal jaundice requires investigation to identify liver disease
- The earlier in life biliary atresia is diagnosed and treated surgically, the better the prognosis.
- Chronic hepatitis B virus (HBV) infection in children can be prevented.
- Hepatitis C is now curable with oral antiviral drugs

- Liver transplantation is an effective therapy for acute or chronic liver failure.
- Liver disease in children is uncommon and should be managed by, or in conjunction with national centres.
- If prolonged (persistent) jaundice, always look to see if the stools are pale, which suggests bile duct obstruction.

The symptoms and signs of hepatic disfunction

Encephalopathy
Jaundice
Epistaxis
Cholestasis:
- fat malabsorption
- deficiency of fat-soluble vitamins
- pruritus
- pale stools
- dark urine

Ascites
Hypotonia
Peripheral neuropathy
Rickets secondary to vitamin D deficiency
Varices with portal hypertension
Spider nevi
Muscle wasting from malnutrition
Bruising and petechiae
Splenomegaly with portal hypertension
Hypersplenism
Hepatorenal failure
Palmar erythema
Clubbing
Loss of fat stores secondary to malnutrition

Viral hepatitis

The clinical features of acute viral hepatitis include nausea, vomiting, abdominal pain, lethargy, and jaundice.

Hepatitis A

Hepatitis A virus is an RNA virus which is spread by faecal-oral transmission. Vaccination is required for travellers to endemic areas. There is no treatment and no evidence that bed rest or change of diet is effective.

Hepatitis B

Hepatitis B (HBV) is a DNA virus that is an important cause of acute and chronic liver disease worldwide.

- perinatal transmission from carrier mother
- inoculation with infected blood via blood transfusion, needlestick injuries, or renal dialysis
- among adults it can also be transmitted sexually

Asymptomatic carrier children can develop chronic HBV liver disease which may progress in cirrhosis.

Exercise 5
Study the following summary and then interpret basic information in English.

1. Genital conditions in male infants
Inguinal hernia/hydrocele
Cause inguinoscrotal swellings: clinically one can get above a hydrocele
Expedient surgical repair of inguinal hernias is required in infants to prevent bowel strangulation or after reduction of an irreducible hernia
2. Genital conditions in female infant
Vulvovaginitis in infants is usually due to nappy rash
Labial adhesions tend to recur; no treatment is indicated unless symptomatic
3. Hepatitis B virus (HBV)
Perinatal transmission from carrier mothers should be prevented by maternal screening and giving the infant a course of hepatitis B vaccine with hepatitis B immunoglobulin if indicated. Universal hepatitis B immunization is given in many countries.
Infection may result in chronic HBV liver disease, which may progress to cirrhosis and hepatocellular carcinoma.

Hepatitis C

Hepatitis C virus (HCV) is an RNA virus that was responsible for 90% of post-transfusion hepatitis until the screening of donor blood was introduced. The prevalence is high among intravenous drug users. Six percent of transmission occurs from infected mothers. It seldom causes an acute infection, but the majority become chronic carriers.

Hepatitis D virus

Hepatitis D virus (HDV) is a defective RNA virus that depends on hepatitis B virus for replication. It occurs as coinfection with hepatitis B virus.

Hepatitis E virus

This is an RNA virus that is enterally transmitted, usually by contaminated water. Hepatitis E virus causes a mild, self-limiting illness in most people and is known to be transmitted by blood transfusion or eating infected pork. In pregnant women it causes fulminant hepatic failure with a high mortality rate.

Acute liver failure (fulminant hepatitis)

Acute liver failure in children is the development of massive hepatic necrosis with subsequent loss of liver function, with or without hepatic encephalopathy. The child may present within hours or weeks with jaundice, encephalopathy, coagulopathy, hypoglycaemia, and electrolyte disturbance. Early signs of encephalopathy include alternate periods of irritability and confusion with drowsiness. Older children may be aggressive and unusually difficult. Complications include cerebral oedema, haemorrhage from gastritis or coagulopathy, sepsis and pancreatitis.

Management

Early referral to a national paediatric liver centre is essential. Steps to stabilize the child prior to transfer include:

- maintaining the blood glucose
- preventing sepsis
- preventing haemorrhage
- prevent cerebral oedema

Liver disease in older children
Autoimmune hepatitis and sclerosing cholangitis

The mean age of presentation is 7 years to 10 years. It is more common in girls. It may present as an acute hepatitis, as fulminant hepatic failure or chronic liver disease with autoimmune features such as skin rash, arthritis, haemolytic anaemia, or nephritis. Autoimmune hepatitis may occur in association with inflammatory bowel disease, coeliac disease, or other autoimmune diseases.

Exercise 6
Answer the following questions. Prepare short talks and/or dialogues on these topics

1. What are features of liver disorders in children?
2. What are the symptoms and signs of hepatic disfunction?

3. Characterize Hepatitis A, Hepatitis B, Hepatitis C, Hepatitis D, and Hepatitis E.
4. What can you say about liver disease in older children?

Translation 3

1. The symptoms and signs of hepatic disfunction are encephalopathy, jaundice, epistaxis, cholestasis, ascites, hypotonia, peripheral neuropathy, rickets, varices, spider nevi, muscle wasting, bruising and petechiae, splenomegaly, hypersplenism, hepatorenal failure, palmar erythema, clubbing, loss of fat stores. 2. The clinical features of acute viral hepatitis include nausea, vomiting, abdominal pain, lethargy, and jaundice. 3. Acute liver failure in children is the development of massive hepatic necrosis with subsequent loss of liver function, with or without hepatic encephalopathy. 4. The child may present within hours or weeks with jaundice, encephalopathy, coagulopathy, hypoglycaemia, and electrolyte disturbance. 5. Early signs of encephalopathy include alternate periods of irritability and confusion with drowsiness. 6. Complications include cerebral oedema, haemorrhage from gastritis or coagulopathy, sepsis and pancreatitis. 7. Steps to stabilize the child prior to transfer include: maintaining the blood glucose, preventing sepsis, haemorrhage and cerebral oedema. 8. Liver disease in older children may present as an acute hepatitis, as fulminant hepatic failure or chronic liver disease with autoimmune features such as skin rash, arthritis, haemolytic anaemia, or nephritis. 9. Autoimmune hepatitis may occur in association with inflammatory bowel disease, coeliac disease, or other autoimmune diseases.

Text 4
Cystic fibrosis

Liver disease is the second most common cause of death after respiratory disease in cystic fibrosis. The most common liver abnormality is hepatic steatosis (fatty liver). Liver transplantation may be considered for those in end-stage disease, either alone or in combination with a heart-lung transplant.

Wilson disease

Wilson disease is an autosomal recessive disorder. Many mutations have been identified. Neurological improvement may take up to 12 months of therapy. About 30% of children with Wilson disease will die from hepatic complications if untreated. Liver transplantation is considered for children with acute liver failure or severe end-stage liver disease.

Non-alcoholic fatty liver disease

It is a spectrum of disease, ranging from simple fatty deposition (steatosis) through to inflammation (steatohepatitis), fibrosis, cirrhosis, and end-stage liver failure. In childhood, it may be associated with a metabolic syndrome or with obesity. Some children complain of vague right upper quadrant pain or lethargy. Treatment targets weight loss through diet and exercise, which may lead to liver function tests returning to normal.

Complications of chronic liver disease
Nutrition

Effective nutrition is essential. Barriers to effective nutrition include:

- fat malabsorption — long chain fat is not effectively absorbed without bile. Fat-soluble vitamins are supplemented.
- protein malnutrition — common at presentation of liver disease. Protein intake should not be restricted unless the child is encephalopathic.
- anorexia — when unwell children will require nasogastric tube feeding or occasionally parenteral nutrition.

Fat-soluble vitamins

All fat-soluble vitamins can be given orally. In severe deficiency, intramuscular administration may be required.

The effects of fat-soluble vitamin deficiency

Fat-soluble vitamin	Effect of deficiency
Vitamin K	Bleeding diathesis including intracranial bleeding
Vitamin A	Retinal changes in infants and night blindness in older children
Vitamin E	Peripheral neuropathy, haemolysis, and ataxia
Vitamin D	Rickets and fractures

Pruritus

Severe pruritus is associated with cholestasis. Treatment includes:

- Loose cotton clothing, avoiding overheating, keep nail short
- Moisturizing the skin with emollients
- Medication to stimulate bile flow

Encephalopathy

This occurs in end-stage liver disease and may be precipitated by gastrointestinal haemorrhage, sepsis, sedatives, renal failure, or electrolyte imbalance. Infants present with irritability and sleepiness, while older children present with abnormalities in mood, sleep rhythm, intellectual performance, and behaviour.

Cirrhosis and portal hypertension

Cirrhosis is the end result of many forms of liver disease. It is defined as extensive fibrosis with regenerative nodules. The main pathophysiological effects of cirrhosis are diminished hepatic function and portal hypertension with splenomegaly, varices, and ascites. Hepatocellular carcinoma may develop. Children with compensated cirrhosis may be asymptomatic if liver function is adequate. As the cirrhosis increases, however, the results of deteriorating liver function and portal hypertension become obvious. Physical signs include jaundice, palmar and plantar erythema, telangiectasia and spider nevi, malnutrition, and hypotonia. Dilated abdominal veins and splenomegaly suggest portal hypertension, although the liver may be shrunken and impalpable.

Investigations include:
- screening for the known causes of chronic liver disease
- upper gastrointestinal endoscopy to detect oesophageal varices and/ or erosive gastritis
- abdominal ultrasound — may show a shrunken liver and splenomegaly with gastric and oesophageal varices
- liver biopsy

Oesophageal varices

These are inevitable consequence or portal hypertension and may develop rapidly in children. They are best diagnosed by upper gastrointestinal endoscopy.

Ascites

Ascites is a major problem. Contributory factors include hypoalbuminemia, sodium retention, renal impairment and fluid redistribution.

Spontaneous bacterial peritonitis

This should always be considered if there is undiagnosed fever, abdominal pain, tenderness, or an unexplained deterioration in hepatic or renal function. A diagnostic paracentesis should be performed and the fluid sent for white cell count and differential and culture.

Liver transplantation

Liver transplantation is an accepted therapy for acute or chronic end-stage liver failure. The indication for transplantation in chronic liver failure are:

- severe malnutrition
- complications (bleeding varices, resistant ascites)
- failure of growth and development
- poor quality of life

Absolute contraindications include sepsis, untreatable cardiopulmonary disease or cerebrovascular disease. There is considerable difficulty in obtaining small organs for children. Most children receive part of an adult's liver.

Complications post-transplantation include:

- primary non-function of the liver
- hepatic artery thrombosis
- biliary leaks and strictures
- rejection
- sepsis, the main cause of death

Children who survive the initial postoperative period usually do well. Long-term studies indicate normal psychosocial development and quality of life in survivors.

Exercise 7
Answer the following questions. Prepare short talks and/or dialogues on these topics

1. Characterize cystic fibrosis, Wilson disease and non-alcoholic fatty liver disease.
2. Describe complications of chronic liver disease.
3. Speak about nutrition.
4. What are the effects of fat-soluble vitamin deficiency?
5. Characterize pruritus and encephalopathy.
6. Characterize cirrhosis and portal hypertension.
7. What do you know about oesophageal varices, ascites, and spontaneous bacterial peritonitis?
8. What can you say about liver transplantation?

Translation 4

1. Liver disease is the second most common cause of death after respiratory disease in cystic fibrosis. 2. The most common liver abnormality is hepatic steatosis (fatty liver). 3. Wilson disease is an autosomal recessive disorder. 4. Liver transplantation is considered for children with acute liver failure or severe end-stage liver disease. 5. Non-alcoholic fatty liver disease is a spectrum of disease, ranging from simple fatty deposition (steatosis) through to inflammation (steatohepatitis), fibrosis, cirrhosis, and end-stage liver failure. 6. Treatment targets weight loss through diet and exercise, which may lead to liver function tests returning to normal. 7. Barriers to effective nutrition include: fat malabsorption, protein malnutrition, and anorexia. 8. The effects of fat-soluble vitamin deficiency are bleeding, bleeding diathesis, including intracranial bleeding, retinal changes in infants and night blindness in older children, peripheral neuropathy, haemolysis, and ataxia, rickets and fractures. 10. Treatment of pruritus includes: loose cotton clothing, moisturizing the skin with emollients, and medication to stimulate bile flow. 11. Encephalopathy occurs in end-stage liver disease and may be precipitated by gastrointestinal haemorrhage, sepsis, sedatives, renal failure, or electrolyte imbalance.

Exercise 8

Match the column A with the column B. Try to learn the expressions and/or sentences by heart.

A

1. Cirrhosis is the end result of …
2. The main pathophysiological effects of cirrhosis are: …
3. As he cirrhosis increases, however, …
4. Physical signs include jaundice, palmar and plantar erythema,
5. Investigations include: …
6. Oesophageal varices are inevitable consequence …
7. Spontaneous bacterial peritonitis should always be considered if there is …
8. Liver transplantation is an accepted therapy …
9. The indication for transplantation in chronic liver failure are: …
10. Absolute contraindications include sepsis, …
11. Complications post-transplantation include: …
12. Children who survive …

B

a.   *... undiagnosed fever, abdominal pain, tenderness, or an unexplained deterioration in hepatic or renal function.*
b.   *... diminished hepatic function and portal hypertension with splenomegaly, varices, and ascites.*
c.   *... untreatable cardiopulmonary disease or cerebrovascular disease.*
d.   *... non-function of the liver, hepatic artery thrombosis, biliary leaks, rejection, sepsis.*
e.   *... the results of deteriorating liver function and portal hypertension become obvious.*
f.   *... for acute or chronic end-stage liver failure.*
g.   *... telangiectasia and spider nevi, malnutrition, and hypotonia.*
h.   *... the initial postoperative period usually do well.*
i.   *... many forms of liver disease.*
j.   *... severe malnutrition, complications, failure of growth and development, poor quality of life.*
k.   *... or portal hypertension and may develop rapidly in children.*
l.   *... screening, upper gastrointestinal endoscopy, abdominal ultrasound, or liver biopsy.*

Key 5
Exercise 2
1c; 2f; 3l; 4j; 5d; 6g; 7i; 8a; 9k; 10e; 11c; 12b

Exercise 4
1c; 2f; 3a; 4i; 5h; 6b; 7e; 8g; 9d

Exercise 8
1i; 2b; 3e; 4g; 5l; 6k; 7a; 8f; 9j; 10c; 11d; 12h

VOCABULARY 5

acquisition /ˌæk.wɪˈzɪ.ʃən/
adhesion /ədˈhiː.ʒən/
adopt /əˈdɒpt/
afford /əˈfɔːd/
alertness /əˈlɜːt.nəs/
alternate /ˈɒl.tə.neɪ.t/
appendage /əˈpen.dɪdʒ/
array /əˈreɪ/
atresia /əˈtriː.ʃə/
attempt /əˈtempt/
attentively /əˈten.tɪv.li/
audiometry /ˌɔːdɪˈɒmɪtrɪ/
auditory /ˈɔːdɪtərɪ/
autoimmune /ˈɔː.təʊ.ɪˈmjuːn/
awareness /əˈweə.nəs/
babble /ˈbæbəl/
balanitis /ˌbal.ə.ˈnaɪ.təs/
balanoposthitis /ˌbælə·nəʊ.pɒsˈθaɪ.tɪs/
bile /baɪl/ duct /dʌkt/
biliary /ˈbɪl.i.ər.i/
blindness /blaɪnd.nɪs/
blink /blɪŋk/
bounce /baʊns/
brainstem /ˈbreɪn.stem/
bulging /ˈbʌl.dʒɪŋ/
Candida /ˈkændɪdə/
carcinoma /ˌkɑːsɪˈnəʊmə/
check /tʃek/
cholangitis /kəˈlændʒaɪ.tɪs/
cholestasis /ˈkɒlə·steɪ.sɪs/
circum- /ˈsɜːkəm/
cognition /kɒɡˈnɪʃ.ən/
cognitive /ˈkɒɡ.nɪ.tɪv/
compensate /ˈkɒm.pən.seɪt/
complex /kɒm.pleks/
conjunction /kənˈdʒʌŋk.ʃən/
consonant /ˈkɒnsənənt/
corticosteroid /ˌkɔːtɪ.kəʊˈstɪə.rɔɪd/
crayon /ˈkreɪən/
cremaster /ˌkriːməsˈter/ muscle /ˈmʌs.ļ/
cremasteric /ˌkriːməsˈter.ɪk/
crumb /krʌm/
cube /kjuːb/
cuff /kʌf/
curvature /ˈkɜː.və.tʃər/

142

deposition /ˌdep.əˈzɪʃ.ən/
detection /dɪˈtekʃən/
diathesis /daɪˈæθɪsɪs/
dipstick /ˈdɪpˌstɪk/
disappear /ˌdɪs.əˈpɪər/
doll /dɒl/
dominant /ˈdɒm.ɪ.nənt/
dorsum /ˈdɔː.səm/ pl **dorsa**
element /ˈelɪmənt/
elicit /ɪˈlɪs.ɪt/
emission /ɪˈmɪʃən/
emit /ɪˈmɪt/
emollient /ɪˈmɒljənt/
emphasize /ˈem.fə.saɪz/
encephalopathic /enˌsefələˈpæθɪk/
endoscopy /enˈdɒskəpɪ/
erosive /ɪˈrəʊ.ʒɪv/
evident /ˈev.ɪ.dənt/
expectation /ˌek.spekˈteɪʃən/
exploration /ˌek.spləˈreɪʃən/
extent /ɪkˈstent/
fertility /ˌfəˈtɪl.ɪ.ti/
finally /ˈfaɪ.nə.li/
fine /faɪn/
fix /fɪks/
fully /ˈfʊl.i/
fulminant /ˈfʊl.mɪ.nənt/
glans /glænz/
gonad /ˈgɒnæd/
gonadal /ˈgɒnædəl/
grasp /grɑːsp/
guesswork /ˈgesˌwɜːk/
hepatocellular /hɪˈpætəˈseljʊlə/
heredity /həˈred.ə.ti/
highlight /ˈhaɪ.laɪt/
hydrocele /ˈhaɪdrəʊˌsiːl/
hymen /ˈhaɪmen/
hymenotomy /ˈhaɪmen.ɒtəmɪ/
hypersplenism /ˌhaɪpəˈspliːnɪzəm/
hypoalbuminemia /ˌhaɪpəʊˈælbjʊmɪniːmɪə/
identification /aɪˌden.tɪ.fɪˈkeɪʃən/
imaginative /ɪˈmædʒɪnətɪv/
immature /ˌɪm.əˈtʃʊər/
impairment /ɪmˈpeərˌmənt/
imperforate /ɪmˈpɜːfərɪt/
impossible /ɪmˈpɒsəbəl/
improve /ɪmˈpruːv/

inanimate /ɪˈnæn.ɪ.mət/
incarceration /ɪnˌkɑːsəˈreɪʃən/
incompetence /ɪnˈkɒmpɪtəns/
independently /ˌɪn.dɪˈpen.dənt.li/
indeterminate /ˌɪndɪˈtɜːmɪnɪt/
inevitable /ɪnˈevɪt.əbəl/
inguinal /ˈɪŋ.gwɪ.nəl/
inoculation /ɪˌnɒk.jʊˈleɪ.ʃən/
interact /ˌɪn.təˈrækt/
interactive /ˌɪntərˈæktɪv/
introitus /ɪntrɔɪtəs/
investigate /ɪnˈves.tɪ.geɪt/
irreducible /ˌɪrɪˈdjuːsɪbəl/
ketone /ˈkiː.təʊn/
labial /ˈleɪbɪəl/
labium /ˈleɪbɪəm/
laparoscopy /ˌlæpəˈrɒskəpɪ/
letter /ˈletə/
leucocyte /ˈljuː.kə.saɪt/
limit /ˈlɪm.ɪt/
linear /ˈlɪn.i.ər/
locate /ləʊˈkeɪt/
locomotion /ˌləʊkəˈməʊʃən/
lump /lʌmp/
magical /ˈmædʒ.ɪ.kəl/
match /mætʃ/
mean /miːn/
meaning /ˈmiː.nɪŋ/
meatus /mɪˈeɪtəs/
midteens /ˈmɪd.tiːnz/
migrate /maɪˈgreɪt/
mode /məʊd/
motor /ˈməʊ.tər/
mutation /mjuːˈteɪʃən/
muzzle /ˈmʌz.l̩/
needlestick /ˈniːdəlˌstɪk/
nevus /ˈniː.vəs/ pl **naevi**
nipple /ˈnɪp.l̩/
nitrite /ˈnaɪtreɪt/
notice /ˈnəʊ.tɪs/
oesophageal /iːˌsɒfəˈdʒiːəl/
operational /ˌɒpərˈeɪʃənəl/
orchidopexy /ˌɔːkɪˈdopəksɪ/
orderly /ˈɔː.dəl.i/
otoacoustics /ˌəʊ.təʊˌəˈkuː.stɪks/
outstretched /ˌaʊtˈstretʃt/
overall /ˌəʊ.vəˈrɔːl/

palmar /ˈpælm.ər/
paracentesis /ˌpærəˈsenˈtiː.sɪs/
parachute /ˈpærəˌʃuːt/
parallel /ˈpær.ə.lel/
paraphimosis /ˌpær.ə.faɪˈməʊ.səs/
patent /ˈpeɪ.tənt/
peddle /ˈpedəl/
perform /pəˈfɔːm/
permission /pəˈmɪʃ.ən/
phimosis /faɪˈməʊ.səs/
phrase /freɪz/
pincer /ˈpɪnsə/
point /pɔɪnt/
polysyllabic /ˌpɒl.i.sɪˈlæb.ɪk/
portal /ˈpɔː.təl/
postural /ˈpɒst.ʃər.əl/
preference /ˈpref.ər.ənt s/
preschool /priːˈskuːl/
presenter /prɪˈzentə/
primitive /ˈprɪmɪtɪv/
procedure /prəˈsiːdʒə/
promotion /prəˈməʊˌʃən/
prop /prɒp/
protein /ˈprəʊ.tiːn/
push /pʊʃ/ **up** /ʌp/
quieten /ˈkwaɪə.tᵊn/
random /ˈrændəm/
reach for /riːtʃ/
recognition /ˌrek.əgˈnɪʃ.ən/
redistribution /ˌriːdɪstrɪˈbjuːʃən/
reflex /ˈriː.fleks/
reinforcement /ˌriːɪnˈfɔːsmənt/
rejection /rɪˈdʒekˌʃən/
render /ˈren.dər/
repair /rɪˈpeər/
replication /ˌrep.lɪˈkeɪˌʃən/
responsive /rɪˈspɒn.sɪv/
retention /rɪˈtenˌʃən/
rooting /ˈruːt ɪŋ/
saving /ˈlaɪfˌseɪ.vɪŋ/
scribble /ˈskrɪb.ļ/
scrotal /ˈskrəʊ.təl/
sentence /ˈsen.təns/
shadow /ˈʃæd.əʊ/
sign /saɪn/
slam /slæm/
smell /smel/

spermatogenesis /spər.mat.ə'dʒen.ə.səs/
sphygmomanometer /ˌsfɪg.məʊ.mɪ.tər/
spider /'spaɪ.dər/
spirometry /spaɪ'rɒ.m.ɪ.tri/
startle /'stɑː.tl̩/
steadily /'sted.ɪ.li/
steatohepatitis /ˌstɪətə.he.pə.'taɪ.təs/
step /step/
stranger /'streɪn.dʒər/
suitable /'sjuː.tə.bl̩/
summarize /'sʌm.ər.aɪz/
supplement /'sʌp.lɪ.mənt/
surgical /'sɜː.dʒɪ.kəl/
survivor /sə'vaɪ.vər/
suspend /sə'spend/
target /'tɑː.gɪt/
taxi /'tæksɪ/
teat /tiːt/
telangiectasia /tɪˌlændʒɪek'teɪ.zɪə/
thought /θɔːt/
torsion /'tɔː.ʃən/
uncircumcised /'sɜː.kəm.saɪzd/
undescended /ˌʌn.dɪ'sen.dɪd/
unpleasant /ʌn'plez.ənt/
urinalysis /ˌjʊə.rɪ.'næl.ə.sɪs/
vacuum /'væk.juːm/ **cleaner** /'kliː.nər/
varicocele /'vær.ɪ.koʊˌsil/
varix /'veə.rɪks/ pl **varices** /'vær.ɪ.siːz/
vas /væs/
vertically /'vɜː.tɪ.kəl.i/
vocalization /ˌvəʊ.kəl.aɪ'zeɪ.ʃᵊn/
voluntary /'vɒl.ən.tər.i/
wave /weɪv/
xerotic /zɪ'rɒtɪk/

Malignant disease; Radiotherapy; Leukaemia; Brain tumours; Soft tissue sarcomas; Haematological disorders; Clinical manifestations of sickle cell disease; Bleeding disorders

Text 1
Malignant disease
Features of malignant disease in children are:
- the pattern of malignant disease varies
- early diagnosis often optimises outcome
- management is conducted by specialist centres
- prognosis for many types of malignant disease has improved markedly

The types of disease are very different from those in adults, where carcinomas of the lung, breast, gut, and prostate predominate. The age at presentation varies:
- leukaemia affects children at all ages
- neuroblastoma and Wilms tumour are almost always seen in the first 6 years of age
- Hodgkin lymphoma and bone tumours have their peak incidence in adolescence

For children in the developed world, leukaemia is the most common malignancy followed by brain tumours.

Aetiology
In most cases, the aetiology of childhood cancer is unclear, but it is likely to involve an interaction between environmental factors (e.g. viral infection) and host genetic susceptibility. Cancer is usually sporadic but may be inherited.

Clinical presentation
Cancer in children can present with:
- a localized mass
- the consequences of disseminated disease, e.g. bone marrow infiltration, causing systemic ill-health

- the consequences of pressure from a mass on local structures or tissue, e.g. airway obstruction secondary to enlarged lymph nodes in the mediastinum

Investigations

Once a diagnosis of malignancy is suspected, the child should be referred to a specialist centre for further investigation.

Radiology

The location of solid tumours and evidence of any metastases are identified and localised, using a combination of ultrasound, plain X-rays, CT and MRI scans. Nuclear medicine imaging may be useful to identify bone or bone marrow disease, or e.g. localise neuroblastoma.

Pathology

Typically, diagnoses are confirmed histologically, either by bone marrow aspiration for cases of leukaemia, or by biopsy for most solid tumours. Histological techniques are routinely used to differentiate tumour types. Molecular and genetic techniques are also used to confirm diagnosis and to predict prognosis.

Management

Once malignancy has been diagnosed, the parents and child need to be seen and the diagnosis explained to them. Detailed investigation to define the extent of the disease is paramount to planning treatment. Specialist centres teams can provide the intensive medical and psychosocial support required. Survival statistics suggest that teenagers and young adults have poorer outcomes than children. This relates both to the specific types and biological behaviour of their tumours and to their particular social/psychological needs.

Treatment

Treatment may involve chemotherapy, surgery, or radiotherapy, alone or in combination.

Chemotherapy

Chemotherapy is used:
- as primary curative treatment
- to control primary or metastatic disease before surgery and/or radiotherapy, e.g. in sarcoma or neuroblastoma

- as adjuvant treatment to deal with residual disease and to eliminate presumed micrometastases.

Short-term side effects of chemotherapy

Bone marrow suppression	Anaemia Thrombocytopenia and bleeding Neutropenia
Immunosuppression	Infection
Gut mucosal damage Nausea and vomiting Anorexia	Undernutrition
Alopecia	

High-dose therapy with stem cell rescue

The limitation of chemotherapy (and radiotherapy) is the risk of irreversible damage to normal tissues, particularly bone marrow. Transplantation of bone marrow stem cells can be used as a strategy to intensify the treatment. The source of stem cells may be allogeneic (from a compatible donor) or autologous (from the patient him/herself, harvested beforehand.

Exercise 1
Answer the following questions. Prepare short talks and/or dialogues on these topics

1. Describe features of malignant disease in children.
2. What do you know about aetiology and clinical presentation of cancer?
3. Speak about investigations, radiology, pathology and management of cancer.
4. When is chemotherapy used?
5. Which are short-term side effects of chemotherapy?
6. What is the limitation of chemotherapy (and radiotherapy)?

Translation 1

1. The pattern of malignant disease varies and management is conducted by specialist centres. 2. The types of disease are very different from those in adults, where carcinomas of the lung, breast, gut, and prostate predominate. 3. Leukaemia affects children at all ages, neuroblastoma and Wilms tumour are almost always seen in the first 6 years of age and Hodgkin lymphoma and bone tumours have their peak incidence in adolescence. 4.

Cancer in children can present with: a localized mass, the consequences of disseminated disease and the consequences of pressure from a mass on local structures or tissue. 5. The location of solid tumours and evidence of any metastases are identified and localised, using a combination of ultrasound, plain X-rays, CT and MRI scans. 6. Typically, diagnoses are confirmed histologically, either by bone marrow aspiration for cases of leukaemia, or by biopsy for most solid tumours. 7. Detailed investigation to define the extent of the disease is paramount to planning treatment. 8. Treatment may involve chemotherapy, surgery, or radiotherapy, alone or in combination. 8. Chemotherapy is used: as primary curative treatment, to control primary or metastatic disease and as adjuvant treatment. 9. The limitation of chemotherapy (and radiotherapy) is the risk of irreversible damage to normal tissues, particularly bone marrow. 10. Transplantation of bone marrow stem cells can be used as a strategy to intensify the treatment.

Text 2
Radiotherapy

Radiotherapy uses high-energy radiation to kill cancer cells. There is growing interest in the use of proton beam radiotherapy that may allow the radiation dose to be delivered in a more controlled fashion, reducing the dose to normal adjacent structures. Radiotherapy has an important role in the treatment of some tumours, but the risk of damage to growth and function of normal tissue is greater in a child than in an adult. The need for adequate protection of normal tissues and for careful positioning and immobilisation of the patient during treatment raises practical difficulties, particularly in young children. Cranial radiotherapy in children under the age of 3 years is particularly problematic.

Surgery

Initial surgery is frequently restricted to biopsy to establish the diagnosis, and more extensive operations are usually undertaken to remove residual tumour after chemotherapy and/or radiotherapy.

Supportive care and side-effects of treatment

Cancer treatment produces frequent, predictable, and often severe multisystem side-effects. Children with cancer are immunocompromised and at risk of serious infection. Children with fever and neutropenia must be admitted promptly to hospital. Most common viral infections are no worse in children with cancer than in other children, but measles and varicella zoster (chickenpox) may have atypical presentation and can be life-threatening. During chemotherapy and from 6 months to a year subsequently, the use of live vaccines is contraindicated due to depressed immunity. After this period, re-immunisation against common childhood infections is recommended. Fever with neutropenia requires hospital admission, investigation and treatment.

Venous access

The discomfort of multiple venepunctures for blood sampling and intravenous infusions can be avoided with central venous catheters. A port is similar to a tunnelled catheter but is left entirely under the skin. Central venous catheters can remain in situ for many months if not years, i.e. the duration of chemotherapy treatment but they carry a risk of infection and can get blocked or split.

Psychosocial support

Most will benefit from the counselling and practical support provided by health professionals. Help with practical issues, including transport, finances, accommodation, and care of siblings, is an early priority. The children themselves, and their siblings, need an age-appropriate explanation of the disease. Families should be encouraged to return to as normal a lifestyle as possible. Early return to school is important and children with cancer should not be allowed to under-achieve the expectations previously held for them.

Exercise 2

Study the following summary and then interpret basic information in English.

1. Malignant disease in children - uncommon
Can present with a localised mass or its pressure effects or disseminated disease.
Treatment may involve chemotherapy, surgery, radiotherapy, or high-dose therapy with stem cell rescue.
Measles and varicella zoster infection are potentially life-threatening.
A multidisciplinary team is required to provide supportive care and psychosocial support.
Supportive care includes not only management of side-effects but also pain management and fertility preservation.
Fever with neutropenia must be investigated and treated urgently.

Leukaemia
Clinical presentation

Presentation of ALL (acute lymphoblastic leukaemia) peaks at 2-5 years of age. Clinical symptoms and signs result from disseminated disease and systemic ill-health from infiltration of the bone marrow or other organs with leukemic blast cells. In most children, leukaemia presents over several weeks but in some children the illness presents and progresses very rapidly. In most but not all children, the full blood count is abnormal. Bone marrow examination is essential to confirm the diagnosis. A lumbar puncture is performed to identify disease in the CSF. Chest X-ray is required to identify a mediastinal mas or characteristic of T-cell disease.

Signs and symptoms of acute leukaemia

General:	Malaise, anorexia
Bone marrow infiltration:	Anaemia Pallor, lethargy Neutropenia Infection Thrombocytopenia Bruising, petechiae, nose bleeds Bone pain
Reticuloendothelial infiltration	Hepatosplenomegaly Lymphadenopathy Superior mediastinal obstruction (uncommon)
Other organ ,infiltration'	Central nervous system Headaches, vomiting, nerve palsies Testes Testicular enlargement

Exercise 3
Answer the following questions. Prepare short talks and/or dialogues on these topics

1. Describe use and risks of radiotherapy in a child.
2. Speak about supportive care and side-effects of treatment.
3. Describe clinical presentation of leukaemia and signs and symptoms of acute leukaemia.

Translation 2

1. Radiotherapy uses high-energy radiation to kill cancer cells. 2. Radiotherapy has an important role in the treatment of some tumours, but the risk of damage to growth and function of normal tissue is greater in a child than in an adult. 3. Initial surgery is frequently restricted to

biopsy to establish the diagnosis. 4. Cancer treatment produces frequent, predictable, and often severe multisystem side-effects. 5. Children with fever and neutropenia must be admitted promptly to hospital. 6. Measles and varicella zoster (chickenpox) may have atypical presentation and can be life-threatening. 7. During chemotherapy and from 6 months to a year subsequently, the use of live vaccines is contraindicated due to depressed immunity. 8. The discomfort of multiple venepunctures for blood sampling and intravenous infusions can be avoided with central venous catheters.

Exercise 4
Match the column A with the column B. Try to learn the expressions and/or sentences by heart.

A
1. Help with practical issues, …
2. The children themselves, and their siblings, …
3. Presentation of acute lymphoblastic leukaemia …
4. In most children, leukaemia presents over several weeks …
5. A lumbar puncture is performed …
6. Signs and symptoms of acute leukaemia are: …

B
a. *… to identify disease in the CSF.*
b. *… bone marrow infiltration (malaise, anorexia, anaemia, pallor, lethargy, neutropenia, infection, thrombocytopenia, bruising, petechiae, nose bleeds, bone pain), b. reticulo-endothelial infiltration (hepatosplenomegaly, lymphadenopathy), and c. other organ 'infiltration' (central nervous system, headaches, vomiting, nerve palsies, testicular enlargement).*
c. *… including transport, finances, accommodation, and care of siblings, is an early priority.*
d. *… peaks at 2-5 years of age.*
e. *… need an age-appropriate explanation of the disease.*
f. *… but in some children the illness presents and progresses very rapidly.*

Text 3
Brain tumours
   In contrast to adults, brain tumours in children are almost always primary rather than metastatic. They are the most common solid tumour in children and are the leading cause of childhood cancer deaths.

Clinical features

The developmental age of the child is important as presentation varies according to age and their ability to report symptoms. Signs and symptoms are often related to evidence of raised intracranial pressure. Spinal tumours, primary or metastatic, can present with back pain, peripheral weakness of arms or legs, or bladder/bowel dysfunction. Persistent back pain in children warrants investigation with MRI scan.

Clinical presentation
All ages
- Persistent or recurrent vomiting
- Problems with balance, coordination or walking
- Behavioural change
- Abnormal eye movements
- Seizures (without fever)
- Abnormal head position — wry neck, head tilt or persistent stiff neck

Child/Adolescent
- Persistent or recurrent headache
- Blurred or double vision
- Lethargy
- Deteriorating school performance
- Delayed or arrested puberty, slow growth

Infants
- Developmental delay/regression
- Progressive increase in head circumference, separation of sutures, bulging fontanelle
- Lethargy

Investigations

Magnetic resonance spectroscopy can be used to examine the biological activity of a tumour. Some tumour types can metastasize within the CSF and a lumbar puncture is therefore required for complete staging of the disease.

Management

Surgery is usually the first treatment and is aimed at treating hydrocephalus. In some cases, the anatomical position of the tumour means biopsy is not safe. Even tumours which are histologically 'benign' can threaten survival. The use of radiotherapy and/or chemotherapy varies with tumour type and the age of the patient.

Late effects

The functional implications of the site of the tumour, the potential hazards of surgery and the importance of radiotherapy in treatment all combine to place children with brain tumours at particular risk of neurological disability and of growth, endocrine, neuropsychological, and educational problems.

Lymphomas

Lymphomas are malignancies of the cells of the immune system and can be divided into Hodgkin and non-Hodgkin lymphoma.

Hodgkin lymphoma

Classically presents with painless lymphadenopathy, most frequently in the neck. Lymph nodes are much larger and firmer than the benign lymphadenopathy commonly seen in young children. The lymph nodes may cause airways obstruction. Lymph node biopsy, radiological assessment and bone marrow biopsy is used to determine treatment.

Non-Hodgkin lymphoma

T cell malignancies may present as acute lymphoblastic leukaemia or non-Hodgkin lymphoma. The mediastinal mass may cause superior vena cava obstruction presenting with dyspnoea, facial swelling and flushing, venous distension in the neck, and distended veins in the upper chest and arms. Abdominal disease presents with pain from intestinal obstruction, a palpable mass or even intussusception in cases with involvement of the ileum.

Neuroblastoma

Neuroblastoma and related tumours arise from neural crest tissue in the adrenal medulla and sympathetic nervous system. There is a spectrum of disease from the benign (ganglioneuroma) to the highly malignant (neuroblastoma). Neuroblastoma is most common before the age of 5 years.

Clinical features

Most children have an abdominal mass, but the primary tumour can lie anywhere along the sympathetic chain from the neck to the pelvis. Classically, the abdominal primary is of adrenal origin, but at presentation the tumour mass is often large and complex, crossing the midline and enveloping major blood vessels and lymph nodes. Paravertebral tumours may cause spinal cord compression requiring emergency intervention to prevent devastating long-term neurological damage. Over the age of 5 years clinical symptoms are mostly from metastatic disease, particularly bone pain, bone marrow suppression causing weight loss, and malaise.

Presentation of neuroblastoma

Common	Less common
Pallor Weight loss Abdominal mass Hepatomegaly Bone pain Limp	Paraplegia Cervical lymphadenopathy Proptosis Periorbital bruising Skin nodules

Management

Localised primaries without metastatic disease can often be cured with surgery alone and in some infants, neuroblastoma (including when metastatic) may resolve spontaneously.

Wilms tumour (nephroblastoma)

Wilms tumour originates from embryonal renal tissue and is the most common renal tumour of childhood. Most children present with a large abdominal mass, often found incidentally in an otherwise well child. Staging is to assess for distal metastases (usually in the lung, initial tumour resectability and function of the contralateral kidney).

Exercise 5
Answer the following questions. Prepare short talks and/or dialogues on these topics

1. What are clinical features of brain tumours?
2. Describe clinical presentation, investigations, management and late effects.
3. Characterize Hodgkin lymphoma and Non-Hodgkin lymphoma.
4. What are clinical features of neuroblastoma?
5. What does common presentation of neuroblastoma include?
6. Speak about Wilms tumour.

Translation 3

1. In contrast to adults, brain tumours in children are almost always primary rather than metastatic. 2. Signs and symptoms are often related to evidence of raised intracranial pressure. 3. Spinal tumours can present with back pain, peripheral weakness of arms or legs, or bladder/bowel dysfunction. 4. Clinical presentation includes: persistent or recurrent vomiting, problems with balance, coordination or walking, behavioural change, abnormal eye movements, seizures (without fever), abnormal head position-wry neck, head tilt or persistent stiff neck. 5. Magnetic resonance spectroscopy can be used to examine the biological activity of a tumour. 6. Surgery is usually the first treatment and is aimed at treating hydrocephalus. 7. The use of radiotherapy and/or chemotherapy varies with tumour type and the age of the patient. 8. Hodgkin lymphoma classically presents with painless lymphadenopathy, most frequently in the neck. 9. Lymph node biopsy, radiological assessment and bone marrow biopsy is used to determine treatment.

Exercise 6
Fill in the missing words. Choose the correct ones.

1. T cell _____ may present as acute lymphoblastic _____ or non-Hodgkin _____.	a leukaemia b lymphoma c malignancies
2. The mediastinal mass may cause _____ ____ ____ obstruction presenting with dyspnoea, facial _____ ___ _____, venous distension in the neck, and _____ _____ in the upper chest and arms.	a swelling and flushing b distended veins c superior vena cava
3. Abdominal disease presents with pain from _____ _____, _____ ____ or even intussusception in cases with _____ of the ileum.	a involvement b intestinal obstruction, c palpable mass
4. _____ and related tumours arise from _____ _____ _____ in the _____ _____ and sympathetic nervous system.	a neural crest tissue b adrenal medulla c Neuroblastoma

5. Most children have an abdominal mass, but the _____ _____ can lie anywhere along the _____ _____ from the _____ __ ___ _____.	a neck to the pelvis b sympathetic chain c primary tumour
6. Classically, the abdominal primary is of _____ _____, but at presentation the tumour mass is often _____ ___ _____, crossing the midline and enveloping major _____ _____ __ _____ _____.	a large and complex b blood vessels and lymph nodes c adrenal origin
7. Paravertebral tumours may cause _____ ____ compression requiring _____ _____ to prevent _____ ____-____ neurological damage.	a emergency intervention b devastating long-term c spinal cord
8. Wilms tumour originates from _____ _____ _____ and is the most common _____ _____ of childhood.	a renal tumour b embryonal renal tissue

Text 4
Soft tissue sarcomas

Sarcomas are cancer of connective tissue such as muscle or bone. There are a wide variety of primary sites, resulting in varying presentations and prognosis.

- Head and neck are the most common site of disease, causing e.g. proptosis, nasal obstruction, or bloodstained nasal discharge.
- Genitourinary tumours may involve the bladder, paratesticular structures, or the female genitourinary tract. Symptoms include dysuria and urinary obstruction, scrotal mass, or bloodstained vaginal discharge.
- Metastatic disease (lung, liver, bone, or bone marrow) is associated with a particularly poor prognosis.

Management

Multimodality treatment (chemotherapy, surgery, and radiotherapy) is used, dependent on the age of the patient and the site, size, and extent of disease. The tumour margins are deceptively ill-defined, and attempts at primary surgical excision are often unsuccessful and are not attempted unless this can be achieved without mutilation or irreversible organ damage.

Bone tumours

The limbs are the most common site. Persistent localised bone pain is the characteristic symptom, usually preceding the detection of a mass, and is an indication for early X-ray. A bone X-ray shows destruction and variable periosteal new bone formation.

Retinoblastoma

Retinoblastoma is a malignant tumour of retinal cells. It may affect one or both eyes. All bilateral tumours are hereditary. Most children present within the first 3 years of life. The most common presentation of unsuspected disease is when a white pupillary reflex is noted to replace the normal red one or with a squint. The aim is to cure, yet preserve vision. Enucleation of the eye may be necessary for more advanced disease. Chemotherapy is used to shrink the tumour, followed by local laser treatment to the retina. Most patients are cured, although many are visually impaired. There is a significant risk of second malignancy (especially sarcoma).

Kaposi sarcoma

Kaposi sarcoma is a low-grade cancer that arises from the cells of the blood or lymph vessels and is triggered by human herpes virus. Treatment involves a combination of chemotherapy and antiretroviral therapy.

Long-term survivors

Improved survival rates mean an ever-increasing population of adult survivors of childhood cancer. Over half have at least one residual problem as a consequence of either the disease or its treatment. All survivors need regular long-term follow-up to provide appropriate treatment or advice. Some survivors will require specific counselling for problems such as poor or asymmetric growth, infertility and sexual dysfunction, and advances in the use of adult growth hormone.

Some problems that may occur following cure of childhood cancer

Problem	Cause
Specific organ dysfunction	Nephrectomy for Wilms tumour Toxicity from chemotherapy
Growth/endocrine problems	Growth hormone deficiency from pituitary irradiation Bone growth retardation at sites of irradiation
Infertility	Gonadal irradiation Alkylating agent chemotherapy

Neuropsychological problems	Cranial irradiation (particularly at age <5 years Brain surgery
Second malignancy	Irradiation
Social/educational disadvantage	Chronic ill health Absence from school

Palliative and end-of-life care

Palliative care assists with symptom management, psychosocial support for the child and family, attention to practical needs and spiritual care throughout the child's illness. If a child relapses, further treatment may be considered. A reasonable number can still be cured and others may have a further significant remission with good-quality life. However, for some children, a time comes when death is inevitable and the staff and family must make decision to concentrate on end-of-life care. Pain control and symptom relief are a serious source of anxiety for parents, but they can often be achieved successfully at home. Health professionals with experience in palliative and end-of-life care for children work together with the family. After the child's death, families should be offered continuing contact with an appropriate member of the team who looked after their child, and be given support through their bereavement. With adequate support from health professionals, end-of-life care for children can often be provided at home.

Exercise 7
Study the following summary and then interpret basic information in English.
Presentation of malignant disease in children

Brain tumours	Raised intracranial pressure Neurological signs — depends on anatomical position
Retinoblastoma	Screening if positive family history White pupillary reflex or squint
Lymphomas	Enlarged lymph nodes in the neck or abdomen Mediastinal mass — may cause superior vena cava obstruction
Wilms tumour	Large abdominal mass in a well child Occasionally anorexia, abdominal pain, haematuria
Langerhans cells histiocytosis	Seborrheic rash Widespread soft tissue infiltration Bone pain, swelling or fracture Diabetes insipidus
Soft tissue sarcomas	Mass any site

Neuroblastoma	Abdominal mass
	Malaise, anorexia
	Pallor, lethargy
	Bone pain
Acute lymphoblastic leukaemia (ALL)	Malaise, anorexia
	Pallor, lethargy
	Infections
	Bruising, petechiae, nose bleeds
	Lymphadenopathy
	Hepatosplenomegaly
	Bone pain
Malignant bone tumours	Localised bone pain

Exercise 8
Answer the following questions. Prepare short talks and/or dialogues on these topics

1. Characterize soft tissue sarcomas, bone tumours, retinoblastoma, and Kaposi sarcoma.
2. What can you say about problems that may occur following cure of childhood cancer?
3. Speak about palliative and end-of-life care.

Translation 4

1. Sarcomas are cancer of connective tissue such as muscle or bone. 2. Head and neck are the most common site of disease, causing, e.g. proptosis, nasal obstruction, or bloodstained nasal discharge. 3. Genitourinary tumours may involve the bladder, para-testicular structures, or the female genitourinary tract. 4. Metastatic disease (lung, liver, bone, or bone marrow) is associated with a particularly poor prognosis. 5. Multimodality treatment (chemotherapy, surgery, and radiotherapy) is used, dependent on the age of the patient and the site, size, and extent of disease. 6. Persistent localised bone pain is the characteristic symptom, usually preceding the detection of a mass, and is an indication for early X-ray. 7. Retinoblastoma is a malignant tumour of retinal cells. 8. The most common presentation of unsuspected disease is when a white pupillary reflex is noted to replace the normal red one or with a squint. 9. Chemotherapy is used to shrink the tumour, followed by local laser treatment to the retina.

Exercise 9
Match the column A with the column B. Try to learn the expressions and/or sentences by heart.

A

1. Kaposi sarcoma is a low-grade cancer …
2. All survivors need regular long-term follow-up …
3. Causes of some problems that may occur following cure of childhood cancer …
4. Palliative care assists with symptom management, psychosocial support …
5. A reasonable number can still be cured …
6. However, for some children, a time comes …

B

a.   … *are nephrectomy for Wilms tumour, toxicity from chemotherapy, growth hormone deficiency from pituitary irradiation, bone growth retardation at sites of irradiation, gonadal irradiation, alkylating agent, chemotherapy, cranial irradiation, and brain surgery.*
b.   … *that arises from the cells of the blood or lymph vessels and is triggered by human herpes virus.*
c.   … *when death is inevitable and the staff and family must make decision to concentrate on end-of-life care.*
d.   … *for the child and family, attention to practical needs and spiritual care throughout the child's illness.*
e.   … *to provide appropriate treatment or advice.*
f.   … *and others may have a further significant remission with good-quality life.*

Text 5
Haematological disorders

Features of haematological disorders in children are:
- the composition and concentration of haemoglobin changes during childhood
- iron deficient anaemia
- causes of haemolytic anaemia include sickle disease, thalassemia, G6PD deficiency and hereditary spherocytosis
- the most common inherited causes of abnormal bleeding are haemophilia A and B and von Willebrand disease (vWD)
- Petechiae or purpura may be nonthrombocytopenic or thrombocytopenic

Hemopoiesis is the process which maintains lifelong production of haemopoietic (blood) cells. The main site of hemopoiesis in foetal life is the liver, whereas throughout postnatal life it is the bone marrow. Haemopoietic stem cells can also be used for treatment, e.g. cells from healthy donors can be transplanted into children with bone marrow failure. Understanding the developmental changes in haemoglobin helps to explain the patterns of abnormal haemoglobin production in some inherited childhood anaemias.

Anaemia

Anaemia results from one or more of the following mechanisms:
- reduced red cell production
- increased red cell destruction (haemolysis)
- blood loss — relatively uncommon in children

Causes of anaemia in infants and children

Impaired red cell production ⇒	Red cell aplasia ⇒	Parvovirus B19 infection Diamond-Black fan anaemia (congenital red cell aplasia) Transient erythroblastopenia of childhood Rarities: Fanconi anaemia,
	Ineffective erythropoiesis ⇒	aplastic anaemia, leukaemia Iron deficiency Folic acid deficiency Chronic inflammation (juvenile idiopathic arthritis) Chronic renal failure Rarities: myelodysplasia, lead poisoning
Increased red cell destruction (haemolysis) ⇒	Red cell membrane disorders ⇒ White cell membrane disorders ⇒ Haemoglobinopathies⇒ Immune ⇒	Hereditary spherocytosis Glucose-6-phosphate dehydrogenase deficiency Thalassemia, sickle cell disease Haemolytic disease of the newborn Autoimmune haemolytic anaemia
Blood loss ⇒	Feto-maternal bleeding ⇒ Chronic gastrointestinal blood loss ⇒ Inherited bleeding disorders ⇒	Meckel diverticulum von Willebrand disease

Infants should not be fed unmodified cow's milk as its iron content is low and poorly absorbed. Treatment of iron deficiency anaemia is with dietary advice and oral iron therapy for several months.

Dietary sources of iron
High in iron
- Red meat — beef, lamb
- Liver, kidney
- Oily fish — pilchards, sardines, etc.

Average iron
- Pulses, beans, and peas
- Fortified breakfast cereal with added vitamin C
- Wholemeal products
- Dark green vegetables — broccoli, spinach, etc.
- Dried fruit — raisins, sultanas
- Nuts and seeds — cashews, peanut butter, etc.

Foods to avoid in excess in toddlers
- Cow's milk
- Tea: tannin inhibits iron uptake
- High-fibre foods: phytates inhibit iron absorption

Exercise 10
Answer the following questions. Prepare short talks and/or dialogues on these topics

1. What are features of haematological disorders in children?
2. Explain the term hemopoiesis.
3. What are causes of anaemia in infants and children?
4. Which are dietary sources of iron?
5. Which foods should be avoided in excess in toddlers?

Translation 5
1. Features of haematological disorders in children are: the composition and concentration of haemoglobin changes, iron deficient anaemia, haemolytic anaemia, inherited causes of abnormal bleeding, petechiae or purpura. 2. Hemopoiesis is the process which maintains lifelong production of haemopoietic (blood) cells. 3. The main site of hemopoiesis in foetal life is the liver, whereas throughout postnatal life it is the bone marrow. 4. Anaemia results from one or more of the following mechanisms: reduced red cell production, increased red cell destruction, and blood loss. 5. Infants should not be fed unmodified cow's milk as its iron content is low and poorly absorbed. 6. Dietary sources of iron are: red meat, liver, kidney, oily fish, pulses, beans, and peas, fortified breakfast cereal with added vitamin C,

wholemeal products, dark green vegetables, dried fruit, and nuts and seeds.
7. Foods to avoid in excess in toddlers are: cow's milk, tea, and high-fibre
foods.

Text 6
Clinical manifestations of sickle cell disease

Anaemia ⇒	All have moderate anaemia with clinically detectable jaundice from chronic haemolysis
Infection ⇒	All have marked increase in susceptibility to infection from encapsulated organisms such as pneumococci and Haemophilus influenzae. There is also an increased incidence of osteomyelitis caused by Salmonella and other organisms. This susceptibility to infection is due to hyposplenism secondary to chronic sickling and microinfarction in the spleen in infancy. The risk of overwhelming sepsis is greatest in early childhood.
Painful crises ⇒	Vaso-occlusive crises causing pain affect many organs of the body with varying frequency and severity. A common mode of presentation in late infancy is the hand-foot syndrome, in which there is dactylitis with swelling and pain of the fingers and/or feet from Vaso-occlusion. The bones of the limbs and spine are the most common sites. The most serious type of painful crisis is acute chest syndrome, which can lead to severe hypoxia and the need for mechanical ventilation and emergency transfusion. Avascular necrosis of the femoral heads may also occur. Acute Vaso-occlusive crisis may be precipitated by exposure to cold, dehydration, excessive exercise or stress, hypoxia or infection.
Acute anaemia ⇒	Sudden drop in haemoglobin from: Haemolytic crises — sometimes associated with infection Aplastic crises — haemoglobin may fall precipitously. Parvovirus infection causes complete, though temporary, cessation of red blood cell production. Sequestration crises — sudden splenic of hepatic enlargement, abdominal pain and circulatory collapse from accumulation of sickled cells in spleen.
Priapism ⇒	needs to be treated promptly with exchange transfusion as it may lead to fibrosis of the corpora cavernosa and subsequent erectile impotence.
Splenomegaly ⇒	common in young children, but becomes much less frequent in older children.

Long-term problems ⇒	Short stature and delayed puberty Stroke and cognitive problems — although 1 in 10 children with sickle cell disease have a stroke, twice that number develop more subtle neurological damage, often manifest with poor concentration and school performance Adeno tonsillar hypertrophy — causing sleep apnoea syndrome leading to nocturnal hypoxaemia, which can cause Vaso-occlusive crises and/or stroke Cardiac enlargement from chronic anaemia Heart failure — from uncorrected anaemia Renal dysfunction
	Pigment gallstones — due to increased bile pigment production Leg ulcers — uncommon in children Psychosocial problems — difficulties with education and behaviour exacerbated by time off school may occur.

Causes of anaemia:
- Reduced red cell production
- Increased red cell destruction (haemolysis)
- Combination of causes (e.g. anaemia of prematurity)
- Blood loss (uncommon)

Reduced red cell production

Iron deficiency anaemia	Red cell aplasia
• Common in infants and toddlers • Usually dietary in origin • Occurs because of high iron requirement • Will not occur if infants are weaned at 6 months of age or onto a mixed diet including iron-rich food • Is diagnosed from a hypochromic microcytic anaemia and low serum ferritin	• Congenital red cell aplasia • Transient erythroblastopenia of childhood • Parvovirus B19 infection
• Is treated with dietary advice and oral iron therapy for at least 3 months.	

Exercise 11
Answer the following questions. Prepare short talks and/or dialogues on these topics

1. Describe clinical manifestations of sickle cell disease.
2. What are causes of anaemia?
3. Speak about iron deficiency anaemia.

Translation 6

1. Clinical manifestations of sickle cell disease are: anaemia, infection, painful crises, acute anaemia, priapism, splenomegaly, and long-term problems. 2. Iron deficiency anaemia is common in infants and toddlers. 3. Iron deficiency anaemia occurs because of high iron requirement. 4. Iron deficiency anaemia is diagnosed from a hypochromic microcytic anaemia and low serum ferritin. 5. It is treated with dietary advice and oral iron therapy for at least 3 months. 6. Reduced red cell production is also caused by congenital red cell aplasia, transient erythroblastopenia of childhood and Parvovirus B19 infection.

Text 7
Bleeding disorders

Age of onset	Neonate — in 20% of haemophilias, bleeding occurs in the neonatal period, usually with intracranial haemorrhage or bleeding after circumcision Toddler — haemophilias may present when starting to walk Adolescent — von Willebrand disease may present with menorrhagia
Family history	Family tree — detailed family tree required Gender of affected relatives (if all boys, suggest haemophilia)
Bleeding history	Previous surgical procedures and dental extractions — if uncomplicated, suggest bleeding tendency is acquired rather than inherited Presence of systemic disorders Drug history, e.g. anticoagulants Unusual pattern or inconsistent history — consider non-accidental injury
Pattern of bleeding	Mucous membrane bleeding and skin haemorrhage — characteristic of platelet disorders or von Willebrand disease Bleeding into muscles or into joints — characteristic of haemophilia Scarring and delayed haemorrhage — suggestive of disorders of connective tissue

Haemophilia
Clinical features

The hallmark of severe disease is recurrent spontaneous bleeding into joints and muscles, which can lead to crippling arthritis if not properly treated. Most children present towards the end of the first year of life, when they start to crawl or walk (and fall over). Bleeding episodes are most frequent in joints and muscles. Almost 40% of cases present in the neonatal period, particularly with intracranial haemorrhage, bleeding post circumcision or prolonged oozing from head stick and venepuncture sites.

Severity of haemophilia

Severity	Bleeding tendency
Severe	Spontaneous joint/muscle bleeds
Moderate	Bleed after minor trauma
Mild	Bleed after surgery

Exercise 12
Study the following summary and then interpret basic information in English.

1. The child with abnormal bleeding – into soft tissues, mucocutaneous or following surgery
Acquired disorders
Vitamin K deficiency:
mainly neonates or early infancy
Liver disease
Thrombocytopenia:
immune, DIC etc.
Consider:
Age of onset
Family history
Bleeding history
Pattern of bleeding
Inherited disorders
Haemophilia A and haemophilia B
von Willebrand disease
Thrombosis
All children with thrombosis should be screened for inherited or acquired predisposing disorders

Exercise 13
Study the following summary and then interpret basic information in English.

The child with petechiae or purpura

Non-thrombocytopenic

Henoch-Schönlein purpura	Lesions confined to buttocks, extensor surfaces of legs, and arms Swollen painful knees and ankles Abdominal pain Haematuria
Sepsis	Meningococcal or viral Clinical features — fever, septicaemia, meningitis Rash in meningococcal sepsis — positive glass test (rash does not blanch when pressed) If suspected, give parenteral penicillin immediately
Trauma	Accidental or non-accidental
Other causes (rare)	

Thrombocytopenia

Immune thrombocytopenia (ITP)	2-10 years Widespread petechiae and purpura and superficial bruising Distinguish from acute leukaemia and aplastic anaemia — clinical features, full blood count and blood film Bone marrow examination not required if only the platelet count is low, characteristic clinical features and no steroid treatment given
	Is acute, benign and self-limiting in about 80% of children Treatment — controversial, usually not required unless there is bleeding
Leukaemia	Clinical features — malaise, infection, pallor, hepatosplenomegaly, lymphadenopathy Blood count — also low Hb, blast on film, confirmed on bone marrow
Disseminated intravascular coagulation	Critically ill — severe sepsis or shock or extensive tissue damage
Other causes (uncommon)	

Exercise 14
Answer the following questions. Prepare short talks and/or dialogues on these topics

1. Speak about bleeding disorders.
2. What are clinical features of haemophilia?
3. Describe acquired disorders and inherited disorders.
4. Give characteristics of Henoch-Schönlein purpura, sepsis, and trauma.

5. Explain the term thrombocytopenia.

Translation 7

1. Bleeding disorders can start in neonates, toddlers or adolescents. 2. Family history describes gender of affected relatives (if all boys, suggest haemophilia). 3. Bleeding history includes previous surgical procedures and dental extractions, presence of systemic disorders, drug history, and inconsistent history. 4. Pattern of bleeding characterizes mucous membrane bleeding and skin haemorrhage – characteristic of platelet disorders or von Willebrand disease. 5. Bleeding into muscles or into joints is characteristic of haemophilia, scarring and delayed haemorrhage is suggestive of disorders of connective tissue. 6. The hallmark of severe haemophilia is recurrent spontaneous bleeding into joints and muscles, which can lead to crippling arthritis if not properly treated. 7. Most children present towards the end of the first year of life, when they start to crawl or walk. 8. Almost 40% of cases present in the neonatal period, particularly with intracranial haemorrhage, bleeding post circumcision or prolonged oozing from head stick and venepuncture sites.

Exercise 15

Fill in the missing words. Choose the correct ones.

1. _____ _____ are: vitamin K _____, liver disease, and _____.	a thrombocytopenia b deficiency c Acquired disorders
2. _____ _____ are: haemophilia A and _____ B, and ___ _____ _____.	a haemophilia b Inherited disorders c von Willebrand disease.
3. In Henoch-Schönlein purpura lesions ___ _____ to buttocks, extensor surfaces of legs, and arms, _____ _____ knees and ankles, abdominal pain, and _____.	a haematuria b swollen painful c are confined
4. Clinical features of _____ ___ _____ sepsis are fever, _____, meningitis, and rash in meningococcal _____.	a sepsis b septicaemia c meningococcal or viral

5. _____ thrombocytopenia (ITP) is acute, _____ and _____-_____ in about 80% of children.	a self-limiting b benign c Immune
6. Distinguish from acute leukaemia and _____ _____: clinical features are full _____ _____ and _____ _____.	a blood count b blood film c aplastic anaemia
7. In leukaemia clinical features include, _____ , infection, _____, hepatosplenomegaly, and _____.	a lymphadenopathy b pallor c malaise
8. In disseminated intravascular _____ the child is _____ ____ with severe sepsis or shock or extensive _____ _____.	a critically ill b coagulation c tissue damage

Key 6
Exercise 4
1c; 2e; 3d; 4f; 5a; 6b

Exercise 6
1c, a, b; 2 c, a, b; 3c, b, a; 4 c, a, b; 5 c, b, a; 6 c, a, b; 7 c, a, b; 8 b, a

Exercise 9
1b; 2e; 3a; 4d; 5f; 6c

Exercise 15
1c, b, a; 2 b, a, c; 3 c, b, a; 4 c, b, a; 5 c, b, a; 6 c, a, b; 7 c, b, a; 8 b, a, c

VOCABULARY 6

acquire /əˈkwaɪər/
adenotonsillar /ˌædɪnəʊˈtɒn.sələ/
adjacent /əˈdʒeɪ.sənt/
adrenal /əˈdriː.nəl/ **medulla** /meˌdʌl.ə/
alkylating /ˌælkəˈleɪtɪŋ/
allogeneic /ˈæləʊdʒɪˌneɪɪk/
alopecia /ˌə.lə.ˈpiː.ʃiː.ə/
anticoagulant /ˌæn.ti.kəʊˈæg.jʊ.lənt/
aplasia /əˈpleɪ.zɪə/
aplastic /əˈplæs.tɪk/
arrest /əˈrest/
autologous /ɔːˈtɒl.ə.gəs/ **transplant** /trænˈsplɑːnt/
avascular /əˈvæskjʊlə/
balance /ˈbæl.əns/
beam /biːm/
beef /biːf/
benign /bɪˈnaɪn/
bereavement /bɪˈriː.vmənt/
bladder /ˈblæd.ər/
blanch /blɑːntʃ/
blast /ˌblæst/ **cell** /sel/
blood /blʌd/ **vessel** /ˈves.əl/
blood-stained /blʌd steɪnd/
bone /bəʊn/ **marrow** /ˈmær.əʊ/
broccoli /ˈbrɒk.əl.i/
bruising /ˈbruː.zɪŋ/
cashews /ˈkæʃuː/
cereal /ˈsɪə.ri.əl/
cessation /sesˈeɪ.ʃən/
circumference /səˈkʌm.fər.əns/
compatible /kəmˈpæt.ɪ.bļ/
compression /kɒm.ˈpreʃˌen/
concentration /ˌkɒn.sənˈtreɪ.ʃən/
conduct /kənˈdʌkt/
confined /kənˈfaɪnd/
connective tissue /kəˌnek.tɪvˈtɪʃ.uː/
contraindicate /ˌkɒn.trəˈɪn.dɪ.keɪt/
contralateral /ˌkɒn.trəˈlæt.ər.əl/
corpus /ˈkɔː.pəs/ pl **corpora** /ˈkɔː.pər.ə/
counselling /ˈkaʊnt.səl.ɪŋ/
cranial /ˈkreɪ.ni.əl/
crawl /krɔːl/
crest /krest/
crippling /ˈkrɪp.lɪŋ/
cross /krɒs/

curative /ˈkjʊərətɪv/

dactylitis /ˈdæktɪ.laɪ.tɪs/

deceptively /dɪˈseptɪvlɪ/

depressed /dɪˈprest/

deteriorate /dɪˈtɪə.ri.ə.reɪt/

devastating /ˈdev.ə.steɪ.tɪŋ/

diabetes /ˌdaɪəˈbiː.ti:z/ **insipidus** /ɪn.sɪpˈɪ.dəs/

Diamond-Blackfan anaemia /ˈdaɪəmənd blakˈfan əˈniː.mi.ə/

disorder /dɪˈsɔː.dər/

disseminated /dɪˈsem.ɪ.neɪt.ɪd/

distal /ˈdɪs.təl/

diverticulum /ˌdaɪ.vəˌtɪk.jʊ.ləm/ pl **diverticula**

dysuria /dɪˈsju.ə.riə/

eliminate /ɪˈlɪm.ɪ.neɪt/

encapsulate /ɪnˈkæp.sjʊ.leɪt/

enlargement /ɪnˈlɑːdʒ.mənt/

entirely /ɪnˈtaɪə.li/

enucleation /ɪˈnjʊklɪˈeiʃˠn/

envelope /ɪnˈveləp/

erectile /ɪˈrek.taɪl/

erythroblastopenia /e.riθˈrəʊ.blasˈtəʊ.piːˈniː.æ/

exacerbate /ɪgˈzæs.ə.beɪt/

excision /ˌekˈsi.ʃən/

extensive /ɪkˈsten.sɪv/

extensor /ɪkˈsten.sər/

failure /ˈfeɪ.ljər/

Fanconi /faːn.kəʊˈniː/ **anaemia** /əˈniː.mi.ə/

fashion /ˈfæʃ.ən/

femoral /ˈfem.ər.əl/ **head** /hed/

ferritin /ˈfer.ə.tən/

follow-up /ˈfɒl.əʊ.ʌp/

fortified /ˈfɔː.tɪˌfaɪd/

gallstone /ˈɡɔːl.stəʊn/

ganglioneuroma /ˈɡæŋɡlɪəʊnjʊˈrəʊmə/

gender /ˈdʒen.dər/

genitourinary /ˌdʒen.ɪ.təʊˈjʊə.rɪ.nər,i/

Glucose-6-phosphate dehydrogenase (G6PD) /gluˈkəʊs fosfəɪt diːˈhaɪ.drodʒ'en.eɪs/

deficiency /dɪˈfɪʃ.ənt .si/

haemoglobinopathy ˌhiː.məʊɡləʊbɪˈnɒpəθɪ/

haemolysis /ˌhiː.məˈlɪ.sɪs/

haemophilia /ˌhiː.məˈfɪl.i.ə/

Haemophilus /hiːˈmɑː.fə.ləs/

haemorrhage /ˈhem.ər.ɪdʒ/

hallmark /ˈhɔːl.mɑːk/

harvest /ˈhɑː.vɪst/

hemopoiesis /ˌhiː.məʊpəˈiːsɪs/

Henoch-Schönlein purpura /ˈhen.əḵ ˌʃœn.laɪn ˈpər.pjə.rə/

173

hereditary /həˈred.ɪ.tər.i/
herpes /ˈhɜː.piːz/
histiocytosis /ˈhɪstɪəˌsaɪtəʊ.sis/
histological /ˌhɪstəˈlɒdʒɪkəl/
Hodgkin /hɒdʒkɪn/ **lymphoma** /lɪmˈfəʊ.mə/
hydrocephalus /ˌhaɪ.drəˈsef.ə.ləs/
hypertrophy /haɪˈpɜː.trə.fi/
hypochromic /ˈhaɪpəˈkrəm.ɪk/
hyposplenism /ˈhaɪ.pəʊ ˈspliː.nɪzm/
hypoxaemia /ˌhai.pɒkˈsiː.mi.ə/
ileum /ˈɪl.i.əm/ pl **ilea**
implication /ˌɪm.plɪˈkeɪ.ʃən/
impotence /ˈɪm.pə.təns/
in situ /ɪn ˈsɪt.juː/
incidence /ˈɪnt.sɪ.dənt s/
incidentally /ˌɪnsɪˈdentəlɪ/
inconsistent /ˌɪn.kənˈsɪs.tənt/
inevitable /ɪnˈevɪt.əbəl/
infiltration /ˌɪn.fɪlˈtreɪ.ʃən/
influenza /ˌɪn.fluˈen.zə/
infusion /ɪnˈfjuː.ʒən/
inherit /ɪnˈher.ɪt/
intensify /ɪnˈtensɪˌfaɪ/
interaction /ˌɪn.təˈræk.ʃən/
intestinal /ˌin.ˈtes.tin.əl/
intussusception /ˌɪn.təs.səsˈsep.ʃən/
involvement /ɪnˈvɒlv.mənt/
irradiation /iˌrei.di.eiˈʃən/
irreversible /ˌɪr.ɪˈvɜː.sɪ.b̩l/
Kaposi sarcoma /kæpəʊˈziː saːˈkəʊmə/
lamb /læm/
Langerhans /ˈlæŋəˌhæns/ **cells** /sels/
limp /lɪmp/
lumbar /ˈlʌm.bər/ **punction** /ˈpʌŋk.ʃən/
lymph /lɪmf/ **node** /nəʊd/
lymphoblastic /ˌlɪmfəʊˈblæs.tɪk/
mediastinum /ˌmiː.di.əˈstaɪn.əm/
menorrhagia /ˌmenɔːˈreɪdʒ.ɪə/
metastasis /metˈæs.təs.ɪs/
metastatic /ˌmet.əˈstæt.ɪk/
microcytic /ˌmai.krəʊˈsɪt.ɪk/
microinfarction /ˌmaɪkrə.ɪnˈfɑːk.ʃən/
midline /ˈmɪd.laɪn/
mucocutaneous /mjuːkəʊ.kjuːˈteɪn.ɪəs/
mucous membrane /ˌmjuː.kəsˈmem.breɪn/
mutilation /ˌmjuː.tɪˈlei.ʃən/
neuroblastoma /ˌnjʊə.rəʊˈblaː.stəʊ.mə/

neutropenia /njuːtrəˈpiːnɪə/
ooze /uːz/
optimise /ˈɒptɪˌmaɪz/
osteomyelitis /ˌɒs.ti.əʊ.maɪ.əˈlaɪ.tɪs/
overwhelming /ˌəʊ.vəˈwel.mɪŋ/
palliative /ˈpæl.i.ə.tɪv/
pallor /ˈpæl.ər/
paramount /ˈpær.ə.maʊnt/
paratesticular /ˈpɑː.r.ə tesˈtɪk.jə.ləʳ/
paravertebral /ˈpɑː.r.ə ˈvɜː.tɪ.brˀl/
parvovirus /ˈpɑː.r.vəʊˌvaɪ.rəs/
peanut /ˈpiː.nʌt/
performance /pəˈfɔː.məns/
periosteum /ˌper.ɪˈɒs.ti.əm/ pl **periostea**
phytate /ˈfaɪˌteɪt/
pigment /ˈpɪgmənt/
pilchard /ˈpɪltʃəd/
platelet /ˈpleɪt.lət/
pneumococcus /ˌnuː.moʊˈkɑː.kəs/ pl **pneumococci** /ˌnuː.moʊˈkɒkaɪ/
precipitate /prɪˈsɪp.ɪ.teɪt/
precipitously /prɪˈsɪp.ɪ.təs.li/
predict /prɪˈdɪkt/
predominate /prɪˈdɒm.ɪ.neɪt/
presentation /ˌprez.ənˈteɪ.ʃən/
preservation /ˌprez.əˈveɪ.ʃən/
presume /prɪˈzjuːm/
priapism /ˈpraɪ.əˌpɪz.əm/
prognosis /prɒgˈnəʊ.sɪs/
promptly /ˈprɒmpt.li/
proptosis /prɑːpˈtəʊ.səs/
proton /ˈprəʊtɒn/
pupillary /pjuːˈpɪl.ər.i/
purpura /ˈpər.pjə.rə/
raisin /ˈreɪzən/
rash /ræʃ/
regression /rɪˈgreʃ.ən/
relapse /rɪˈlæps/
remission /rɪˈmɪʃ.ən/
renal /ˈriː.nəl/
requirement /rɪˈkwaɪə.mənt/
rescue /ˈreskjuː/
resectability /rɪsektəˈbɪlɪtɪ/
residual /rɪˈzɪd.ju.əl/
resolve /rɪˈzɒlv/
retardation /ˌriː.tɑːˈdeɪ.ʃən/
reticulo-endothelial /rɪˈtɪkjʊlə ˌendəʊˈθiːlɪəl/
retinal /ˈret.ɪ.nəl/

retinoblastoma /ˌre.tə.nəʊˌbla.ˈstəʊ.mə/
sarcoma /sɑːˈkəʊ.mə/
scarring /skɑːr.ɪŋ/
seborrheic /ˌsebərˈriːɪk/
sequestration /ˌsiː.kwesˈtreɪˌʃᵊn/
side /saɪd/ **effect** /ɪˈfekt/
skin /skɪn/
spectroscopy /ˈspektrəˌskə.pɪ/
spherocytosis /ˌsfɪərəʊsaɪˈtəʊsɪs/
spinach /ˈspɪn.ɪtʃ/
spinal /ˈspaɪ.nəl/ **cord** /kɔːd/
spiritual /ˈspɪr.ɪ.tju.əl/
split /splɪt/
sporadic /spəˈrædɪk/
squint /skwɪnt/
stage /steɪdʒ/
stature /ˈstætʃ.ər/
stem /stem/ **cell** /sel/
stroke /strəʊk/
sultana /sʌlˈtɑːnə/
superior /suːˈpɪə.ri.ər/ **vena cava** /ˌviː.nəˈkeɪ.və/
suppression /səˈpreʃən/
susceptibility /səˌsep.tɪˈbɪl.ɪ.ti/
sympathetic /ˌsɪm.pəˈθe.tɪk/
tannin /ˈtænɪn/
testicular /tesˈtɪk.jə.lər/
thalassemia /ˌθæl.əˈsiː.mi.ə/
threaten /ˈθret.ən/
thrombocytopenia /ˌθrɒm.bəʊ.saɪt.əˈpiː.ni.ə/
thrombocytopenic /ˌθrɒm.bəʊˌsaɪt.əʊˈpiː.nik/
tilt /tɪlt/
tissue /ˈtɪʃ.uː/
tumour /ˈtjuː.mər/
ulcer /ˈʌl.sər/
undertake /ˌʌn.dəˈteɪk/
unsuccessful /ʌn.səkˈses.fʊl/
unsuspected /ʌnˈsə.ˈspekt.ɪd/
vaso-occlusion /veɪˈzəʊ.əˈkluː.ʒən/
vaso-occlusive /veɪˈzəʊ.əˈkluː.siv/
venepuncture /viːˈnɪ.pʌŋk.tʃə/
von Willebrand disease (vWD) /fɒn wɪlˈə.brænd dɪˈziːz/
wholemeal /ˈhəʊlˌmiːl/
widespread /ˌwaɪdˈspred/
Wilms' /wɪlmz/ **tumour** /ˈtjuː.mər/
wry /raɪ/

Child and adolescent mental health; Early relationships; Strategy for meal refusal; Disobedience, defiance, and tantrums; Problems in middle childhood; Antisocial behaviour

Text 1
Features of child mental health are:
- good emotional health in childhood is a stronger predictor of high satisfaction in adult life than any other factor
- suicide is the second most common cause of death in adolescents
- more than 50% of adult mental illness is apparent by age 15 years
- mental illness is the single biggest cause of morbidity in adults.

How to ask about emotional and behavioural problems
Effective history taking must be open, explorative, non-judgemental and empathic. It is best to interview both parents if possible. Ask open questions where possible and feel able to ask directly about feelings. Interview the child and ask to see the older child alone as part of the assessment. They may have things they may feel too embarrassed to discuss with parents present. Keep your questions very simple and specific. This also applies to adolescents, who you need to ask about use of drugs and alcohol, experience of abuse, thoughts of self-harm and suicide.

The following questions may be useful:
- How does the problem affect the child and family?
- Who is in the family?
- Has the child themselves suffered any adversity?
- How did the current difficulties start?
- What else was happening at the time?
- The next set of questions will reveal more:
- How do people respond to the problem?
- What do you think about the problem?
- What worries everyone most?
- What are you doing about it already?
- Are there any times when it gets better?

How mental health problems evolve in childhood?

The process by which mental health problems evolve is closely related to the process of child development. Genetic factors are important in the aetiology of many mental health problems. For developmental problems in which emotion and behaviour are integral to the presentation, such as autism spectrum disorder (ASD) and attention deficit hyperactivity disorder (ADHD), genetic factors are predominant in determining the neurobiology that underpins them.

Early biological adversity is an important risk factor both for developmental conditions and mental health problems. These include:

- prematurity
- exposure to toxins in utero, most commonly alcohol
- serious illness in infancy (e.g. meningitis)

In addition, later illness and chronic conditions (e.g. epilepsy) can represent a biological psychological and social challenge all in one.

Effects of chronic illness on mental health

- Biological: direct effect on neurobiology, either from conditions itself (e.g. epilepsy) or treatment (e.g. steroids for asthma).
- Psychological: often marked by a similar psychological process to bereavement, with both denial and over-acceptance possible adverse results.
- Social: effect on family wide-ranging and complex. Difference from peers becomes increasingly important and difficult in adolescence.

Developmental problems and behavioural responses

- Language impairment: child unable to verbalize feelings, so expresses them in behaviour problem — if this is not appreciated early on, this will escalate
- Autism spectrum disorder (ASD): difficulty by the child understanding and accepting even quite subtle changes can lead to avoidant and often extreme behaviours
- Attention deficit hyperactivity disorder (ADHD): child 'acts before thinking' and so frequently lashes out or shouts when frustrated

Psychological factors
Self-esteem

Most children experience praise and success in enough areas of their lives to develop a sense of inner self-confidence and self-worth. Children who lack a belief in their own worth may adopt extraordinary and problematic behaviours in order to attract the attention and acclaim of others. It may also be a vulnerability factor for depression and anxiety disorders. Repeated failure, academically or socially, will undermine self-esteem, as will some disorders themselves (dyspraxia, enuresis and faecal soiling in particular).

Cognitive style

During middle childhood, the dominant mode of thought is practical and orderly but tied to immediate circumstances and specific experiences, rather than hypothetical possibilities. Adjust the way you talk to children to be compatible with their thinking style.

Social factors
Early relationships and attachment

In the first 2 months of a baby's life, infants are not fussy about who responds to their needs. From 3-6 months of age they become more selective, demanding comfort from one or two caregivers. By age 6-8 months they are particular about who responds to their needs or holds them. They show tearful separation anxiety if their main caregiver, usually mother, is not there. If tired, fearful, unhappy, or in pain they will cling to her and be comforted by her presence. Children who have never had the opportunity for a close, secure attachment relationship in their early years are at risk of growing up as self-centred individuals who seek the affection and attention of others but have difficulty with close personal relationships and with learning to conform with social rules of conduct. In the second year of life children extend their emotional attachments to other family members and carers. By school age, they can tolerate separations from their parents for several hours. With entry into school, the importance of teachers and other children in shaping psychological development increases.

Exercise 1
Answer the following questions. Prepare short talks and/or dialogues on these topics

1. What are features of child mental health?
2. How to ask about emotional and behavioural problems?
3. How mental health problems evolve in childhood?
4. Describe effects of chronic illness on mental health.
5. Characterize developmental problems and behavioural responses.
6. What can you say about psychological factors and social factors?

Translation 1

1. Good emotional health in childhood is a stronger predictor of high satisfaction in adult life than any other factor. 2. Suicide is the second most common cause of death in adolescents. 3. Mental illness is the single biggest cause of morbidity in adults. 4. Effective history taking must be open, explorative, non-judgemental and empathic. 5. The following questions may be useful: how does the problem affect the child and family; has the child themselves suffered any adversity; how did the current difficulties start; are there any times when it gets better? 6. The process by which mental health problems evolve is closely related to the process of child development. 7. For developmental problems such as autism spectrum disorder (ASD) and attention deficit hyperactivity disorder (ADHD), genetic factors are predominant. 8. Early biological adversity is an important risk factor both for developmental conditions and mental health problems (prematurity, exposure to toxins in utero, serious illness in infancy). 9. Effects of chronic illness on mental health can be: biological, psychological and social.

Exercise 2

Fill in the missing words. Choose the correct ones.

1. Developmental problems and behavioural responses are: _____ _____, _____ _____ _____ (ASD), and attention deficit hyperactivity disorder (_____).	a ADHD b autism spectrum disorder c language impairment
2. Children who _____ _ _____ in their own worth may _____ extraordinary and problematic behaviours in order to _____ ____ _____ and acclaim of others.	a lack a belief b attract the attention c adopt
3. _____ _____, academically or socially, will undermine, _____-_____ as will some disorders themselves (_____, enuresis and faecal soiling in particular).	a Repeated failure b dyspraxia c self-esteem
4. In the first 2 months of a baby's life, infants ____ ___ _____ about who _____ __ _____ _____ but from 3-6 months of age they, _____ ____ _____ and by age 6-8 months	a become more selective b are not fussy c responds to their needs
5. They show tearful _____ anxiety if their mother, is not there.	a separation

6. If tired, fearful, unhappy, or ___ ___ they will _____ ___ her and ___ _____ by her presence.	a be comforted b cling to c in pain
7. In the second year of life children _____ their emotional _____ to other family members and _____	a carers b attachments c extend
8. With entry into school, the _____ of teachers and other children in _____ psychological development _____.	a increases b shaping c importance

Text 2
Early relationships
Young children:

- develop a close attachment relationship with their mother (or main caregiver)
- if separated from their mother, may develop separation anxiety
- if admitted to hospital, should be able to have their parents stay with them.

Adversities in the family

Families are generally the most potent environmental influence on a child's mental health. A predisposition to particular childhood emotional and behavioural problems can be inherited, but family influences interact with this so that overt disorder may or may not emerge. The following are some of the known risk factors:

- angry discord between family members
- parental mental ill health, especially maternal depression
- bereavement
- divorce and subsequent loss of parent figure (in some cases)
- intrusive overprotection
- lack of parental authority
- physical and sexual abuse
- emotional rejection or excessive criticism
- inconsistent, unpredictable discipline
- using the child to fulfil unreasonable personal emotional needs of a parent

- inappropriate responsibilities or expectations for the child's level of maturity.

Bullying is a known adversity, and other forms of peer-mediated persecution. Conversely, having a number of steady, good-quality peer relationships is a marker for good prognosis in an emotional or behavioural problem. The majority of older children and adolescents have internet access, and utilize social media websites regularly, often using smartphone devices. Social media platforms are transforming the way young people communicate with one another. There is increasing evidence that vulnerable adolescents can be harmed by exposure to websites which may promote eating disorders or addictive behaviour. There are many online fora where discussions about self-harm and suicide can have a toxic effect on the adolescent. Cyberbullying over the internet is usually carried out by the same people as conventional bullying, but appears to be more damaging.

Regarding adversities
- The child's family is the most potent influence on the child's mental health
- Adversities outside the family, e.g. bullying, may aggravate the situation.

Resilience
There are some specific resilience factors that should be enquired about:
- time spent together as a family
- meals eaten as a family
- regular exercise
- regular and sufficient sleep
- absence of bullying

The biopsychosocial formulation
It is useful to split factors into:
- predisposing — which usually can't be helped
- precipitating — which are useful in explaining the situation
- perpetuating factors — which are ongoing
- protective factors (resilience)

Specific paediatric mental health problems
Problems of the preschool years
Meal refusal

A common scenario is a mother complaining that her child refuses to eat any or much of what she provides. Examination reveals a healthy, well-nourished child whose height and weight are securely within normal limits on a centile growth chart. An account of what goes on at a typical mealtime may reveal:

- A past history of force-feeding
- Irregular meals
- Unsuitable meals
- Unreasonably large portions
- Multiple opportunities for distraction, e.g. TV
- Most importantly, how much does the child eat between meals? Not all parents regard sweets and crisps as being food.

Exercise 3
Answer the following questions. Prepare short talks and/or dialogues on these topics

1. Speak about early relationships in young children.
2. Explain adversities in the family and outside the family.
3. Characterize specific paediatric mental health problems.

Translation 2

1. Young children develop a close attachment relationship with their mother (or main caregiver). 2. A predisposition to particular childhood emotional and behavioural problems can be inherited, but family influences interact with this so that overt disorder may or may not emerge. 3. The risk factors are: angry discord between family members, maternal depression, bereavement, divorce, intrusive overprotection, physical and sexual abuse, emotional rejection, unpredictable discipline, inappropriate responsibilities or expectations. 4. Adversities outside the family include bullying and other forms of peer-mediated persecution. 5. There is increasing evidence that vulnerable adolescents can be harmed by exposure to websites which may promote eating disorders or addictive behaviour. 6. Cyberbullying over the internet is usually carried out by the same people as conventional bullying. 7. There are some specific resilience factors that should be enquired about: time spent together as a family, meals eaten as a family, regular exercise, regular and sufficient sleep, absence of bullying. 8. An account of what goes on at a typical mealtime may reveal: a past history of force-feeding, irregular

meals, unsuitable meals, unreasonably large portions, multiple opportunities for distraction.

Text 3
Strategy for meal refusal
- Mealtime history
- What is the parent most concerned about?
- Nutrition?
- Refer to growth chart
- Discipline and parenting?
- Family history of eating problems
- Parenting style
- What do others say?
- Is it part of a broader behavioural problem?
- How much food is eaten between meals?
- Food diary to record child's intake over a number of days

Advice
- As long as offered wholesome food with adequate range, children are remarkably good at eating an appropriate quantity of food when allowed a reasonable choice
- As it is impossible to force a child to eat, avoid confrontation at mealtimes
- Develop a relaxed atmosphere
- Use favourite foods as a reward. Introduce other rewards for compliance at mealtimes (e.g. additional privileges such as extra TV time)
- Reduce eating between meals if necessary, although many young children prefer small, frequent snacks.

Sleep-related problems
Difficulty in settling to sleep at bedtime
This is a common problem in the toddler years. Many cases will respond to simple advice:
- creating a bedtime routine which cues the child to what is required
- telling the child to lie quietly in bed until he/she falls asleep
- having a period of an hour before sleep time when the child is not involved with screens.

A more active intervention involves parents imposing a graded pattern of lengthening periods between tucking their child up in bed and coming back after a few minutes to visit. The object is to provide the opportunity for the child to learn how to sleep alone.

Reasons for a child not settling at night

- Too much sleep in the late afternoon
- Displaced sleep/wake cycle — not waking child in morning because did not settle until late on the previous night
- Separation anxiety
- Overstimulated or overwrought in the evening
- Kept awake by siblings or noisy neighbours or TV in the bedroom
- Erratic parental practices: no bedtime or routine to cue child into sleep readiness, sudden removal from play to go to bed without prior warning to wind down
- Use of bedroom as punishment
- Dislike of darkness and silence — night light and playing story tapes can be helpful
- Some chronic physical conditions may be associated with sleep problems, e.g. painful crisis in sickle cell disease.

Waking at night

Some children cry because they cannot settle themselves back to sleep without their parent's presence. The circumstances are different — it is quieter, darker, etc. The graded approach described above for evening settling can also be used in the middle of the night.

Nightmares

These are bad dreams which can be recalled by the child. They are common, rarely requiring professional attention unless they occur frequently or are stereotype in content, indicating a morbid preoccupation or symptomatic of a psychiatric disorder such as posttraumatic stress disorder.

Night (sleep) terrors

These are different from nightmares, occurring about 1.5 hours after settling. The parents find the child sitting up in bed, eyes open, seemingly awake but obviously disorientated, confused and distressed, and unresponsive to their questions and reassurances. The child settles back to sleep after a few minutes and has no recollection of the episode in the morning. A night terror is a parasomnia, a disturbance of the structure of sleep wherein a very rapid emergence from the first period of deep slow-wave sleep produces a state or high arousal and confusion. Sleepwalking has similar origins. The most important intervention for sleepwalking is to make the environment safe to prevent injury to the child (e.g. not sleeping on the upper bunk of a double-bunk bed, putting gates before the staircase, locking the kitchen, etc.)

Exercise 4
Answer the following questions. Prepare short talks and/or dialogues on these topics
Explain strategy for meal refusal.

1. Describe sleep-related problems.
2. Speak about difficulty in settling to sleep at bedtime.
3. What are reasons for a child not settling at night and waking at night?
4. Differentiate between nightmares and night (sleep) terrors.

Translation 3
1. Mealtime history includes: nutrition, discipline and parenting, family history of eating problems, food diary to record child's intake over a number of days. 2. Children are remarkably good at eating an appropriate quantity of food when allowed a reasonable choice. 3. Avoid confrontation at mealtimes, develop a relaxed atmosphere, use favourite foods as a reward, reduce eating between meals. 4. Difficulty in settling to sleep at bedtime is a common problem in the toddler years. 5. Reasons for a child not settling at night are: too much sleep in the late afternoon, separation anxiety, overstimulated or overwrought in the evening, kept awake by noisy neighbours or TV, erratic parental practices, use of bedroom as punishment, dislike of darkness and silence, some chronic physical conditions e.g. painful crisis in sickle cell disease.

Exercise 5
Fill in the missing words. Choose the correct ones.

1. Some children cry because they cannot _____ themselves _____ to sleep without their parent's _____.	a presence b settle back
2. _____ are bad dreams which can be _____ by the child.	a recalled b Nightmares
3. They occur frequently or are _____ in content, indicating a _____ _____ or symptomatic of a _____ _____.	a psychiatric disorder b stereotype c morbid preoccupation

4. Night (sleep) _____ are different from _____.	a terrors b nightmares
5. The parents find the child sitting up in bed, eyes open, but _____ _____ obviously disorientated, _____ ___ _____, and unresponsive to their questions and _____.	a reassurances b confused and distressed c seemingly awake
6. The child has ___ _____ of the _____ in the morning.	a no recollection b episode
7. The most important _____ for _____ is to _____ the environment _____ to prevent injury to the child.	a sleepwalking b make safe c intervention

Text 4
Disobedience, defiance, and tantrums

Normal toddlers often go through a phase of refusing to comply with parent's demands, sometimes angrily. This is an understandable reaction to the discovery that the world is not organized around them. That is one reason why children play their parents up but may be fine with others. Temper tantrums are ordinary responses to frustration, especially at not being allowed to have or to do something. They are common in young preschool children. Examine the child to identify potential medical or psychological factors. Medical factors include global or language delay, hearing impairment (e.g. glue ear), and medication with bronchodilators or anticonvulsants. The easiest course of action is to distract the child of, to let tantrum burn itself out while the parent leaves the room, returning a few minutes later when things quieten down. This should be done in a calm, neutral manner and certainly not accompanied by threats of abandonment. An alternative course is to 'time out', which is a form of structured ignoring. Disobedience can be dealt with by using a star chart to reward the child for complying with parental requests. The chart needs to be where the child can see it and the child must know what to do in order to get a star. However, if a tangible reward had been promised for a certain number of stars, it is important to follow through with this.

Managing toddler disobedience

- Ensure your demand is reasonable for the developmental stage of the child

- Tell the child what you want him/her to do rather than nagging about what you do not want him/her to do
- Praise for compliance, especially when it is spontaneous
- Use simple incentives to reward good behaviour
- Use instructions like 'If you do this or that ... then I can do such and such'
- Avoid threats that cannot be carried out
- Follow through with any consequences you indicated for noncompliance
- Ignore some episodes of defiance if they are not significant

Analysing a tantrum
- Antecedents — what happened in the minutes before the episode
- Behaviour — exactly what did the episode consist of
- Consequences — what happened as a result, including what you did and the outcome

Tantrums: management strategies
- Affection and attention before the tantrum
- Distraction
- Avoiding antecedents

Ignoring:
- effective but can be difficult
- no surrender (when parents give in, tantrums become harder to deal with over time)

Time out from positive reinforcement:
- walk away, returning when quietens down
- separate from siblings
- holding firmly if the child is putting themselves or others in danger
- star chart to prevent future episodes.

For temper tantrums:
- Analyse according to antecedents, behaviour and consequences
- Consider distraction, avoiding antecedents, ignoring and time out

Aggressive behaviour
Small children can be aggressive for a host of reasons, ranging from spite to exuberance. Much aggressive behaviour is learned, either by being rewarded (often inadvertently) or by copying parents, siblings or

peers. Many instances of aggressive, demanding behaviour are provoked or intensified by a parent shouting at or smacking their child. A tired or stressed child will be irritable and prone to angry outbursts, as will children whose communication skills are compromised by deafness or a developmental language disorder. Once established, an aggressive behavioural style is remarkably persistent over a period of years. There are several parenting programmes for teaching parents to manage aggression in their children.

Exercise 6
Answer the following questions. Prepare short talks and/or dialogues on these topics

1. What is meant by disobedience, defiance, and tantrums?
2. How to manage toddler disobedience?
3. What can you say about analysing a tantrum?
4. What are management strategies of tantrums?
5. How to manage aggressive behaviour?

Translation 4
1. Normal toddlers often go through a phase of refusing to comply with parent's demands, sometimes angrily. 2. Temper tantrums are ordinary responses to frustration, especially at not being allowed to have or to do something. 3. Medical factors include global or language delay, hearing impairment (e.g. glue ear), and medication with bronchodilators or anticonvulsants. 4. The easiest course of action is to distract the child of, to let tantrum burn itself out while the parent leaves the room, returning a few minutes later when things quieten down. 5. Managing toddler disobedience: ensure your demand is reasonable for the developmental stage of the child, tell the child what you want him/her to do, praise for compliance, reward good behaviour, ignore some episodes of defiance if they are not significant. 6. Management strategies of tantrums: ignoring, time out from positive reinforcement. 7. Small children can be aggressive for a host of reasons, ranging from spite to exuberance. 8. Many instances of aggressive, demanding behaviour are provoked or intensified by a parent shouting at or smacking their child. 9. A tired or stressed child will be irritable and prone to angry outbursts, as will children whose communication skills are compromised by deafness or a developmental language disorder.

Text 5
Problems in middle childhood
Nocturnal enuresis

In colloquial speech, 'enuresis' is synonymous with bed-wetting. Small children need reasonable freedom from stress in order to learn night-time continence. Emotional stress can interfere and cause secondary enuresis (relapse after a period of dryness). Organic causes of enuresis include:

- urinary tract infection
- faecal retention causes bladder neck dysfunction
- polyuria from osmotic diuresis, e.g. diabetes mellitus, or renal concentrating disorders, e.g. chronic kidney disease

It may also be associated with developmental, attention or learning difficulties. Investigation with urinalysis is only indicated if the bed wetting occurs during the day, if there are features of urinary tract infection, diabetes mellitus or ill health. The parents should stop punitive procedures, as these are counterproductive. Excessive or insufficient fluid intake and abnormal toileting patterns should be addressed. The child earns praise and a star can be awarded for agreed behaviour. If a child does not respond to a star chart, it may be supplemented with an enuresis alarm. This is a sensor, usually placed in the child's pants which sounds an alarm when it becomes wet. The alarm method takes several weeks to achieve dryness but is effective in most cases so long as the child is motivated. Desmopressin, a synthetic analogue of antidiuretic hormone, may be used in children over 7 years of age, e.g. for holidays or sleep overs. It can be taken as tablets or sublingually. Fluid intake should be restricted after use.

Faecal soiling

It is abnormal for a child to soil after the age of 4 years. Children who soil fall into two broad groups: those with and those without a rectum loaded with faeces. There are a number of factors:

- constipation, possibly following dehydration during an illness
- inhibition of defecation because of pain from a fissure
- inhibition because of fear of punishment for incontinence
- anxieties about using the toilet

Any reason for faecal retention, such as an anal fissure, should be identified and treated, but the most important thing is to empty the rectum as soon as possible. A stool softener is given for a couple of weeks, followed, if necessary, by a stimulant laxative. Rarely, an enema is required. The child can be encouraged to defecate regularly in the toilet, which earns stars on a star chart. Such retraining may take a number of weeks while the distended rectum shrinks to normal size. Soiling may occur in conjunction with an empty rectum for various reasons. Similarly, diarrhoea can overwhelm bowel control. Lastly, the child may defecate intentionally as a hostile act. Such children may have other behavioural problems requiring psychiatric referral.

Recurrent unexplained somatic symptoms

Somatization is the term used for the communication of emotional distress, troubled relationships, and personal predicaments through bodily symptoms. The prepubertal child may experience affective distress as recurrent abdominal pain and headaches. With increasing age, limb pain, aching muscles, fatigue, and neurological symptoms become more prominent. In the majority of cases, no organic cause can be objectively demonstrated, yet the child is obviously in pain. Some of these children have clinically significant anxiety. The child should be interviewed about school, friends and family, noting the general level of anxiety and ability to communicate. This should be an integral part of the interview. A thorough physical examination is important to reassure the child and family that there is no underlying organic cause. It is sensible to ask the child to point to where the pain is. The pain may be limited to school days or coincide with upsetting events in the home, such as parental conflict, or other specific situations. Problems at school, particularly bullying and teasing, or difficulties with a teacher or class work may only be known by the child. Learning pain-coping skills, such as relaxation, may be helpful, especially for headaches.

Ticks

A tick is a quick, sudden, coordinated movement, which is apparently purposeful and recurs in the same part of the child's body. It can be purposefully suppressed to some extent. About 1 in 10 children develop a tic at some stage, typically around the face and head — blinking, frowning, head flicking, sniffing, throat clearing and grunting. Boys are more commonly affected. Ticks are most likely to occur when the child is inactive and often disappear when actively concentrating. Transient tic disorder clears up over the next few months, although they may recur from time to time. Less commonly, the child has ticks from which he/she is hardly ever free. If the tics continue for more than 12 months, they are considered chronic, although most cases still resolve in adulthood. If there is both multiple motor ticks and vocal tics such as grunting, coughing, humming, squeaking, the condition is known as Tourette syndrome. The first line of treatment is cognitive behavioural therapy with habit reversal techniques.

Exercise 7

Answer the following questions. Prepare short talks and/or dialogues on these topics

- What can you say about nocturnal enuresis?
- Speak about faecal soiling.
- What is meant by recurrent unexplained somatic symptoms?
- Characterize ticks.

Translation 5

1. Small children need reasonable freedom from stress in order to learn night-time continence. 2. Emotional stress can interfere and cause secondary enuresis (relapse after a period of dryness). 3. Investigation with urinalysis is only indicated if the bed wetting occurs during the day, if there are features of urinary tract infection, diabetes mellitus or ill health. 4. A sensor is usually placed in the child's pants which sounds an alarm when it becomes wet. 5. The alarm method takes several weeks to achieve dryness but is effective in most cases so long as the child is motivated. 6. Desmopressin, a synthetic analogue of antidiuretic hormone, may be used in children over 7 years of age, e.g. for holidays or sleep overs. 7. Children who soil fall into two broad groups: those with and those without a rectum loaded with faeces. 8. There are a number of factors: constipation, pain from a fissure, fear of punishment for incontinence, or anxieties about using the toilet. 9. Any reason for faecal retention, such as an anal fissure, should be identified and treated. 10. Diarrhoea can overwhelm bowel control or the child may defecate intentionally as a hostile act.

Exercise 8

Match the column A with the column B. Try to learn the expressions and/or sentences by heart.

A

1. Somatization is the term used for the communication of ...
2. The prepubertal child may experience affective distress ...
3. With increasing age, limb pain, aching muscles, fatigue, and neurological symptoms ...
4. The child should be interviewed about school, friends and family, ...
5. The pain may be limited to school days ...
6. Problems at school, particularly bullying and teasing, or difficulties with a teacher or class work ...
7. A tick is a quick, sudden, coordinated movement, ...

8. About 1 in 10 children develop a tic at some stage, ...
9. If the tics continue for more than 12 months ...
10. If there is both multiple motor ticks and vocal tics ...

B

a. ... *such as grunting, coughing, humming, squeaking, the condition is known as Tourette syndrome.*

b. ... *which is apparently purposeful and recurs in the same part of the child's body.*

c. ... *may only be known by the child.*

d. ... *they are considered chronic, although most cases still resolve in adulthood.*

e. ... *noting the general level of anxiety and ability to communicate.*

f. ... *as recurrent abdominal pain and headaches.*

g. ... *become more prominent.*

h. ... *typically around the face and head – blinking, frowning, head flicking, sniffing, throat clearing and grunting.*

i. ... *emotional distress, troubled relationships, and personal predicaments through bodily symptoms.*

j. ... *or coincide with upsetting events in the home, such as parental conflict.*

Text 6
Antisocial behaviour

Children steal, lie, disobey, light fires, destroy things, and pick fights for various reasons:

- failure to learn when to exercise social restraint
- lack of social skills, such as the ability to negotiate a disagreement
- they may be responding to the challenges of their peers
- they may be chronically angry and resentful
- they may find their own notions of good behaviour overwhelmed by emotion such as sadness or temptation.

When serious antisocial behaviour is the dominant feature and is so severe as to represent a handicap to general functioning, a diagnosis of conduct disorder is made. Children with conduct disorder may not have necessarily broken the law, although their behaviour excites strong social disapproval. A milder form, characterized by angry, defiant behaviour to authority figures such as parents and teachers, is known as oppositional-defiant disorder. Poor parental cooperation and motivation can result in minimal benefit. Affected children often do not have the level of motivation required.

Exercise 9
Study the following summary and then interpret basic information in English.

1. Nocturnal enuresis
Common, males more than females.
Most affected children are psychologically and physically normal
Treatment usually considered only at > 5 years of age
Management – explanation, star charts, enuresis alarm, sometimes desmopressin.
2. Faecal retention
Present in most children who soil
May be due to constipation or reluctance to use the toilet
When present, the rectum needs to be emptied, initially with a stool softener and laxative, followed by retraining.
3. Somatic symptoms
May be a means of communicating emotional distress
Sources of stress should be identified and ameliorated if possible
In many children with unexplained recurrent abnormal pain or headaches, no significant sources of stress are identified.
4. Antisocial behaviour
It is important to exclude any coexisting psychiatric condition and treat this directly, e.g. ADHD or depression.
Parenting groups are an evidence-based treatment for these disorders, but require motivation.

Anxiety

Pathological anxiety exists in two forms: specific and general. In phobias there is fear of a specific object or situation. Most children have a number of irrational fears (the dark, ghosts, kidnappers, dogs, spiders, bats, snakes) which are common. Some of these persist into adulthood. Treatment by cognitive behavioural therapy with graded exposure to the feared event may be successful. Often, it is first manifested as physical complaints: nausea, headache or pain. It may take the form of health worries. Some children with generalized anxiety may develop unusual coping strategies in an attempt to gain control over their parents and the world in general. It may be a justifiable reaction to an event, or be disproportionate. Children rarely say spontaneously that they are anxious — instead they tend to complain of aches and pains or behave in apparently manipulative ways to cope with or avoid the feared situation.

School refusal

A child may be absent from school because of illness, because parents keep the child off school, or because of truancy. In truancy, a child leaves to go to school but never arrives or leaves early. It is often accompanied by other behavioural difficulties. A few non-attendees at school suffer from school refusal, an inability to attend school on account of overwhelming anxiety. Anxiety may present as complaints of nausea, headache or otherwise not being well.

Treatment of school refusal

- Advise and support parents and school about the condition
- Treat any underlying emotional disorder
- Plan and facilitate an early and graded return to school at a pace tolerable for the child with all involved (child, family, teachers, educational psychologist and educational welfare officers)
- Help the parents make it more rewarding for the child to return to school than stay at home
- Address bullying or educational difficulties if present

Educational underachievement

Children who achieve less well at school than expected are sometimes brought to doctors. Core medical responsibilities include checking sight and hearing and attempting to elicit the cause of underachievement.

Causes of underachievement at school

- Long-standing problem
- Visual problems
- Hearing problems
- Dyslexia
- Generalized or specific learning problems
- Hyperactivity
- Antieducation family background
- Chaotic family background

Exercise 10
Answer the following questions. Prepare short talks and/or dialogues on these topics

1. Characterize antisocial behaviour and anxiety.
2. What is treatment of school refusal?
3. What are causes of underachievement at school?
4. Give the names of long-standing problems.

Translation 6

1. Children steal, lie, disobey, light fires, destroy things, and pick fights for various reasons. 2. When serious antisocial behaviour is the dominant feature and is so severe as to represent a handicap to general functioning, a diagnosis of conduct disorder is made. 3. Angry, defiant behaviour to authority figures such as parents and teachers, is known as oppositional-defiant disorder. 4. Pathological anxiety exists in two forms: specific and general. 5. Most children have a number of irrational fears (the dark, ghosts, kidnappers, dogs, spiders, bats, snakes) which are common. 6. Treatment by cognitive behavioural therapy with graded exposure to the feared event may be successful. 7. Often, anxiety is first manifested as physical complaints: nausea, headache or pain. 8. Some children with generalized anxiety may develop unusual coping strategies in an attempt to gain control over their parents. 9. Children tend to complain of aches and pains or behave in apparently manipulative ways to cope with or avoid the feared situation. 10. A child may be absent from school because of illness, because parents keep the child off school, or because of truancy. 11. Plan and facilitate an early and graded return to school at a pace tolerable for the child. 12. Core medical responsibilities include checking sight and hearing and attempting to elicit the cause of underachievement. 13. Causes of underachievement at school are: visual problems, hearing problems, dyslexia, generalized or specific learning problems, hyperactivity, and chaotic family background.

Key 7
Exercise 2
1c, b, a; 2a, c, b; 3a, c, b; 4b, c, a; 5a; 6c, b, a; 7c, b, a; 8c, b, a

Exercise 5
1b, a; 2b, c, a; 3 a, b; 4 a, b; 5 c, b, a; 6 a, b; 7 c, a, b

Exercise 8
1i; 2f; 3g; 4e; 5j; 6c; 7b; 8h; 9d; 10a

VOCABULARY 7

abandonment /əˈbæn.dən.mənt/
abrasion /əˈbreɪ.ʒən/
abuse /əˈbjuːz/
access /ˈæk.ses/
accident /ˈæk.sɪ.dənt/
acclaim /əˈkleɪm/
acyclovir /əˈsaɪkləʊvɪr/
adaptation /ˌæd.əpˈteɪ.ʃən/
addictive /əˈdɪk.tɪv/
adduction /əˈdəkt.ʃən/
adenectomy /ad.en.əʊm.ek.tə.mi/
adherence /ədˈhɪə.rənts/
adjacent /əˈdʒeɪ.sənt/
adulthood /ˈæd.ʌlt.hʊd/
adverse /ˈæd.vɜːs/
adversely /ˈæd.vɜː.sli/
affection /əˈfek.ʃən/
afford /əˈfɔːd/
albumin /ˈæl.bjʊ.mɪn/
alkylating /ˌælkəˈleɪtɪŋ/
allogeneic /ˈæləʊdʒɪ.neɪɪk/
alopecia /ˌəˈ.ləˈpiː.ʃiː.ə/
ambient /ˈæm.bi.ənt/
ameliorate /əˈmiːljəˌreɪt/
amicable /ˈæm.ɪk.ə.bəl/
anaemia /əˈniː.mi.ə/
analogue /ˈænəˌlɒg/
anaphylaxis /ˌæn.ə.frˈlæk.sɪs/
aneurysm /ˌæn.jʊə.rɪ.zəm/
antecedent /ˌæntɪˈsiːdənt/
antenatal /ˌæn.tiˈneɪ.təl/
anterior /ænˈtɪə.ri.ər/
anti /ˈæntɪ/
anticonvulsant /ˌæn.ti.kənˈvʌl.sənt/
antidiuretic /ˌæn.ti.ˌdaɪ.jʊˈret.ɪk/
antigen /ˈæn.tɪ.dʒən/
antiretroviral /æn.tiˌret.rəʊˈvaɪə.rəl/
anus /ˈeɪ.nəs/
aplasia /əˈpleɪ.zɪə/
aplastic /əˈplæs.tɪk/
apparently /əˈpær.ənt.li/
appreciate /əˈpriː.ʃi.eɪt/
aqueduct /ˈækwɪˌdʌkt/
arch /ɑːtʃ/
arousal /əˈraʊzəl/

197

arrest /əˈrest/
arteriosus /ɑː.tɪə.riːˈəʊ.səs/
arthralgia /aːˈθræl.dʒɪ.ə/
aspect /ˈæs.pekt/
aspiration /ˌæspɪˈreɪʃən/
assay /əˈseɪ/
assistance /əˈsɪs.tənt s/
atopic /əˈtɒp.ɪk/ **eczema** /ˈek.sɪ .mə/
atresia /əˈtriː.ʒɪə/
attachment /əˈtætʃmənt/
attendee /əˌtenˈdiː/
attention /əˈten.ʃən/
attract /əˈtrækt/
audiologist /ˈɔː.dɪ ɒ.lə.dʒɪst/
augmentation /ˌɔːgmenˈteɪʃən/
auricle /ˈɔː.rɪkəl/
auricular /ɔːˈrɪkjʊlə/
availability /əˌveɪ.ləˈbɪl.ɪ.ti/
avascular /əˈvæskjʊlə/
avoid /əˈvɔɪd/
Bartonella henselae /bahr,təʊ.nelˈæ henˈse.li:/
bartonellosis /ˈbɑː.tᵊn.eəʊ.sɪs/
bat /bæt/
beam /biːm/
bed-wetting /ˈbed ˌwet.iŋ/
beef /biːf/
benzylpenicillin /ben.zɪl ˌpen.əˈsɪl.ɪn/
beware /bɪˈweə/
biased /ˈbaɪ.əst/
bilateral /baɪˈlæt.ər.əl/
bilirubin /ˌbɪl.ɪˈruː.bɪn/
bladder /ˈblæd.ər/
blade /bleɪd/
blanch /blɑːntʃ/
blast /ˌblæst/ **cell** /sel/
blepharitis /ˌblef.əˈraɪ.təs/
blink /blɪŋk/
blood /blʌd/ **vessel** /ˈves.əl/
blotchy /blɒtʃ.i/
blueberry /ˈbluːbərɪ/
boggy /ˈbɒgɪ/
bone /bəʊn/ **marrow** /ˈmær.əʊ/
booster /ˈbuː.stər/
brachial /ˈbreɪ.ki.əl/
breakdown /ˈbreɪk.daʊn/
breech /briːtʃ/ **delivery** /dɪˈlɪv.ər.i/
broad /brɔːd/

bronchopulmonary /ˈbrɒŋ.kəˈpʊl.mə.ner.i/
bronchus /ˈbrɒŋ.kəs/ pl **bronchi** /ˈbrɒŋ.kaɪ/
brow /braʊ/
Brucella /bruːsɪˈllə/
Brudzinski sign /bruː.dʒinˈskiː saɪn/
buccal /ˈbʌk.əl/
bullous /ˈbʊ.ləs/
bullying /ˈbʊlɪɪŋ/
bunk /bʌŋk/
burn /bɜːn/
caesarean section /sɪˌzeə.ri.ənˈsek.ʃən/
calcification /ˌkæl.sɪ.fɪˈkeɪ.ʃən/
callus /ˈkæl.əs/
candidiasis /ˌkan.dəˈdaɪ.ə.səs/ pl. **candidiases** /ˌkan.dəˈdaɪ.ə.ˌsiːz/
cannula /ˈkæn.jʊ.lə/ pl **cannulae**
caput /ˈkeɪp.ˌuːt/
cardiomegaly /ˌkɑːr.diəˈmeg.ə.laɪ/
carditis /kɑːˈdaɪ.tɪs/
caregiver /ˈkeəˌgɪv.ər/
carriage /ˈkær.ɪdʒ/
cashews /ˈkæʃuː/
catering /ˈkeɪtərɪŋ/
cavernous /ˈkævənəs/
cellular /ˈsel.jʊ.lər/
central /ˈsen.trəl/ **venous** /ˈviː.nəs/ **line** /laɪn/
cephalhaematoma /ˌsefəlˌhiːməˈtəʊmə/
cerebral /ˈser.ɪ.brəl/ **artery** /ˈɑːtərɪ/
cerebral /ˈser.ɪ.brəl/ **infarction** /ɪnˈfɑːk.ʃən/
cerebrospinal /ˌser.ɪ.brəʊˈspaɪ.nəl/
cessation /sesˈeɪ.ʃən/
chaotic /keɪˈɒtɪk/
chart /tʃɑːt/
chickenpox /ˈtʃɪk.ɪn.pɒks/
chignon /ˈʃiːnjɒn/
child /tʃaɪld/ **rearing** /rɪər.ɪŋ/
chin-lift /tʃɪn lɪft/
choana /ˈkəʊ.ə.nə/
circuit /ˈsɜːkɪt/
clavicle /ˈklæv.ɪ.kļ/
clearing /ˈklɪə.rɪŋ/
cling /klɪŋ/
clitoridis /klɪˈtɒr.ɪ.dɪs/
clonic /ˈkləʊ.nɪk/
coagulopathy /kəʊˌæg.juˈlɒ.pə.θi/
cohesive /kəʊˈhiː.sɪv/
coincide /ˌkəʊɪnˈsaɪd/
colitis /kəˈlɪ.tɪs/

colloquial /kəˈləʊkwɪəl/
commence /kəˈmens/
compatible /kəmˈpæt.ɪ.b̩l/
comply /kəmˈplaɪ/ **with** /wɪð/
compression /kɒm.ˈpreʃ.en/
compromise /ˈkɒmprəˌmaɪz/
concentration /ˌkɒn.sənˈtreɪ.ʃən/
confined /kənˈfaɪnd/
confluent /kənˈfluːənt/
conform /kənˈfɔːm/
confrontation /ˌkɒnfrʌnˈteɪʃən/
confused /kənˈfjuːzd/
conjugated /ˈkɒn.dʒə.geɪt.ɪd/
conjunctiva /ˌkɒn.dʒʌŋkˈtaɪ.və/ pl **conjunctivae**
conjunctivitis /kənˌdʒʌŋk.tɪˈvaɪ.tɪs/
connective tissue /kəˌnek.tɪvˈtɪʃ.uː/
consequence /ˈkɒn.sɪ.kwəns/
considerable /kənˈsɪd.ər.ə.b̩l/
contagiosum /kənˈteɪdʒɪəsəm/
contraction /kənˈtræk.ʃən/
contraindicate /ˌkɒn.trəˈɪn.dɪ.keɪt/
contraindication /ˌkɒn.trəˌɪn.dɪˈkeɪ.ʃən/
contralateral /ˌkɒn.trə.ˈlæt.ər.əl/
contribute /kənˈtrɪbjuːt/
controversy /ˈkɒntrəˌvɜːsɪ/
convection /kənˈvekˌʃən/
conversely /kɒnˈvɜːslɪ/
conversion /kənˈvɜːˌʃən/
cope /kəʊp/
cornea /ˈkɔːnɪə/ pl **corneae**
corpora /ˈkɔːpər.ə/ **carvenosa** /ˈkæv.ən.əʊs ə/
corporal /ˈkɔːpər.əl/
coryza /kəˈraɪ.zə/
coughing /ˈkɒf.ɪŋ/
counterproductive /ˌkaʊn.tə.prəˈdʌk.tɪv/
court /kɔːt/
crawl /krɔːl/
crest /krest/
crippling /ˈkrɪp.lɪŋ/
crop /krɒp/
crossing /ˈkrɒs.ɪŋ/
crust /krʌst/
crusted /ˈkrʌs.tɪd/
cue /kjuː/
cutaneous /kjuːˈteɪ.ni.əs/
cyberbullying /ˈsaɪbəˈbʊlɪɪŋ/
cyst /sɪst/

dactylitis /ˈdæktɪ.laɪ.tɪs/
darkness /ˈdɑːknɪs/
day-care /ˈdeɪˌkeə/
deafness /ˈdef.nəs/
deceptively /dɪˈseptɪvlɪ/
decision /dɪˈsɪʒ.ən/
decline /dɪˈklaɪn/
defecate /ˈdef.ə.keɪt/
defective /dɪˈfek.tɪv/
defiance /dɪˈfaɪəns/
defiant /dɪˈfaɪənt/
delivery /dɪˈlɪv.ər.i/
dendritic /denˈdrɪ.tɪk/
dengue /ˈdeŋgɪ/ **fever** /ˈfiːvə/
denial /dɪˈnaɪ.əl/
denude /dɪˈnjuːd/
dependency /dɪˈpen.dənt .si/
depigmented /deˈpɪg.mənt.ɪd/
depress /dɪˈpres/
desaturation /dɪˈsætʃərˈeɪʃən/
desquamate /ˈdeskwəˈmeɪt/
desquamation /ˌdeskwəˈmeɪ.ʃən/
determinant /dɪˈtɜː.mɪ.nənt/
devastating /ˈdev.ə.steɪ.tɪŋ/
diabetes /ˌdaɪ.əˈbiː.tiːz/
diamond /ˈdaɪəmənd/
differentiate /ˌdɪfəˈrenʃieɪt/
digit /ˈdɪdʒ.ɪt/
dilatation /ˌdɪl.əˈteɪ.ʃən/
diphtheria /dɪfˈθəɪr.i.ə/
disadvantage /ˌdɪs.ədˈvɑːn.tɪdʒ/
disapproval /ˌdɪs.əˈpruː.vəl/
disaster /dɪˈzɑː.stər/
discipline /ˈdɪsɪplɪn/
disconnected /ˌdɪs.kəˈnek.tɪd/
discord /ˈdɪs.kɔːd/
discredit /dɪsˈkredɪt/
discreet /dɪˈskriːt./
disfigure /dɪsˈfɪgə/
disobedience /ˌdɪsəˈbiːdɪəns/
disobey /ˌdɪsəˈbeɪ/
displaced /dɪˈspleɪst/
disseminate /dɪˈsem.ɪ.neɪt/
dissemination /dɪˌsem.əˈneɪ.ʃən/
distortion /dɪ ˈstɔː.ʃən/
distract /dɪˈs.trækt/
donor /ˈdəʊ.nər/

dorsiflexion /ˌdɔːsɪˈflekʃən/
double-bunk /ˈdʌbəl bʌŋk/
drainage /ˈdreɪ.nɪdʒ/
draught /drɑːft/
droplet /ˈdrɒp.lət/
drowsiness /ˈdraʊ.zɪ.nəs/
duct /dʌkt/
dural /ˈdjʊə.rəl/
dysentery /ˈdɪs.ənˌter.i/
dysfunction /dɪsˈfʌŋk.ʃən/
earache /ˈɪə.reɪk/
eczema /ˈek.sɪ.mə/
eczematous /ekˈsem.ə.təs/
education /ˌedjʊˈkeɪʃən/
efficiently /ɪˈfɪʃ.ənt.li/
electrode /ɪˈlekˌtroʊd/
electrolyte /ɪˈlek.trə.laɪt/
eliminate /ɪˈlɪm.ɪ.neɪt/
embarrassed /ɪmˈbær.əst/
emerge /ɪˈmɜːdʒ/
emergence /ɪˈmɜːdʒəns/
emotional /ɪˈməʊ.ʃən.əl/
empathy /empəθɪ/
encapsulate /ɪnˈkæp.sjʊ.leɪt/
encompass /ɪnˈkʌm.pəs/
endemic /enˈdem.ɪk/
engender /ɪnˈdʒendə/
enlarge /ɪnˈlɑːdʒ/
enlargement /ɪnˈlɑːdʒ.mənt/
enormous /ɪˈnɔːməs/
Entamoeba /ˌentəˈmiːbə/ histolytica /ˌhɪs.təˈlɪ.tɪ.kə/
enterocolitis /ˌen.tə.rəʊ.kə.ˈlaɪ.təs/
enterovirus /ˌɛn.tə.roʊˈvaɪ.rəs/
epidermis /ˌep.ɪˈdɜː.mɪs/
epiglottitis /ˌep.ɪ.gləˈtaɪ.tɪs/
Epstein /ˈepˌstaɪn/ pearls /pər.ə.lz/
Epstein-Barr virus, EBV /ˈepˌstaɪn bɑː ˈvaɪrəs/
epulis /əˈpjʊ.ləs/
eradication /ɪˌrædiˈkeɪ.ʃən/
Erb palsy /erb ˈpɔː.l.zi/
erectile /ɪˈrek.taɪl/
erratic /ɪˈræt.ɪk/
erythema /ˌer.ɪˈθiː.mə/ infectious /ɪnˈfek.ʃəs/
erythroblastopenia /e.riθˈrəʊ.blasˈtəʊ.piːˈniː.æ/
escalate /ˈes.kə.leɪt/
evaporative /ɪˈvæp.ər.eɪ.tɪv/
event /ɪˈvent/

Ewing sarcoma /sɑːˈkəʊ.mə/
exacerbate /ɪɡˈzæs.ə.beɪt/
excessively /ɪkˈsesɪvlɪ/
excision /ˌekˈsiʃən/
excite /ɪkˈsaɪt/
exercise /ˈeksəˌsaɪz/
exert /ɪɡˈzɜːt/
exfoliative /eksˈfeʊlɪˌeɪ.tɪv/
exhausted /ɪɡˈzɔː.stɪd/
expand /ɪkˈspænd/
explorative /ek.spləˈrə.tɪv/
exposure /ɪkˈspəʊ.ʒər/
extensive /ɪkˈstent.sɪv/
extensor /ɪkˈstent.sər/
extraordinary /ɪkˈstrɔː.dɪn.ər.i/
extremely /ɪkˈstriːm.li/
extremity /ɪkˈstrem.ɪ.ti/
exuberance /ɪɡˈzjuː.bər.əns/
exudation /ˌek.sjuːˈdəɪˌʃən/
face /feɪs/
facility /fəˈsɪl.ə.ti/
fade /feɪd/
faecal /ˈfiː.kəl/
fall /ˈfɔːl/ **asleep** /əˈsliːp/
fan /fæn/
Fanconi /faːn.kəʊˈniː/ **anaemia** /əˈniː.mi.ə/
fasciitis /ˈfeɪʃ.ɪaɪ.tɪs/
fashion /ˈfæʃ.ən/
fatal /ˈfeɪ.təl/
fatigue /fəˈtiːɡ/
fearful /ˈfɪə.fəl/
fight /faɪt/
flaccid /ˈflæksɪd/
flame /fleɪm/
flection /ˈflek.ʃən/
flee /fliː/
flexed /flekst/
flick /flɪk/
fluctuate /ˈflʌk.tju.eɪt/
flulike /ˈfluː.laɪk/
foetal /ˈfiː.təl/
follicle /ˈfɒl.ɪ.kl̩/
force-feeding /fɔːs ˌfiː.dɪŋ/
forceps /ˈfɔː.seps/
fortified /ˈfɔː.tɪˌfaɪd/ **cereal** /ˈsɪə.ri.əl/
frontonasal /ˈfrʌntə ˈneɪzəl/
frown /fraʊn/

frustration /frʌsˈtreɪ.ʃən/

fungal /ˈfʌŋ.gəl/

fusion /ˈfjuː.ʒən/

fussy /ˈfʌsɪ/

G6PD, Glucose-6-phosphate dehydrogenase /gluˈkəʊs fosfəɪt diːˈhaɪ.drodʒ'en.eɪs/ **deficiency** /dɪˈfɪʃ.ən.si/

gamma /ˈgæmə/

ganglion /ˈgæŋ.gli.ən/ pl **ganglia**

gender /ˈdʒen.dər/

genitourinary /ˌdʒen.ɪ.təʊˈjʊə.rɪ.nər,i/

germinal /ˈdʒɜː.mə.nᵊl/

ghost /gəʊst/

gingival /dʒɪnˈdʒaɪ.vəl/

gingivostomatitis /ˈdʒɪn.dʒɪ.vəˈstəʊmə'taɪ.tɪs/

glandular /ˈglæn.djʊ.lər/

glomerulonephritis /glɒˌmer.jʊ.ləʊ.nɪˈfraɪ.tɪs/

Glucose-6-phosphate dehydrogenase /gluˈkəʊs fosfəɪt diːˈhaɪ.drodʒ'en.eɪs/

granulomatous /ˌgrænjʊˈlɒm.ə.təs/

grimace /ˈgrɪ.məs/

gross /grəʊs/ **national** /ˈnæʃənəl/ **income** /ˈɪnkʌm/

growth /grəʊθ/

gum /gʌm/

haemangioma /ˌhiːmˌænˌdʒɪˈəʊ.mə/

haematocrit /hiːˈmə.tə.krɪt/

haematoma /hiːˈmə.təʊ.mə/ pl **haematomata**

haemoglobinopathy /ˌhiːməʊgləʊbɪˈnɒpəθɪ/

haemolysis /ˌhiːˈmɒ.lɪ.sɪs/

haemophagocytosis /ˌhiːməˌfægəsaɪˈtəʊ.sɪs/

haemophilia /ˌhiːˈmə'fɪl.i.ə/

haemopoiesis /ˌhiːməʊpəˈiːsɪs/

haemorrhage /ˈhem.ər.ɪdʒ/

hailed /heɪld/

hallmark /ˈhɔːl.mɑːk/

hand /hænd/

handicap /ˈhændɪˌkæp/

hardship /ˈhɑːdʃɪp/

harm /hɑːm/

harvest /ˈhɑː.vɪst/

hepatomegaly /ˌhep.ə.toʊˈmeg.ə.li/

hereditary /həˈred.ɪ.tər.i/

hernia /ˈhɜː.nɪə/

herpangina /ˈhɜːpænˈdʒaɪ.nə/

herpetic /hɜːˈpetɪk/ **whitlow** /ˈwɪtləʊ/

Hib /ˈhɪb/ **Haemophilus** /hiːˈmɑː.fə.ləs/ **influenzae** /ˌɪnˌflʊˈen.zə/ **type B**

histiocytosis /ˈhɪstɪəˌsaɪtəʊ.sɪs/

histological /ˌhɪstəˈlɒdʒɪkᵊl/

Hodgkin /ˈhɒdʒkɪn/ **lymphoma** /lɪmˈfəʊ.mə/

holding /ˈhoʊl.dɪŋ/
homelessness /ˈhəʊm.ləs.nəs/
hostile /ˈhɒs.taɪl/
household /ˈhaʊs.həʊld/
hum /hʌm/
human /ˈhjuː.mən/ papilloma virus /ˌpa.pə.ˈləʊ.mə ˈvaɪə.rəs/
humidity /hjuːˈmɪd.ɪ.ti/
hydrops /haɪdrɒps/
hypernatremia /ˌhaɪ.pə.neɪ.ˈtriː.mi.ə/
hypertonia /ˌhaɪ.pə.ˈtəʊ.niə/
hyperventilation /ˌhaɪ.pə.ven.tɪˈleɪ.ʃən/
hypocalcaemia /ˌhaɪ.pəʊ.kælˈsiː.mi.ə/
hypocalcaemic/ˌhaɪ.pəʊ.ˌkal.ˈsiː.mik/
hypochromic /ˈhaɪpəˈkrəm.ɪk/
hypomagnesaemia /ˌhaɪ.pəʊ.ˌmæg.nəˈsiː.mi.ə/
hyponatraemia /ˌhaɪ.pɒ.nəˈtriː.mɪ.ə/
hyposplenism /ˈhaɪ.pəʊ ˈspliː.nɪzm/
hypoxic /haɪˈpɒk.sɪk/
imbalance /ˌɪmˈbæl.ənt s/
immaturity /ˌɪm.əˈtʃʊə.rɪ.ti/
immunosupressive /ˌimjʊnəʊ.səˈpresiv/
impact /ˈɪm.pækt/
imperative /ɪmˈper.ə.tɪv/
implication /ˌɪm.plɪˈkeɪ.ʃən/
impose /ɪmˈpəʊz/
impotence /ˈɪm.pə.təns/
in /ɪn/ particular /pəˈtɪk.jʊ.lər/
in situ /ɪn ˈsɪt.juː/
in spite of /spaɪt/
in utero /in.juːˈtər.əʊ/
inactive /ɪnˈæk.tɪv/
inadvertently /ˌɪn.ədˈvɜː.tənt.li/
incentive /ɪnˈsentɪv/
incidentally /ˌɪnsɪˈdentəlɪ/
incisor /ɪnˈsaɪ.zər/
inconsistent /ˌɪn.kənˈsɪs.tənt/
incorrect /ˌɪnkəˈrekt/
indentation /ˌɪn.denˈteɪ.ʃən/
inequality /ˌɪnɪˈkwɒlɪtɪ/
inevitable /ɪnˈevɪt.əbəl/
infective /ɪnˈfek.tɪv/
infested /ɪnˈfest.ɪd/
inflation /ɪnˈfleɪ.ʃən/
influence /ˈɪn.flʊ.əns/
infusion /ɪnˈfjuː.ʒən/
inguinal /ˈɪŋ.gwɪ.nəl/
inherit /ɪnˈherɪt/

inhibition /ˌɪn.hɪˈbɪʃ.ən/
inoculation /ɪˌnɒk.jʊˈleɪ.ʃən/
inotropes /inˈəʊ.trəʊps/
insect /ˈɪn.sekt/
insecurity /ˌɪn.sɪˈkjʊə.rɪ.ti/
insidious /ɪnˈsɪdɪəs/
insipid /ɪnˈsɪpɪd/
intensify /ɪnˈtensɪˌfaɪ/
intentionally /ɪnˈten.ʃən.əl.i/
interaction /ˌɪn.təˈræk.ʃən/
interferon /ˌɪntəˈfɪə.rɒn/
interstitial /ˌɪn.təˈstɪʃ.əl/
intraabdominal /ɪn.trə.æbˈdɒm.ɪ.nəl/
intracerebral /ˌɪn.trəˈser.ə.brəl/
intraosseous /ˌɪn.trəˈɒs.i.əs/
intravascular /ˌɪn.trəˈvæs.kjʊ.lər/
intravenously /ˌɪn.trəˈviː.nəs.li/
intrusive /ɪnˈtruː.sɪv/
invariably /ɪnˈveə.ri.ə.bli/
involvement /ɪnˈvɒlv.mənt/
irrational /ɪˈræʃ.ən.əl/
irritability /ˌɪr.ɪ.təˈbɪl.ɪ.ti/
ischaemia /ɪˈskiː.mi.ə/
issue /ˈɪʃ.uː/
itchy /ˈɪtʃ.i/
jaw-thrust /dʒɔː θrʌst/ **manoeuvre** /məˈnuː.vər/
jerk /dʒɜːk/
junction /ˈdʒʌŋk.ʃən/
justifiable /ˈdʒʌstɪˌfaɪəbəl/
Kawasaki disease /kɑːwəˈsɑːki dɪˌziːz/
keep /kiːp/ **awake** /əˈweɪk/
keratin /ˈker.ət.ɪn/
kernicterus /kɜːnˈɪk.tər.əs/
kidnapper /ˈkɪdnæpə/
kidney /ˈkɪd.ni/
Koplik spots /kopˈlik spots/
labour /ˈleɪ.bər/
lace /leɪs/
lactate /lækˈteɪt/
Langerhans cells /ˈlæŋəˌhæns/
large /ˌlɑːdʒ/ **bowel** /ˈbaʊ.əl/
lash /læʃ/ **out** /aʊt/
latency /ˈleɪ.tən.si/
laxative /ˈlæks.ə.tɪv/
lengthen /ˈleŋkθən/
leukomalacia /ˈljuː.kə.mə.ˈleɪ.ʃiː.ə/
lie /laɪ/

ligation /lɪˈɡeɪˌʃən/
limp /lɪmp/
load /ləʊd/
localize /ˈləʊ.kəl.aɪz/
loose /luːs/
lupus /ˈluː.pəs/
lupus /ˈluː.pəs/ **erythematosus** /ˌer.ə.ˌthiː.məˈtəʊ.səs/
Lyme's disease /ˈlaɪmz dɪˌziːz/
lymph /lɪmf/
lymphoblastic /ˌlɪm.fəʊˈblæs.tɪk/
lymphocyte /ˌlɪm.fəʊˈsaɪt/
lymphocytic /ˌlɪm.fəʊˈsit.ɪk/
macular /ˌmæk.jʊ.lər/
macule /ˈmækjuːl/
maculopapular /ˌmæk.jʊ.lə.pæp.ju.lər/
malacia /məˈleɪˌʃɪə/
malaise /mælˈeɪz/
malnutrition /ˌmæl.njuːˈtrɪ.ʃən/
management /ˈmæn.ɪdʒ.mənt/
manoeuvre /məˈnuː.vər/
mark /mɑːk/
mastitis /mæˈstaɪ.tɪs/
maturity /məˈtjʊə.rɪ.ti/
maxillary /mæk.sɪl.ə.ri/
meconium /mɪˈkəʊ.nɪ.əm/
mediastinum /ˌmiː.di.əˈstaɪn.əm/
mediator /ˈmiː.di.eɪ.tər/
medulla /meˌdʌl.ə/
menorrhagia /ˌmenɔːˈreɪ.dʒɪə/
metastasis /metˈæs.təs.ɪs/
metastatic /ˌmet.əˈstæt.ɪk/
microcephalus /ˌmai.krəʊˈse.fəl.əs/
microcytic /ˌmai.krəʊˈsɪt.ɪk/
microinfarction /ˌmaɪkrə.ɪnˈfɑːkˌʃən/
middle /ˌmɪd.l̩/
midforehead /ˈmɪd.ˈfɒrɪd/
midline /ˈmɪd.laɪn/
midshaft /ˈmɪd.ˈʃaft/
milium /ˈmi.li.əm/ pl **milia** /ˈmi.li.ə/
minder /ˈmaɪndə/
mnemonic /nɪˈmɒn.ɪk/
modality /məʊˈdælɪtɪ/
molluscum /mɒˈlʌskəm/
monospot /ˈmɒnəʊ.spɒt/
mucocutaneous /mjuːkəʊ.kjuːˈteɪn.ɪəs/
mucositis /mjuːˈkəʊ.saɪ.tɪs/
mucous membrane /ˌmjuː.kəsˈmem.breɪn/

muffin /ˈmʌf.ɪn/

multi /ˈmʌltɪ/

muscle /ˈmʌsəl/ **tone** /təʊn/

myalgia /maɪˈæl.dʒi.ə/

mycobacterium /ˌmai.kəʊ.bækˈtɪə.rɪəm/

myelodysplasia /ˌmaɪə.ləʊˈdɪsˈpleɪ.zɪə/

myocarditis /ˌmaɪ.əʊ.kɑːdˈaɪ.tɪs/

nag /næg/

nape /neɪp/

necessitate /nəˈses.ɪ.teɪt/

necrosis /ˈnek.rəʊ.sɪs/

negative /ˈneg.ə.tɪv/

neglect /nɪˈglekt/

negotiate /nɪˈgəʊʃɪˌeɪt/

neighbourhood /ˈneɪbəˌhʊd/

nephritis /nɪˈfraɪ.tɪs/

nephroblastoma /nɪˈfrəʊˌblæsˈtəʊ.mə/

nephrotic /nɪˈfrɒ.tɪk/

neuroma /njʊˈrəʊ.mə/

neurotoxic /ˌnjʊə.rəʊˈtɒk.sɪk/

neutropenia /njuːtrəˈpiːnɪə/

neutrophil /njuːtrə.fɪl/

nevus /ˈniː.vəs/ pl **nevi**

nightmare /ˈnaɪt.meər/

nonblanching /ˌnɒn.blɑːntʃ.ɪŋ/

non-judgemental /ˌnɒn.dʒʌdʒˈmen.təl/

nonpurulent /ˌnɒn.ˈpjʊə.rʊ.lənt/

nontuberculous /ˌnɒn.tjʊˌbɜːkjʊˈləs/

notable /ˈnəʊ.tə.bl̩/

notion /ˈnəʊʃən/

nurse /nɜːs/

nursery /ˈnɜːsrɪ/

nurture /ˈnɜːtʃə/

obstetrician /ˌɒb.stəˈtrɪʃ.ən/

obviously /ˈɒb.vi.əs.li/

oesophageal /iːˌsɒfəˈdʒiːəl/

oesophagus /ɪˈsɒf.ə.gəs/

oophoritis /ˌəʊvə.fəˈraɪ.tɪs/

oozing /uːz.ɪŋ/

opacity /əʊˈpæsɪtɪ/

opisthotonus /ˌɒpɪsθɒtə.nəs/

opposition /ˌɒpəˈzɪʃən/

optimize /ˈɒp.tɪ.maɪz/

orchitis /ˈɔː.kaɪ.tɪs/

orthodontist /ˌɔːθəˈdɒntɪst/

osteopenia /ˌɒstɪəʊˈpiːnə/

outbreak /ˈaʊtˌbreɪk/

outburst /ˈaʊt.bɜːst/
outcome /ˈaʊtˌkʌm/
outline /ˈaʊt.laɪn/
overt /əʊˈvɜːt/
overwhelm /ˌəʊ.vəˈwelm/
overwrought /ˌəʊvəˈrɔːt/
owing to /ˈəʊ.ɪŋ ˌtuː/
paediatrician /ˌpiː.dɪəˈtrɪ.ʃən/
pain-coping /peɪn.kəʊp.ɪŋ/
palate /ˈpæl.ət/
palatine /ˈpælə.tan/
palliative /ˈpæl.i.ə.tɪv/
palm /pɑːm/
palsy /ˈpɔːl.zi/
pancreatic /ˌpæŋ.krɪˈæ.tɪk/
panencephalitis /pænˌen.kef.əˈlaɪ.tɪs/
papule /ˈpæpjuːl/
paranasal /ˌpær.əˈneɪ.zəl/ sinus /saɪ.nəs/
parasomnia /ˌpar.əˈsɑːm.niː.ə/
paratesticular /ˈpɑːr.ə tesˈtɪk.jə.lər/
paratyphus /ˌpærəˈtaɪfəs/
paravertebral /ˈpɑːr.ə ˈvɜː.tɪ.brəl/
parenchymal /pəˈreŋ.kə.məl/
parental /pəˈren.təl/
parenteral /pəˈren.tə.rəl/
parenthood /ˈpeərənthʊd/
parenting /ˈpeərəntɪŋ/
parietal /pəˈraɪə.təl/
parotid /pəˈrɒt.ɪd/ gland /glænd/
participate /pɑːˈtɪs.ɪ.peɪt/
particularly /pəˈtɪk.jʊ.lə.li/
parvovirus /ˈpɑːr.vəʊ.ˌvaɪ.rəs/
patency /ˈpeɪ.tən.si/
pathogen /ˈpæθ.ə.dʒən/
pathognomonic /ˌpæθə.gnəˈmɒnɪk/
pearl /pɜːl/
pedestrian /pəˈdes.tri.ən
peel /piːl/
peer /pɪər/
performing /pəˈfɔːm.ɪŋ/
pericarditis /ˌper.ɪ.kɑːdˈaɪ.tɪs/
periosteum /ˌper.iˈɑs.ti.əm/
periventricular /ˌper.ɪ.venˈtrɪk.jə.lər/
permissive /pəˈmɪsɪv/
pernasal /ˈpər.ˈneɪ.zəl/
perpetuate /pəˈpetʃ.u.eɪt/
persecution /ˌpɜː.sɪˈkjuː.ʃən/

pertussis /pəˈtʌ.sɪs/
petechial /pɪˈtiːkɪ.əl/
pharyngitis /ˌfær.ɪnˈdʒaɪ.tɪs/
phobia /ˈfəʊ.bi.ə/
phosphate /ˈfɒs.feɪt/
physical /ˈfɪz.ɪ.kəl/
phytate /ˈfaɪ.ˌteɪt/
pick /pɪk/
pigment /ˈpɪɡmənt/
pilchard /ˈpɪltʃəd/
pilosebaceous /ˌpaɪ.ləʊ.siˈbeɪ.ʃəs/
pimple /ˈpɪm.pl̩/
pinpoint /ˈpɪn.pɔɪnt/
placental /pləˈsen.təl/ **abruption** /əˈbrʌp.ʃən/
platelet /ˈpleɪt.lət/
play /pleɪ/ **up** /ʌp/
plethoric /pləˈθɔːr.ik/
plot /plɒt/
pneumococcus /ˌnuː.məʊˈkɑː.kəs/ pl **pneumococci** /ˌnuː.məʊˈkɒkaɪ/
Pneumocystis /njuːməʊˈsɪstɪs/ **jiroveci** /dʒaɪ.rəʊ.viːˈsaɪ/ **(carinii)** /kæ.raɪ.niːaɪ/
pneumonitis /ˌnu.məˈnaɪ.tɪs/
polio /ˈpəʊ.li.əʊ/
porosis /ˈpɔːrəsɪs/
Port /pɔːt/ **wine** /waɪn/
postexposure /ˈpəʊst.ɪkˈspəʊ.ʒər/
postpone /pəʊstˈpəʊn/
potent /ˈpəʊ.tənt/
poverty /ˈpɒv.ə.ti/
powerful /ˈpaʊə.fəl/
precipitating /prɪˈsɪp.ɪ.teɪt.ɪŋ/
precipitously /prɪˈsɪp.ɪ.təs.li/
predicament /prɪˈdɪk.ə.mənt/
predict /prɪˈdɪkt/
predictor /prɪˈdɪk.tər/
predominate /prɪˈdɒm.ɪ.neɪt/
pregnancy /ˈpreg.nən.si/
prelabour /ˌpriː.ˈleɪ.bər/
premature /ˈprem.ə.tʃər/
preoccupation /priːˌɒkjʊˈpeɪʃən/
presenting /prɪˈzent.ɪŋ/ **part** /pɑːt/
preservation /ˌprez.əˈveɪ.ʃən/
pressure /ˈpreʃ.ər/
preventable /prɪˈven.tə.bl̩/
priapism /ˈpraɪ.əˌpɪz.əm/
privilege /ˈprɪvɪlɪdʒ/
process /ˈprəʊ.ses/
proficient /prəˈfɪʃənt/

profoundly /prəˈfaʊnd.li/

prognosis /prɒgˈnəʊ.sɪs/

prolong /prəˈlɒŋ/

prominent /ˈprɒm.ɪ.nənt/

prophylaxis /ˌprɒf.ɪˈlæk.sɪs/

proptosis /prɑːpˈtəʊ.səs/

protective /prəˈtek.tɪv/

proton /ˈprəʊtɒn/

punishment /ˈpʌn.ɪʃ.mənt/

purpose /ˈpɜː.pəs/

purposefully /ˈpɜːpəsfəlɪ/

purulent /ˈpjʊə.rʊ.lənt/

pustular /ˈpʌs.tjuː.l.ər/

pustule /ˈpʌstjuːl/

pyridoxine /ˌpir.əˈdɑːk.ˌsiːn/

radiant /ˈreɪ.di.ənt/

ranula /ˈran.jə.lə/

reactant /riˈæk.tənt/

reassurance /ˌriːəˈʃʊə.rəns/

recheck /ˌriːˈtʃek/

recollection /ˌrekəˈlekʃən/

reconstitute /ˌriːˈkɒn.stɪ.tjuːt/

recurrent /rɪˈkʌrənt/

reduction /rɪˈdʌk.ʃən/

reference /ˈref.ər.ənt s/

refugee /ˌrefjʊˈdʒiː/

regular /ˈreg.jʊ.lər/

relationship /rɪˈleɪ.ʃən.ʃɪp/

release /rəˈliːs/

rely /rɪˈlaɪ/ **on** /ɒn/

remarkably /rɪˈmɑːkəblɪ/

remission /rɪˈmɪʃ.ən/

renitis /rɪˈnaɪ tɪs /

replacement /rɪˈpleɪs.mənt/

rescue /ˈreskjuː/

resectability /rɪˌsektəˈbɪlɪtɪ/

resentful /rɪˈzentfə/

resilience /rɪˈzɪlɪəns/

resolve /rɪˈzɒlv/

resorption /ˌriːˈsɔːrp.ʃən/

restraint /rɪˈstreɪnt/

retardation /ˌriː.tɑːˈdeɪ.ʃən/

reticuloendothelial /rɪˈtɪkjʊlə ˌendəʊˈθiːlɪəl/

retina /ˈret.ə.nə

retinitis /ˌre.təˈnaɪ.təs/

retraining /ˌriːˈtreɪn.ɪŋ/

retroperitoneal /ˌret.rə ˌper.ɪ.təˈni.əl/

reversal /rɪˈvɜː.səl/
reward /rɪˈwɔːd/
rheumatic /ruːˈmætɪk/
rhythmic /ˈrɪðmɪk/
road /rəʊd/ **traffic** /ˈtræf.ɪk/
rotavirus /ˈrəʊtəˌvaɪrəs/
rural /ˈrʊərəl/
salmonella /ˌsæl.məˈnel.ə/ pl **salmonellae**
sarcoidosis /ˌsɑr.kɔɪˈdoʊ.sɪs/
sarcoma /sɑːˈkəʊ.mə/
scratch /skrætʃ/
scrotum /ˈskrəʊ.təm/
sebaceous /sɪˈbeɪʃəs/
seborrheic /ˌsebərˈriː.ɪk/
seborrhoea /sɪˈb.əˈri.ə/
secretory /ˈsek.rə.tər.i/
security /sɪˈkjʊə.rɪ.ti/
seek /siːk/ **(sought, sought)**
seemingly /ˈsiː.mɪŋ.li/
selective /sɪˈlek.tɪv/
self-autonomy /ˌself.ɔːˈtɒn.ə.mi/
self-confidence /ˌself ˈkɒn.fɪ.dəns/
self-limiting /self.ˈlɪm.ɪ.tɪŋ/
self-resolving /ˌself rɪˈzɒlv.ɪŋ/
self-worth /ˌselfˈwɜːθ/
sensible /ˈsensɪbəl/
separate /ˈsep.ər.ət/
septum /ˈsep.təm/
sequestration /ˌsiː.kwesˈtreɪ.ʃən/
seroconversion /sɪˈrɒ.kənˈvɜː.ʃən/
settle /ˈsetəl/ **back** /bæk/
shape /ʃeɪp/
shelter /ˈʃel.tər/
shoulder /ˈʃəʊl.dər/
shout /ʃaʊt/ **at** /ət/
shouting /ˈʃaʊ.tɪŋ/
shunt /ʃʌnt/
sibling /ˈsɪb.lɪŋ/
side /saɪd/ **effect** /ɪˈfekt/
silence /ˈsaɪ.ləns/
single-parent /ˈsɪŋgəl ˈpeə.rənt/
sinus /ˈsaɪ.nəs/ pl **sinuses**
sinusitis /ˌsaɪ.nəˈsaɪ.tɪs/
sleepwalk /ˈsliːpˌwɔːk/
smack /smæk/
small /smɔːl/ **bowel** /ˈbaʊ.əl/
smallpox /ˈsmɔːl.pɒks/

snap /snæp/
sniffing /ˈsnɪf.ɪŋ/
soft /sɒft/ **palate** /ˈpæl.ət/
softener /ˈsɒfənə/
sole /səʊl/
somatization /səʊˈmæ.taɪ.zeɪˈʃən/
species /ˈspiː.ʃiːz/
specific /spəˈsɪf.ɪk/
spectroscopy /ˈspektrəˌskə.pɪ/
speech /spiːtʃ/ **therapist** /ˈθer.ə.pɪst/
spherocytosis /ˌsfɪərəʊsaɪˈtəʊsɪs/
spite /spaɪt/
spleen /spliːn/
splenectomy /spləˈnek.tə.mi/
spread /spred/
squeak /skwiːk/
stain /steɪn/
steal /stiːl/
strawberry /ˈstrɔː.bər.i/
subaponeurotic / ˌsəb.ˌap.ə.ˌnjʊə.rəʊ.tɪk/
subclinical /sʌbˈklɪn.ɪ.kəl/
subconjunctival /ˌsʌbˌkɒn.dʒaŋkˈtɪ.vəl/
subcutaneously /ˌsʌb.kjʊˈteɪ.ni.əs.li/
sublingually /ˌsʌbˈlɪŋ.gwəli/
submucous /ˌsʌb.ˈmjuː.kəs/
suboccipital /ˌsʌb.ɒkˈsɪp.ɪ.təl/
subsequent /ˈsʌb.sɪ.kwənt/
substandard /sʌbˈstændəd/
succedaneum /sʌkse.deɪniː.um/
suicide /ˈsuː.ɪ.saɪd/
sultana /sʌlˈtɑː.nə/
support /səˈpɔːt/
supportive /səˈpɔː.tɪv/
suppress /səˈpres/
suppression /səˈpreʃən/
surfactant /sərˈfakˈtənt/
surrender /səˈrendə/
surrogate /ˈsʌr.ə.gət/
survive /səˈvaɪv/
swelling /ˈswel.ɪŋ/
syncitial virus /sin.ˈsiˌʃiː.əl ˈvaɪ.rəs/
syphilis /ˈsɪf.ɪ.lɪs/
tag /tæg/
take /ˈteɪk/ **a history** /ˈhɪs.tər.i/
tangible /ˈtæn.dʒə.bl̩/
tannin /ˈtæn.ɪn/
tantrum /ˈtæntrəm/

tearful /ˈtɪə.fəl/

teenage /ˈtiːnˌeɪdʒ/

temptation /tempˈteɪʃən/

tense /tens/

term /tɜːm/ **infant** /ˈɪn.fənt/

tetanus /ˈtet.ən.əs/

thick /θɪk/

threat /θret/

threaten /ˈθret.ən/

threshold /ˈθreʃ.h əʊld/

throat /θrəʊt/

thrombocytopenia /ˌθrɒm.bəʊ.saɪt.əˈpiː.ni.ə/

thrombocytopenic /ˌθrɒm.bəʊ.saɪt.əˈpiː.nik/

tick /tɪk/

tied /taɪd/

tilt /tɪlt/

time /taɪm/ **out** /aʊt/

Tourette syndrome /tʊəˈrets ˌsɪn.drəʊm/

toxocariasis /ˌtɒks əkəˈraɪə.sɪs/

toxoplasma gondii /tokˈsəʊ.plazˈmæ gonˈdiːaɪ/

trace /treɪs/

tracheooesophageal /ˈtreɪkɪəʊˈiːˌsɒfəˈdʒiːəl/

truancy /ˈtruːənsɪ/

tuberculin /tjuːˈbɔː.kjə.lɪn/

tuck /tʌk/ **up** /ʌp/

tuft /tʌft/

typhus /ˈtaɪfəs/

ulceration /ˌʌl.sərˈeɪ.ʃən/

ulcerative /ˈʌl.sər.ə.tɪv/ **colitis** /kəʊ ˈlaɪ.təs/

ultimately /ˈʌl.tɪ.mət.li/

umbilical /ʌmˈbɪl.ɪ.kəl/

unconjugated /ˈkɒn.dʒə.geɪt.ɪd/

underachievement /ʌn.də.rəˈtʃiː.v.mənt/

underestimate /ˌʌn.dəˈres.tɪ.meɪt/

undermine /ˌʌndəˈmaɪn/

underpin /ˌʌndəˈpɪn/

undertake /ˌʌn.dəˈteɪk/

undue /ʌnˈdjuː/

unexpected /ˌʌn.ɪkˈspek.tɪd/

unpredictable /ˌʌn.prɪˈdɪk.tə.bl̩/

unreasonable /ʌnˈriː.zən.ə.bl̩/

unresponsive /ˌʌn.rɪˈspɒnt .sɪv/

unrest /ʌnˈrest/

unsuccessful /ˌʌn.səkˈses.fəl/

unsuitable /ʌnˈsuː.təbəl/

unsuspected /ʌnˈsə.ˈspekt.ɪd/

unusually /ʌnˈjuːʒʊəl.i/

update /ʌpˈdeɪt/
uproot /ʌpˈruːt/
upsetting /ʌpˈsetɪŋ/
uptake /ˈʌp.teɪk/
urethral /jʊəˈriː.θrəl/
urticaria /ˌɔː.tɪˈkeə.ri.ə/
uterus /ˈjuː.tər.əs/ pl **uteri**
valve /vælv/
variation /ˌveə.riˈeɪ.ʃən/
varicella /ˌvær.ɪˈsel.ə/ **zoster** /zɒ.stər/
vaso occlusion / veɪˈzəʊ.əˈkluː.ʒən/
vector /ˈvek.tər/
vehicle /ˈviː.ɪ.kl/
venous /ˈviː.nəs/
ventouse /ven.tuːˈs/
verbalize /ˈvɜːbəˌlaɪz/
vertebra /ˈvɜː.tɪ.brə/ pl **vertebrae** /ˈvər.təˌbreɪ/
vesicular /veˈsɪk.jʊlə/
vigilance /ˈvɪdʒ.ɪ.ləns/
vigorous /ˈvɪg.ər.əs/
violence /ˈvaɪə.ləns/
viraemic /vaɪˈri.mik/
von Willebrand disease (vWD) /fɒn wɪlˈə.brænd dɪˈziːz/
wealth /welθ/
well-being /ˌwelˈbiː.ɪŋ/
wholemeal /ˈhəʊlˌmiːl/

Recent onset of problem; Chronic fatigue syndrome;
Drug misuse; Dermatological disorders; Atopic eczema
(atopic dermatitis); Infections and infestations

Text 1
Recent onset of problem

- Preoccupations (parental divorce, bullying, etc.)
- Fatigue
- Depression
- Rebellion against teacher, parents, or 'swot' label
- Unsuspected poor attendance at school
- Sexual abuse
- Drug abuse
- Prodromal period of a psychotic illness (rare)
- Degenerative brain condition, rare but important

Problems of adolescence

Although a popular image of adolescence is one of angry, rebellious teenagers, alienated their parents and embroiled in emotional turmoil, studies show that most adolescents maintain good relationship with their parents. Minor psychological symptoms such as moodiness or social sensitivity are quite common, but serious psychiatric problems are no more prevalent than in adult life. Family relationships are often influenced by teenagers' negotiation of their own autonomy.

Formal operational thought

- The ability to form abstract thoughts
- Comparing implications of hypotheses
- Thinking about one's own thinking
- Testing the logic that links propositions
- Manipulating interactive abstract concepts

Anorexia nervosa and other eating disorders

Dieting to slim is endemic among teenage girls. Part of the reason for this is the contemporary equation between thinness and attractiveness. In some girls, however, the slimming process takes over, typically with a phobic horror of normal body weight and shape. This is anorexia nervosa, and the features are:

- self-induced weight loss
- a distorted perception of her body
- a determined attempt to lose weight or avoid weight gain, by either restricting food intake, self-induced vomiting, laxative abuse, excessive exercising or using a combination of these methods
- when body weight falls below a critical point, pubertal development is halted, and menstruation ceases
- the discovery by a girl that through self-starvation she can control her shape and development increases her sense of self-worth and self-effectiveness
- pre-occupations and dreams of food and cooking come to dominate mental life
- there ensues a tremendous mental struggle not to give in and eat
- the dramatic and visible effects of self-starvation on the girl can unite some parents in caring for their daughter and safe a discordant marriage from divorce.

An affected person will often deny hunger, reassure everyone that she is in the peak of health, exercise to lose weight and disagree frequently that she is too thin. She will conceal her poor eating by secretly disposing of her meals or lying about her weight. She will show obsessional, perfectionist character traits. As a result of starvation, her body develops a low metabolic rate with slow-to-relax tendon reflexes, reduced peripheral circulation, bradycardia and amenorrhoea. Fine lanugo hair appears over her trunk and limbs. Plasma proteins are sometimes low and ankle oedema is not uncommon. Some discover that self-restraint in carbohydrate intake can be bypassed by self-induced vomiting following repeated bouts of overeating. And that further weight loss can be achieved by diuretics and laxatives. This can cause wide fluctuations in weight and metabolic abnormalities such as hypokalaemia and alkalosis. This condition is bulimia which can occur at normal body weight or in association with low body weight.

Management

The initial management of anorexia nervosa is to restore near-normal body weight by refeeding. The emergence of physical complications may necessitate admission to hospital. The cornerstone of treatment is family therapy.

Medical aspects

Anorexia has a high mortality rate compared with other psychiatric disorders. Some of the excess mortality arise from medical complications such as malnutrition, electrolyte imbalance and infection. 'Refeeding syndrome', the metabolic abnormalities on reinstituting nutrition, can be life-threatening, but is manageable if standard guidelines are followed. In addition to medical complications, the next important cause of mortality is suicide. Eating disorders have become a major problem in adolescent girls.

Exercise 1
Answer the following questions. Prepare short talks and/or dialogues on these topics

1. Characterize problems of adolescence.
2. Describe anorexia nervosa and other eating disorders (management, medical aspects).

Translation 1

1. Most adolescents maintain good relationship with their parents. 2. Minor psychological symptoms such as moodiness or social sensitivity are quite common, but serious psychiatric problems are no more prevalent than in adult life. 3. In some girls, however, the slimming process takes over, typically with a phobic horror of normal body weight and shape. 4. The features of anorexia nervosa are: self-induced weight loss, self-induced vomiting, laxative abuse, excessive exercising. 5. When body weight falls below a critical point, pubertal development is halted, and menstruation ceases. 6. Pre-occupations and dreams of food and cooking come to dominate mental life. 7. An affected person will often deny hunger, she will conceal her poor eating by secretly disposing of her meals or lying about her weight.

Exercise 2
Fill in the missing words. Choose the correct ones.

1. As a result of _____, her body develops a low _____ _____ with slow-to-relax tendon reflexes, reduced, _____ _____ bradycardia and amenorrhoea.	a peripheral circulation b metabolic rate c starvation
2. Some discover that self-restraint in _____ _____ can be bypassed by _____-_____ vomiting following repeated _____ ___ overeating.	a bouts of b self-induced c carbohydrate intake

3. This condition is _____ which can occur at normal _____ _____ or in _____ with low body weight.	a association b body weight c bulimia
4. The _____ _____ of anorexia nervosa is to _____ near-normal body weight by _____.	a refeeding b restore c initial management
5. _____ has a high _____ _____ compared with other _____ disorders.	a psychiatric b Anorexia c mortality rate
6. Some of the excess mortality arise from _____ _____ such as _____, _____ _____ and infection.	a electrolyte imbalance b malnutrition c medical complications
7. The metabolic abnormalities on _____ nutrition, can be life-threatening (_____ _____), but is _____ if standard guidelines are followed.	a ‚refeeding syndrome' b manageable c reinstituting
8. ___ _____ to medical complications, the next _____ _____ of mortality is _____.	a important cause b suicide c In addition

Text 2
Chronic fatigue syndrome

Chronic fatigue syndrome refers to persisting high levels of subjective fatigue, leading to rapid exhaustion on minimal physical or mental exertion. Some cases have no history or evidence of a precipitating infection. Myalgia, migratory arthralgia, headache, difficulty getting off to sleep, poor concentration and irritability are virtually universal. Stomach pains, scalp tenderness, eye pain and photophobia, and tender cervical lymphadenopathy are frequently encountered. Depressive symptoms are common. The majority of cases will remit spontaneously with time, but this takes months or sometimes years. The recommended treatment involves graded exercise therapy and/or cognitive behavioural therapy. If too much pressure is put upon the child, tantrums or mute withdrawal can occur. The parents and the child need continuing support to maintain as much of a normal life as possible.

Depression

Depression as a clinical condition is more than sadness and misery; it extends to affect motivation, judgement, the ability to experience pleasure and provokes emotions of guilt and despair. It may disturb sleep, appetite and weight. It leads to social withdrawal. Teenagers will, out of loyalty, often pretend to their parents that things are all right if interviewed in their presence. It is necessary to ask specifically about suicidal ideas and plans. Many will recover spontaneously. Alternatively, the child could be offered non-directive supportive therapy or guided self-help. If mild depression does not respond to these measures in 2-3 months, the child should be referred to specialist mental health services. Children with moderate and severe depression should be referred to specialist mental health services for more specific psychological intervention such as cognitive behavioural therapy, family therapy, or interpersonal therapy.

Features of depression in adolescents
More common than adults

- Apathy, boredom and an inability to enjoy oneself rather than depressed mood
- Separation anxiety which reappears, having resolved in earlier life
- Decline in school performance
- Social withdrawal
- Hypochondriacal ideas and complaints of pain in chest, abdomen, and head
- Irritable mood or frankly antisocial behaviour

Less common than adults

- Loss of appetite
- Loss of sleep
- Loss of libido
- Slowing of thought and movement
- Delusional ideas

Deliberate self-harm

Young people deliberately cause themselves harm for multiple reasons and in multiple ways. Self-harm is common and is increasing. Many adolescents do not present to healthcare professions actively, therefore no assessment of an adolescent with emotional or behavioural difficulties is complete without screening for self-harm. Common methods of self-harm include cutting, burning, biting, bruising, or tying ligatures around the neck. Punching of walls should also be considered self-harm. The patient wearing long sleeves, reluctant to show their skin, should raise concern.

How to ask about self-harm:
This involves:
- a history taken with the young person alone
- creating a safe environment
- allowing sufficient time
- setting rules about confidentiality clearly
- validating the young person's distress
- giving assurance that they will be supported
- asking questions directly, but sensitively

Exercise 3
Answer the following questions. Prepare short talks and/or dialogues on these topics

1. What is meant by chronic fatigue syndrome?
2. What are features of depression in adolescents?
3. What do you know about deliberate self-harm?

Translation 2

1. Chronic fatigue syndrome refers to persisting high levels of subjective fatigue, leading to rapid exhaustion on minimal physical or mental exertion. 2. Myalgia, migratory arthralgia, headache, difficulty getting off to sleep, poor concentration and irritability are virtually universal. 3. Stomach pains, scalp tenderness, eye pain and photophobia, and tender cervical lymphadenopathy are frequently encountered. 4. The majority of cases will remit spontaneously with time, but this takes months or sometimes years. 5. The recommended treatment involves graded exercise therapy and/or cognitive behavioural therapy. 6. Depression as a clinical condition is more than sadness and misery; it extends to affect motivation, judgement, the ability to experience pleasure and provokes emotions of guilt and despair. 7. It may disturb sleep, appetite and weight and it leads to social withdrawal. 8. It is necessary to ask specifically about suicidal ideas and plans. 9. Children with moderate and severe depression should be referred to specialist mental health services for more specific psychological intervention such as cognitive behavioural therapy, family therapy, or interpersonal therapy. 10. Features

of depression in adolescents are: apathy, boredom, separation anxiety, social withdrawal, hypochondriacal complaints, irritable mood, slowing of thought and movement, and delusional ideas. 11. Young people deliberately cause themselves harm for multiple reasons and in multiple ways. 12. Common methods of self-harm include cutting, burning, biting, bruising, or tying ligatures around the neck. 13. The patient wearing long sleeves, reluctant to show their skin, should raise concern.

Text 3
Drug misuse

Most teenagers are exposed to illicit drugs at some stage. A number will then experiment with them, some becoming habitual users. A very small number become dependent, psychologically or physically. What is taken varies with culture and opportunity, but alcohol and cannabis are common; solvents, LSD, ecstasy, and amphetamine derivatives somewhat less so; and cocaine or heroin currently least prevalent. Abuse implies heavy misuse. The signs vary with the agent but may include:

- intoxication
- unexplained absences from home or school
- mixing with known users
- high rates of spending or stealing money
- possession of the equipment required for drug use
- medical complications associated with use.

An assessment will involve interviewing the adolescent, possibly combined with taking a urine sample for drug screening. Medical involvement is predominantly focused on users who have other psychopathology or with the physical consequences of intoxication or injection when these threaten health. Solvent abuse (mainly glue and aerosol sniffing) is quite widespread as group activity of young adolescents. It can occasionally give rise to cardiac dysrhythmias, bone marrow suppression or renal failure, and any of these can cause death, as may a fall or road traffic accident when intoxicated. Cannabis and LSD use may trigger anxiety or psychotic disorders. Ecstasy taken at dances or raves can cause dangerous hyperthermia, dehydration and death. 'Legal Highs' are of increasing concern to clinicians. These include chemical substances which produce similar effects to illegal drugs (e.g. cocaine, cannabis, ecstasy). They can have depressant or stimulant, including hallucinogenic properties. They are easily purchased online, often labelled as incense or salts.

Psychosis

Psychosis is a breakdown in the perception and understanding of reality and a lack of awareness that the person is unwell. This can affect ideas and beliefs, and lead to odd behaviour. Speech is hard to follow, leading to thought disorder. Perceptual abnormalities lead to hallucinations. Psychotic disorders include:

- Schizophrenia — there is generally no major disturbance of mood other than blunting or flattening of affect.
- Bipolar affective disorder, where the psychosis is associated with lowered mood as in depression or elevation in mood as in mania.
- Organic psychosis occurs in delirium, substance — induced disorders and dementia.

Both schizophrenia and bipolar affective disorder increase in frequency of presentation during adolescence. Investigations should include a urine drug screen, exclusion of medication — induced psychosis, exclusion of medical causes (i.e. infection, seizures, thyroid abnormalities and sleep disorders) and dementia. Urgent referral to a psychiatrist is needed for comprehensive assessment and treatment with antipsychotic medication, psycho-education, family therapy and individual therapy. Psychosis may be precipitated by or be a consequence of substance abuse.

Management of emotional and behavioural problems

In general, the management of children's emotional and behavioural problems:

- should be psychological rather than pharmacological
- does not need the child to be admitted to hospital (unless required as a place of safety for suicidal children or for child protection)
- involves parents as key participants
- may involve a variety of health and social service professional

Main psychological treatment interventions employed for emotional and behavioural problems
Explanation and formulation

Suitable for mild problems with a good prognosis

Counselling of a child or parents

Used to provide non-directive supporting therapy to aid coping with difficulties (e.g. bereavement counselling).

Parenting groups

Parenting groups have become popular. Parents are given techniques on how to play with their children and respond effectively to their challenging behaviour.

Behavioural therapy

It is particularly effective in the management of behavioural problems in young children.

Family therapy

It uses a series of interviews with the entire household to alter dysfunctional patterns of relationships between family members.

Cognitive therapy

Used by specialists to explore the way thinking affects feelings and behaviour. It helps the young person to identify and challenge unhelpful thinking styles that perpetuate negative feelings and behaviour.

Individual or group dynamic psychotherapy

Counselling, which can help children who have relationship difficulties with a parent. Once the mainstay of child psychiatry, it is now less commonly used.

Exercise 4
Answer the following questions. Prepare short talks and/or dialogues on these topics

1. What do you know about drug misuse?
2. Characterize psychosis.
3. How to manage emotional and behavioural problems?
4. Speak about main psychological treatment interventions (counselling, parenting groups, behavioural therapy, family therapy, cognitive therapy).

Translation 3

1. Most teenagers are exposed to illicit drugs at some stage and a number will then experiment with them, some becoming habitual users. 2. Alcohol and cannabis are common; solvents, LSD, ecstasy, and amphetamine derivatives somewhat less so; and cocaine or heroin currently least prevalent. 3. An assessment will involve interviewing the adolescent, possibly combined with taking a urine sample for drug screening. 4. Solvent abuse (mainly

glue and aerosol sniffing) is quite widespread as group activity of young adolescents. 5. It can occasionally give rise to cardiac dysrhythmias, bone marrow suppression or renal failure. 6. Cannabis and LSD use may trigger anxiety or psychotic disorders. 7. Ecstasy taken at dances or raves can cause dangerous hyperthermia, dehydration and death. 8. 'Legal Highs' include chemical substances which produce similar effects to illegal drugs. 9. They are easily purchased online, often labelled as incense or salts. 10. Psychosis is a breakdown in the perception and understanding of reality and a lack of awareness that the person is unwell.

Exercise 5
Match the column A with the column B. Try to learn the expressions and/or sentences by heart.

A
1. Psychotic disorders include: ...
2. Organic psychosis occurs in ...
3. Investigations should include a urine drug screen, ...
4. In general, the management of children's emotional and behavioural problems: ...
5. Behavioural therapy is particularly effective ...
6. Family therapy uses a series of interviews with the entire household ...
7. Cognitive therapy is used by specialists to explore ...

B
a. ... *exclusion of medication-induced psychosis, exclusion of medical causes (i.e. infection, seizures, thyroid abnormalities and sleep disorders) and dementia.*
b. ... *schizophrenia and bipolar affective disorder.*
c. ... *to alter dysfunctional patterns of relationships between family members.*
d. ... *delirium, substance-induced disorders and dementia.*
e. ... *the way thinking affects feelings and behaviour.*
f. ... *should be psychological, does not need the child to be admitted to hospital, involves parents.*
g. ... *in the management of behavioural problems in young children.*

Exercise 6
Study the following summary and then interpret basic information in English.

1. Anorexia nervosa
Female: male ration is 10:1.
Peak age of onset — 14 years.
Affected girls have a distorted body image, so seldom agree that they are too thin and may deceive everyone by pretending to eat.
Features include: efforts to lose weight, arrest of puberty, cessation of periods.
May be accompanied by bulimia — overeating followed by self-induced vomiting
Management is family therapy and individual therapy to restore body weight.
Some require hospitalization; prognosis is variable, but has a mortality from suicide, malnutrition and infection.
2. In chronic fatigue syndrome
There is exhaustion on minimal exertion.
There is thought to be a combination of physical and psychological factors.
Management is with graded exercise and/or cognitive behavioural therapy, but recovery may take months or years.

Text 4
Dermatological disorders

Features of dermatological disorders in children are:

- in the newborn, transient skin disorders are common but need to be distinguished from serious or permanent conditions
- atopic eczema affects up to 20% of children
- skin infections and infestations, especially viral warts and head lice, are common in school aged children,
- acne is troublesome for many during adolescence

The newborn

The skin at birth is covered with a chalky-white greasy coat — the vernix caseosa. In the preterm infant, the skin is thin, poorly keratinized, and trans epidermal water loss is markedly increased. Thermoregulation is also impaired as the preterm infant lacks subcutaneous fat and is unable to sweat.

Morphology of skin lesions
Primary skin lesions (arise de novo in the skin)

Lesion	Description	Example
Macule	A small flat area of altered colour or texture	Freckles, measles, rubella, roseola, café-au-lait macule of tuberous sclerosis
Patch	Larger flat area of altered colour or texture	Depigmented patch of vitiligo
Pustule	A small raised lesion	Allergic, inflammatory papules of acne
Maculopapular	Combination of macules and papules	Measles, scarlet fever, parvovirus B19 (erythema infectiosum, fifth disease)
Plaque	A larger raised lesion	Scaly plaque of psoriasis
Nodule	A larger raised lesion with a deeper component (involvement of the dermis or subcutaneous fat)	Nodular lesion of erythema nodosum
Vesicle	A small clear blister	Varicella
Bulla	A large clear blister	Skin trauma, bullous impetigo
Wheal/weal	A transient raised lesion due to dermal oedema	Urticaria (hives)
Pustule	A pus-containing blister	Acute paronychia
Purpura	Bleeding into skin or mucosa. Small areas are petechiae, whereas large areas are ecchymoses. Do not blanch on pressure.	Meningococcal septicaemia. Henoch-Schönlein purpura, immune thrombocytopenia, disseminated intravascular coagulation (DIC)

Secondary skin lesions (evolve from primary lesions or from scratching of primary lesions by the patient)

Lesion	Description	Example
Excoriation	Scratch mark, loss of epidermis following trauma	Atopic dermatitis (from acute rubbing)
Lichenification	Roughening of skin with accentuation of skin markings	Atopic dermatitis (chronic rubbing)
Scales	Flakes of dead skin	Cradle cap seborrheic dermatitis

Crust	Dry mass of exudates consisting of serum, dried blood, scales, and pus	Impetigo
Scar	Formation of new fibrous tissue post wound healing	Acne
Erosion	Loss of epidermis and dermis (heals with scarring)	Epidermolysis bullosa
Ulcer	Loss of epidermis and dermis (heals with scarring)	Ulcerating haemangioma

Rashes of infancy
Nappy rashes

Nappy rashes are common. Mild cases respond to the use of a protective emollient, whereas more severe cases may require mild topical corticosteroids. Leaving the child without a napkin will accelerate resolution.

Common causes of nappy rashes
- Irritant (contact) dermatitis
- Infantile seborrheic dermatitis
- Candida infection
- Atopic eczema

Infantile seborrheic dermatitis

It starts on the scalp as an erythematous scaly eruption. The scales form a thick yellow adherent layer, commonly called cradle cap. The scaly rash may spread to the face, behind the ears, and then extend to the flexures and napkin area. It is not itchy, however, it is associated with an increased risk of subsequently developing atopic eczema. Mild cases will resolve with emollients. The scales on the scalp can be cleared with an ointment applied to the scalp daily for a few hours and then washed off. Widespread body eruption will clear with a mild topical corticosteroid, either alone or mixed with an antibacterial and antifungal agent.

Some itchy rashes
- Atopic eczema
- Chickenpox
- Urticaria/allergic reactions
- Contact dermatitis
- Insect bites
- Scabies
- Fungal infections
- Pityriasis rosea

Exercise 7
Answer the following questions. Prepare short talks and/or dialogues on these topics

1. What are features of dermatological disorders in children?
2. Describe morphology of skin lesions in the newborn.
3. Give examples of primary skin lesions (macule, patch, pustule, maculopapular, plaque, nodule, vesicle, bulla, wheal/weal, pustule, purpura)
4. Give examples of secondary skin lesions (excoriation, lichenification, scales, crust, scar, erosion, ulcer).
5. What can you say about nappy rashes?
6. What is meant by infantile seborrheic dermatitis?

Translation 4

1. Features of dermatological disorders in children are: atopic eczema, viral warts and head lice, and acne. 2. The skin at birth is covered with a chalky-white greasy coat – the vernix caseosa. 3. In the preterm infant, the skin is thin, poorly keratinized, and trans epidermal water loss is markedly increased. 4. Primary skin lesions include: a small flat area of altered colour or texture, larger flat area of altered colour or texture, a small raised lesion, combination of macules and papules, a larger raised lesion, a larger raised lesion with a deeper component, a small clear blister, a large clear blister, a transient raised lesion due to dermal oedema, a pus containing blister, bleeding into skin or mucosa. 5. Small areas are petechiae, whereas large areas are ecchymoses. 6. Secondary skin lesions include: scratch mark, loss of epidermis following trauma, roughening of skin with accentuation of skin markings, flakes of dead skin, dry mass of exudates consisting of serum, dried blood, scales, and pus, formation of new fibrous tissue post wound healing, loss of epidermis and dermis. 7. Mild cases of nappy rashes respond to the use of a protective emollient, whereas more severe cases may require mild topical corticosteroids. 8. Infantile seborrheic dermatitis starts on the scalp as an erythematous scaly eruption. 9. The scaly rash may spread to the face, behind the ears, and then extend to the flexures and napkin area. 10. The scales on the scalp can be cleared with an ointment applied to the scalp daily for a few hours and then washed off. 11. Some itchy rashes are: atopic eczema, chickenpox, urticaria/allergic reactions, contact dermatitis, insect bites, scabies, fungal infections, Pityriasis rosea.

Text 5
Atopic eczema (atopic dermatitis)

Onset of atopic eczema is usually in the first year of life. There is often a family history of atopic disorders: eczema, asthma, allergic rhinitis (hay fever). Exclusive breast-feeding may delay the onset of eczema but does not appear to have a significant impact on the prevalence of eczema during later childhood. In atopic eczema, itching (pruritus) is the main symptom at all ages and this results in scratching and exacerbation of the rash. The excoriated areas become erythematous, weeping, and crusted.

Distribution of atopic eczema

The distribution of eczema tends to change with age. In infants, the face and scalp are prominently affected, although the trunk may be involved. In older children, the skin flexures (cubital and popliteal fossae), and frictional areas, such as the neck, wrists, and ankles are characteristically involved.

Causes of exacerbation of eczema
- Bacterial infection, e.g. Staphylococcus, Streptococcus spp.
- Viral infection, e.g. herpes simplex virus
- Ingestion of an allergen, e.g. egg
- Contact with an irritant or allergen
- Environment: heat, humidity
- Change or reduction in medication
- Psychological stress
- Unexplained

Management

It is advisable to avoid soap and biological detergents. Clothing next to the skin should be of pure cotton, avoiding nylon and pure woollen garments. Nails need to be cut short to reduce skin damage from scratching, and mittens at night may be helpful in the very young.

Emollients

These are mainstay of management, moisturizing and softening the skin. They should be applied liberally two or more times a day and after the bath. Ointments are preferable to creams when the skin is very dry. A daily or alternate day bath using emollient oil as a soap substitute is also beneficial.

Occlusive bandages

These are helpful over limbs when scratching and lichenification are a problem. They may be impregnated with zinc paste or zinc and tar paste.

The bandages are worn overnight for 2-3 days, until the skin has improved. For widespread itching in young children, short-term use of wet stockinette wraps may be helpful. Antibiotics with hydrocortisone can be applied topically for mildly infected eczema.

Dietary elimination

Food allergy may be suspected if the child reacts consistently to a food, or in infants and young children with moderate or severe atopic eczema, particularly if associated with gut dysmotility (colic, vomiting, altered bowel habit) or faltering growth. The most common food allergens resulting in eczema are egg and cow's milk. Dietary elimination should be carried out with the advice of a dietician to ensure that the diet remains nutritionally adequate.

Check
- Any evidence of infection — bacterial or herpes simplex virus?
- Problems from other allergic disorders?
- Is growth normal?

Management

Avoiding soap, frequently using emollients?
Avoiding nylon and wool clothes?
Is there a need to give or change medications?
- Topical corticosteroids
- Immunomodulators
- Occlusive bandages
- Antibiotics or antiviral agents
- Antihistamines

Allergy test to egg and other foods?
Dietician supervision?
Need for psychological support?

Exercise 8
Answer the following questions. Prepare short talks and/or dialogues on these topics

1. What can you say about atopic eczema (distribution, causes of exacerbation of atopic eczema, and management)?
2. Speak about emollients, and occlusive bandages.
3. What is meant by dietary elimination?

4. Characterize management of atopic eczema.

Translation 5

1. Onset of atopic eczema is usually in the first year of life. 2. There is often a family history of atopic disorders: eczema, asthma, allergic rhinitis (hay fever). 3. In atopic eczema, itching (pruritus) is the main symptom at all ages and this results in scratching and exacerbation of the rash. 4. In infants, the face and scalp are prominently affected, although the trunk may be involved. 5. In older children, the skin flexures (cubital and popliteal fossae), and frictional areas, such as the neck, wrists, and ankles are characteristically involved. 6. Causes of exacerbation of eczema are: bacterial infection, viral infection, ingestion of an allergen, contact with an irritant or allergen, heat, humidity, change in medication, stress. 7. It is advisable to avoid soap and biological detergents. 8. Clothing next to the skin should be of pure cotton, avoiding nylon and pure woollen garments and nails need to be cut short.

Exercise 9
Fill in the missing words. Choose the correct ones.

1. _____ are _____ of management, _____ and softening the skin.	a moisturizing b Emollients c mainstay
2. _____ are _____ to creams when the skin is very dry.	a preferable b Ointments
3. _____ _____ are helpful over limbs when _____ and lichenification are a problem.	a scratching b Occlusive bandages
4. The _____ are worn _____ for 2-3 days, until the skin has improved.	a overnight b bandages
5. Antibiotics with _____ can be applied _____ for _____ infected eczema.	a topically b hydrocortisone c mildly

| 6. ____ _____ may be suspected if the child reacts consistently to a food, or in infants and young children with _____ __ _____ atopic eczema, particularly if associated with ___ _____ (colic, vomiting, altered bowel habit) or _____ _____ | a faltering growth

b gut dysmotility

c moderate or severe

d Food allergy |
| 7. _____ _____ should be _____ ___ with the advice of a dietician to ensure that the diet remains _____ _____. | a nutritionally adequate

b carried out

c Dietary elimination |

Text 6
Infections and infestations
Viral infections
Viral warts

These are caused by the human papillomavirus. Warts are common in children, usually on the fingers and soles (verrucae). Most disappear spontaneously and treatment is only indicated if the lesions are painful or are a cosmetic problem. Cryotherapy with liquid nitrogen is an effective treatment but can be painful and its use should be reserved for older children.

Fungal infections
Ringworm

Dermatophyte fungi invade the horny layer of skin, nails, and hair. The term 'ringworm' is used because of the ringed appearance of skin lesions. Scalp ringworm sometimes acquired from dogs and cats, causes scaling and patchy alopecia with broken hairs. Treatment of mild infections is with topical antifungal preparations, but more severe infections require systemic antifungal treatment for several weeks. Any animal source of infection also needs to be treated.

Parasitic infestations
Scabies

Scabies is caused by an infection the eight-legged mite, which burrows down the epidermis. Severe itching occurs 2-6 weeks after infestation and is worse in warm conditions and at night. In older children, burrows, papules, and vesicles involve the skin between the fingers and toes, axillae, flexor aspects of the wrists, belt line, and around the nipples, penis, and buttocks. In infants and young children, the distribution often includes the palms, soles, and trunk. Confirmation can be made by microscopic examination of skin scrapings from the lesions to identify mite, eggs, and mite faeces.

Complications

The skin becomes excoriated due to scratching and there may be a secondary eczematous or urticarial reaction masking the true diagnosis. Secondary bacterial infection is common, giving crusted, pustular lesions. As it is spread by close bodily contact, the child and whole family should be treated. If a child and other members of the family are itching, suspect scabies.

Exercise 10
Study the following summary and then interpret basic information in English.

1. Assessment of the child with eczema
Condition of the skin
Distribution of the eczema: is the skin excoriated, weeping, crusted, lichenified?
How troublesome is the itching?
Worse or better than usual?
What causes exacerbation — food or other allergens, irritants, medication, stress?
Does it disturb sleep?
Does it interfere with life?
Family knowledgeable about condition and its management?
2. Tinea capitis (scalp ringworm)
Annular scaling scalp lesions with patchy alopecia with broken hairs.
Fungal hyphae or skin scrapings.
Treated with topical or systemic antifungal.
Treat the dog or cat, if infected.
3. Scabies
Very itchy burrows, papules, and vesicles — distribution varies with age.
Scratching leads to excoriation, secondary eczematous, or urticarial reaction often with secondary bacterial infection.
Not only the child but also the whole family will need treatment

Pediculosis

Pediculosis capitis (head lice infestation) is the most common form of lice infestation in children. It is widespread and troublesome among primary-school children. Presentation may be itching of the scalp and nape or from identifying live lice on the scalp or nits (empty egg cases) on hairs.

Louse eggs are cemented to hair close to the scalp and the nits (small whitish oval capsules) remain attached to the hair shaft as the hair grows. Wet combing with a fine-tooth comb to remove live lice (bug-bursting) every 3-4 days for at least 2 weeks is a useful and safe physical treatment.

Other childhood skin disorders
Psoriasis

This familial disorder rarely presents before the age of 2 years. It often follows a streptococcal or viral sore throat or ear infection. Lesions are small, raindrop-like, round or oval erythematous scaly patches on the trunk and upper limbs, and an attack usually resolves over 3 months to 4 months. However, most get a recurrence of psoriasis within the next 3-5 years. Occasionally, children with chronic psoriasis may have a considerable effect on quality of life.

Acne vulgaris

Acne may begin 1-2 years before the onset of puberty. Obstruction to the flow of sebum in the sebaceous follicle initiates the process of acne. Inflammation is also present. There are a variety of lesions, initially open comedones (blackheads) or closed comedones (whiteheads) progressing to papules, pustules, nodules, and cysts. Lesion occurs mainly on the face, back, chest, and shoulders. The more severe cystic and nodular lesions often produce scarring. Menstruation and emotional stress may be associated with exacerbations. Sunshine in moderation, topical antibiotics or topical retinoids may be helpful.

Urticaria

Urticaria (hives), is characterized by flesh-coloured wheals. Papular urticaria is a delayed hypersensitivity reaction most commonly seen on the legs, following a bite from a flea, bedbug, animal or bird mite. Irritation, vesicles, papules and wheals appear and secondary infection due to scratching is common. It may last for weeks or months and may be recurrent.

Exercise 11
Answer the following questions. Prepare short talks and/or dialogues on these topics

1. Speak about infections (viral, fungal).
2. Speak about parasitic infestations (scabies, pediculosis).

3. Describe other childhood skin disorders (psoriasis, acne vulgaris, urticaria).

Translation 6

1. Viral warts are caused by the human papillomavirus. 2. Most disappear spontaneously and treatment is only indicated if the lesions are painful or are a cosmetic problem. 3. Cryotherapy with liquid nitrogen is an effective treatment but can be painful and its use should be reserved for older children. 4. Dermatophyte fungi invade the horny layer of skin, nails, and hair. 5. The term 'ringworm' is used because of the ringed appearance of skin lesions. 6. Treatment of mild infections is with topical antifungal preparations, but more severe infections require systemic antifungal treatment for several weeks. 7. Scabies is caused by an infection the eight-legged mite, which burrows down the epidermis. 8. In older children, burrows, papules, and vesicles involve the skin between the fingers and toes, axillae, flexor aspects of the wrists, belt line, and around the nipples, penis, and buttocks. 9. Confirmation can be made by microscopic examination of skin scrapings from the lesions to identify mite, eggs, and mite faeces. 10. The skin becomes excoriated due to scratching and there may be a secondary eczematous or urticarial reaction masking the true diagnosis.

Exercise 12
Match the column A with the column B. Try to learn the expressions and/or sentences by heart.

A

1. Pediculosis capitis (head lice infestation) is the most common form of ...
2. Presentation may be itching of the scalp and nape ...
3. Wet combing with a fine-tooth comb ...
4. Psoriasis often follows ...
5. Occasionally, children with chronic psoriasis ...
6. Obstruction to the flow of sebum in the sebaceous follicle ...
7. There are a variety of lesions, ...
8. Menstruation and emotional stress may ...
9. Urticaria (hives), is characterized by ...
10. Papular urticaria is a delayed hypersensitivity reaction most commonly seen on the legs, ...
11. Irritation, vesicles, papules and wheals appear ...

B

a.   ... or from identifying live lice on the scalp or nits (empty egg cases) on hairs.

b.   ... a streptococcal or viral sore throat or ear infection.

c.   ... flesh-coloured wheals.

d.   ... and secondary infection due to scratching is common.

e.   ... to remove live lice (bug-bursting) is a useful and safe physical treatment.

f.   ... initially open comedones (blackheads) or closed comedones (whiteheads) progressing to papules, pustules, nodules, and cysts.

g.   ... following a bite from a flea, bedbug, animal or bird mite.

h.   ... may have a considerable effect on quality of life.

i.   ... be associated with exacerbations.

j.   ... initiates the process of acne.

k.   ... lice infestation in children.

Key 8
Exercise 2
1 c, b, a; 2c, b, a; 3 c, b, a; 4 c, b, a; 5 b, c, a; 6 c, b, a; 7 c, a, b; 8 c, a, b

Exercise 5
1b; 2d; 3a; 4f; 5g; 6c; 7e

Exercise 9
1 b, c, a; 2 b, a; 3 b, a; 4 b, a; 5 b, a, c; 6 d, c, b, a; 7 c, b, a

Exercise 12
1k; 2a; 3e; 4b; 5h; 6j; 7f; 8i; 9c; 10g; 11d

VOCABULARY 8

absence /ˈæb.səns/
accelerate /ækˈse.ləˌreɪt/
accentuation /ækˈsent.ʃʊ.eɪ.ʃən/
advisable /ədˈvaɪ.zə.bl̩/
aerosol /ˈeərəˌsɒl/
affective /əˈfektɪv/ **disorder** /dɪsˈɔːdə/
alienated /ˌeɪl.jəˈneɪ.təd/
alkalosis /ˌælkəˈləʊ.sɪs/
allergen /ˈæl.ə.dʒən/
alter /ˈɒl.tər/
alternatively /ɒlˈtɜː.nə.tɪv.li/
amenorrhoea /ˌeɪ.men.əˈriː.ə/
amphetamine /æmˈfetəˌmiːn/
annular /ˈænjʊələr/
antifungal /æn.tɪˈfʌŋ.gəl/
antihistamine /ˌæn.tiˈhɪs.tə.miːn/
assurance /əˈʃʊərəns/
axilla /ækˈsɪl.ə/ pl **axillae**
bandage /ˈbæn.dɪdʒ/
bedbug /ˈbedˌbʌg/
belt /belt/
bipolar disorder /baɪˈpəʊ.lə dɪˌsɔː.dər/
biting /ˈbaɪ.tɪŋ/
blunt /blʌnt/
boredom /ˈbɔːdəm/
bout /baʊt/
bowel /ˈbaʊ.əl/ **habit** /ˈhæbɪt/
bug /bʌg/ **bursting** /ˈbɜːstɪŋ/
bulla /bulˈæ/ pl **bullae** /iː/
bullous /ˈbʊ.ləs/
burn /bɜːn/
burrow /ˈbʌrəʊ/
buttock /ˈbʌt.ək/
bypass /ˈbaɪˌpɑːs/
cannabis /ˈkænəbɪs/
case /keɪs/
cease /siːs/
cement /sɪˈment/
chalky-white /ˈtʃɔːkɪ waɪt/
coagulation /kəʊˈæg.jʊ.leɪ.ʃən/
cocaine /kəˈkeɪn/
comb /koʊm/
comedo /ˈkɑː.məˌdəʊ/ pl **comedones** /niːz/
comedon /ˈkʌm.daʊn/
comprehensive /ˌkɒm.prɪˈhen.sɪv/

conceal /kənˈsiːl/
confidentiality /ˌkɒn.fɪ.den.tʃiˈæl.ɪ.ti/
consistently /kənˈsɪs.tənt.li/
contemporary /kənˈtem.prə.ri/
cradle /ˈkreɪ.dəl/ **cap** /ˈkap/
cubital /kjuːbət.əl/
cutting /ˈkʌt.ɪŋ/
deceive /dɪˈsiːv/
deep /diːp/
degenerative /dɪˈdʒen.ər.ə.tɪv/
deliberately /dɪˈlɪb.ər.ət.li/
delirium /dɪˈlɪrɪ.əm/
delusional /dɪˈluː.ʒən.əl/
dementia /dɪˈmenʃə/
dependent /dɪˈpen.dənt/
derivative /dɪˈrɪvətɪv/
dermatitis /ˌdɜːməˈtaɪ.tɪs/
dermatophyte /ˌdərˈma.tə.ˌfaɪt/
dermis /ˈdɜː.mɪs/
despair /dɪˈspeər/
detergent /dɪˈtɜː.dʒənt/
discordant /dɪsˈkɔːdənt/
disseminated /dɪˈsem.ɪ.neɪt.ɪd/
distort /dɪˈstɔːt/
disturb /dɪˈstɜːb/
divorce /dɪˈvɔːs/
dominate /ˈdɒmɪˌneɪt/
dysmotility /dɪsˈməʊ.tɪl.ɪ.ti/
ecchymosis /ˌekiˈməʊ.sɪs/ pl **ecchymoses** /ˌe.kiˈməʊ.ˌsiːz/
ecstasy /ˈekstəsɪ/
elevation /ˌel.ɪˈveɪ.ʃᵊn/
embroiled /ɪmˈbrɔɪld/
encounter /ɪnˈkaʊn.tə/
ensue /ɪnˈsjuː/
entire /ɪnˈtaɪə/
epidermolysis /ˌep.ə.ˌdərˈmɑː.l.ə.səs/ pl **epidermolyses** /ˌsiːz/
equation /ɪˈkweɪʒən/
exclusive /ɪkˈskluːsɪv/
excoriate /ɪkˈskɔːrɪˌeɪt/
explore /ɪkˈsplɔːr/
fibrous /ˈfaɪbrəs/
flake /fleɪk/
flea /fliː/
flesh /fleʃ/
flexor /ˈflek.sər/
fossa /fɒs.ə/ pl **fossae** /fɒs.iː/
frankly /ˈfræŋklɪ/

freckle /ˈfrekəl/
frictional /ˈfrɪk.ʃⁿn.ᵊl/
fungus /ˈfʌŋ.gəs/ (pl **fungi**)
garment /ˈgɑːmənt/
get /get/ **off** /ɒf/
glue /gluː/
greasy /griːs.i/
guilt /gɪlt/
habitual /həˈbɪtjʊəl/
hallucinogenic /həˌluːsɪnəʊˈdʒenɪk/
halt /hɔːlt/
hay /heɪ/ **fever** /ˈfiː.vər/
heroin /ˈherəʊɪn/
hives /haɪvz/
horny /ˈhɔːni/
horror /ˈhɒrə/
hypha /ˈhaɪfə/ pl **hyphae** /ˈhaɪfiː/
hypochondriacal /ˌhaɪ.pə.kənˈdraɪ.ə.kəl/
illicit /ɪˈlɪs.ɪt/
immunomodulator /ˌi.mjə.nəʊˈmɒdjʊˌleɪt.tər/
impregnate /ˈɪm.preg.neɪt/
incense /ˈɪn.sens/
intoxication /ɪnˌtɒk.sɪˈkeɪ.ʃən/
intravascular /ˌɪn.trəˈvæsk.jʊ.lər/
judgement /ˈdʒʌdʒ.mənt/
keratinize /ˈker.ə.təˌnaɪz/
lanugo /læˈnjuː.gəʊ/
legal high /ˌliː.gᵊl ˈhaɪ/
liberally /ˈlɪbərəli/
lichenification /laɪˌken.ə.fəˈkeɪˌʃən/
lichenified /laɪˈken.əˌfaɪd/
life-threatening /ˈlaɪfˌθret.ən.ɪŋ/
louse /laʊs/ pl **lice** /ˈlaɪs/
loyalty /ˈlɔɪ.əl.ti/
lying /ˈlaɪ.ɪŋ/
lying /ˈlaɪ.ɪŋ/ **about** /əˈbaʊt/
manageable /ˈmænɪdʒəbəl/
marking /mɑːk.ɪŋ/
misery /ˈmɪz.ər.i/
mite /maɪt/
mittens /ˈmɪt.ᵊnz/
moisturizing /ˈmɔɪstʃəˌraɪzɪŋ/
moodiness /ˈmuːdɪnɪs/
mute /mjuːt/
napkin /ˈnæpkɪn/
nit /nɪt/
nitrogen /ˈnaɪ.trə.dʒən/

nodular /ˈnɒdʒ.ə.ləʳ/
obsessional /əbˈseʃənə/
occlusive /ɒˈkluː.sɪv/
odd /ɒd/
ointment /ˈɔɪnt.mənt/
organic /ɔːˈgæn.ɪk/
oval /ˈəʊ.vəl/
papillomavirus /ˌpa.pə.ˈləʊ.məˈvaɪə.rəs/
paronychia /ˌper.ə.ˈni.kiː.ə/
participant /pɑːˈtɪs.ɪ.pənt/
patch /pætʃ/
patchy /ˈpætʃɪ/
pediculosis /pi.ˌdi.kjə.ˈləʊ.səs/ **capitis** /ˈkap.ət.əs/
perception /pəˈsep.ʃən/
perceptual /pəˈseptjʊəl/
perpetuate /pəˈpetʃ.u.eɪt/
persist /pəˈsɪst/
phobic /fəʊbɪk/
pityriasis /ˌpi.ti.ˈraɪ.ə.səs/
pityriasis /ˌpi.ti.ˈraɪ.ə.səs/ **rosea** /ˈrəʊ.ziː.ə/
popliteal /pɑpˈlɪt̮.i.əl/
pretend /prɪˈtend/
prominently /ˈprɒm.ɪ.nənt.li/
property /ˈprɒp.ə.ti/
proposition /ˌprɒpəˈzɪʃən/
pruritus /prʊəˈraɪ.təs/
psoriasis /səˈraɪəsɪs/
psychosis /saɪˈkəʊ.sɪs/
punch /pʌntʃ/
raindrop /ˈreɪnˌdrɒp/
raise /reɪz/
rave /reɪv/
reappear /ˌriː.əˈpɪəʳ/
rebellion /rɪˈbeljən/
refeeding /rɪˈfiː.dɪŋ/
reinstitution /riːˌɪn.stɪˈtʃuː.ʃən/
remit /rɪˈmɪt/
resolution /ˌrez.əˈluː.ʃən/
restore /rɪˈstɔːʳ/
retinoid /ˈre.tə.ˌnɔːid/
ringworm /ˈrɪŋˌwɜːm/
roseola /rəʊˈzi.ələ/
roughen /ˈrʌfən/
rub /rʌb/
scabies /ˈskeɪ.biːz/
scale /skeɪl/
scaling /skeɪl.ɪŋ/

scaly /ˈskeɪ.li/

schizophrenia /ˌskɪt.səˈfriː.ni.ə/

scraping /ˈskreɪ.pɪŋ/

sebum /ˈsiːbəm/

self-induced /ˌself.ɪnˈdjuːst/

self-starvation /ˌself stɑːˈveɪ.ʃən/

shaft /ʃɑːft/

slim /slɪm/

sniffing /snɪf.ɪŋ/

solvent /ˈsɒl.vənt/

sore /sɔː/ **throat** /θrəʊt/

spending /spendɪŋ/

steal /stiːl/

stockinette /ˌstɒk.əˈnɛt/

struggle /ˈstrʌɡəl/

subsequently /ˈsʌb.sɪ.kwənt.li/

substitute /ˈsʌb.stɪ.tjuːt/

tar /tɑː/

texture /ˈteks.tʃər/

thin /θɪn/

thinness /θɪnnɪs/

tie /taɪ/

trait /treɪt/

transepidermal /trænz.ˌep.ə.ˌdər.mæl/

tremendous /trɪˈmen.dəs/

trigger /ˈtrɪɡ.ər/

validate /ˈvælɪˌdeɪt/

vernix caseosa /vɜːrˈniks kasˈiː.əʊˈsə/

verruca /vəˈruː.kə/pl **verrucae**

vesicle /ˈves.ɪ.kəl/

virtually /ˈvɜː.tju.ə.li/

vitiligo /ˌvɪt.ɪˈlaɪ.ɡəʊ/

wart /wɔːt/

weal /wiːl/

woollen /ˈwʊlən/

Diabetes and endocrinology; Problems in diabetes control; Thyroid disorders; Musculoskeletal disorders; Limp

Text 1
Diabetes mellitus

Its incidence has increased steadily over last 25 years, most likely from changes in environmental risk factors. There is considerable ethnic and geographical variation. Most children have type 1 diabetes (98%) although the number with type 2 diabetes is increasing.

Classification of diabetes according to aetiology
Type 1. Most childhood diabetes
- Destruction of pancreatic β-cells by an autoimmune process

Type 2. Insulin resistance followed later by β-cell failure
- Usually older children, obesity-related, positive family history

Other types
- Maturity onset diabetes of the young
- Drugs, e.g. corticosteroids
- Pancreatic insufficiency
- Endocrine disorders
- Genetic/chromosomal syndromes, e.g. Down and Turner

Neonatal diabetes: transient and permanent
Gestational diabetes

Aetiology of type 1 diabetes

Both genetic predisposition and environmental precipitants play a role. There is an association with other autoimmune disorders such as hypothyroidism, Adison disease, coeliac disease, and rheumatoid arthritis in the patient or family.

Clinical features

Children usually present with only a few weeks of polyuria, excessive thirst (polydipsia), and weight loss; young children may also develop secondary nocturnal enuresis. Diabetic ketoacidosis requires urgent recognition and treatment as it carries a significant risk of mortality in children and young people.

Symptoms and signs of diabetes
Early
Most common — the 'classical triad':
- excessive drinking (polydipsia)
- polyuria
- weight loss

Less common:
- enuresis (secondary)
- skin sepsis
- candida and other infections

Late — diabetic ketoacidosis
- Smell of acetone on the breath
- Vomiting
- Dehydration
- Abdominal pain
- Hyperventilation due to acidosis (Kussmaul breathing)
- Hypovolaemic shock
- Drowsiness
- Coma and death

Initial management of type 1 diabetes
The information provided for the child must be appropriate for age, and updated regularly. An intensive educational programme is needed for the parents and child, which covers:
- a basic understanding of the pathophysiology of diabetes
- injection of insulin: technique and sites
- blood glucose (finger prick) monitoring to allow insulin adjustment and blood ketones when unwell
- healthy diet aiming for a minimum of five portions of fruit and vegetables per day. Patients should be taught estimating the amount of carbohydrate in food.
- encouragement to exercise regularly
- 'sick-day rules' during illness
- the recognition and staged treatment of hypoglycaemia
- where to get advice 24 hours a day

- the help available from voluntary groups
- the psychological impact of a lifelong condition with potentially serious short-term and long-term complications

Insulin

Insulin can be given by continuous infusion of rapid acting insulin from a pump or by injection using a variety of syringe and needle sizes or pen-like devices with insulin-containing cartridges. Insulin may be injected into the subcutaneous tissue of the anterior and lateral aspects of the thigh, the buttocks, and the abdomen. Rotation of the injection sites is essential to prevent lipohypertrophy. The skin should be gently pinched up and the insulin injected at a 45°angle.

Diet

Children and young people with diabetes mellitus are encouraged to eat a healthy diet. The aim is to optimize metabolic control while maintaining normal growth. The diet should be high in fibre.

Blood glucose monitoring

Regular blood glucose measurements are required to adjust the insulin regiment and learn how changes in lifestyle, food and exercise affect control. A record should be kept in a diary or transferred from the memory of blood glucose meter.

Factors affecting blood glucose levels
Increase
- Insufficient insulin
- Food (especially carbohydrates)
- Illness
- Menstruation (shortly before onset)
- Growth hormone
- Corticosteroids
- Sex hormones at puberty
- Stress

Decrease
- Insulin
- Exercise
- Alcohol
- Some drugs
- Marked anxiety/excitement

- Hot weather

Acute complications
Hypoglycaemia

It is inevitable that children and young people who manage their diabetes well will experience hypoglycaemia. Most complain of hunger, tummy ache, sweatiness, feeling faint or dizzy or a 'wobbly feeling' in their legs. If unrecognized or untreated, hypoglycaemia may progress to seizures and coma. Parents can often detect hypoglycaemia in young children by their pallor and irritability. The blood glucose concentration should be checked. Treating a 'hypo' at an early stage requires the administration of easily absorbed glucose in the form of glucose tablets or a sugary drink. Oral glucose gels are quickly absorbed from the buccal mucosa and so are helpful if the child is unable to cooperate. After treatment of 'hypos', parents should give the child some food (usually a biscuit or sandwich) to prevent the blood glucose dropping again.

Long-term management

The aims of long-term management are:
- normal growth and development
- maintaining as normal a home and school life as possible
- good diabetes control
- encouraging children to become self-reliant, but with adult supervision
- anticipating and minimising hypoglycaemia

The long-term complications of diabetes are:
- macrovascular — hypertension, coronary heart disease, cerebrovascular disease
- microvascular — retinopathy, nephropathy, neuropathy

Exercise 1
Answer the following questions. Prepare short talks and/or dialogues on these topics

1. Characterize diabetes mellitus.
2. Describe aetiology of type 1 diabetes (clinical features, symptoms and signs, initial management).
3. What do you know about insulin, diet, and blood glucose monitoring?
4. What are factors affecting blood glucose levels?

5.   Describe long-term management.

Exercise 2
Study the following summary and then interpret basic information in English.

1. The incidence of diabetes mellitus has increased steadily over last 25 years, most likely from changes in environmental risk factors.
2. Most children have type 1 diabetes (98%) although the number with type 2 diabetes is increasing.
3. In type 1 diabetes both genetic predisposition and environmental precipitants play a role.
4. There is an association with other autoimmune disorders such as hypothyroidism, Adison disease, coeliac disease, and rheumatoid arthritis in the patient or family.
5. Children usually present with only a few weeks of polyuria, excessive thirst (polydipsia), and weight loss.
6. Diabetic ketoacidosis requires urgent recognition and treatment as it carries a significant risk of mortality in children and young people.
7. Most common symptoms and signs of diabetes are excessive drinking (polydipsia), polyuria, weight loss.
8. Signs of diabetic ketoacidosis include: smell of acetone, vomiting, dehydration, abdominal pain, hyperventilation, hypovolaemic shock, drowsiness, coma and death.

Translation 1

1. An intensive educational programme is needed for the parents and child, which covers: pathophysiology of diabetes, injection of insulin, blood glucose (finger prick), healthy diet, encouragement to exercise, treatment of hypoglycaemia, and the psychological impact. 2. Insulin can be given by continuous infusion of rapid acting insulin from a pump or by injection using a variety of syringe and needle sizes or pen-like devises with insulin-containing cartridges. 3. Rotation of the injection sites is essential to prevent lipohypertrophy. 4. Children and young people with diabetes mellitus are encouraged to eat a healthy diet. 5. Regular blood glucose measurements are required to adjust the insulin regiment and learn how changes in lifestyle, food and exercise affect control. 6. Factors affecting blood glucose levels are: insufficient insulin, food, illness, menstruation, growth hormone, corticosteroids, sex, stress, hormones, insulin, exercise, alcohol, some drugs, marked anxiety/excitement, and hot weather.

Exercise 3
Fill in the missing words. Choose the correct ones.

1. It is _____ that children and young people who _____ their diabetes well will experience _____.	a hypoglycaemia b manage c inevitable
2. Most complain of hunger, _____ ____, sweatiness, feeling _____ __ _____ or a _____ _____ in their legs.	a 'wobbly feeling' b faint or dizzy c tummy ache
3. Parents can often _____ hypoglycaemia in young children by their _____ and a_____.	a irritability b pallor c detect
4. Oral _____ ____ are quickly absorbed from the _____ _____ and so are helpful if the child is unable __ _____.	a buccal mucosa b to cooperate c glucose gels
5. After treatment of ,_____', parents should give the child some food __ _____ the blood _____ glucose again.	a to prevent b dropping c hypos
6. The _____ __ long-term management are: _____ _____, good diabetes control, and _____ hypoglycaemia.	a anticipating b normal growth c aims of
7. The _____-_____ complications of diabetes are: macrovascular (hypertension, coronary heart disease, _____ _____), or microvascular (_____, nephropathy, neuropathy).	a cerebrovascular disease b long-term c retinopathy

Text 2
Problems in diabetes control

Good blood glucose control is particularly difficult in the following circumstances:

- eating too many sugary foods
- infrequent or unreliable blood glucose testing

- illness — viral illnesses are common in the young
- exercise — vigorous or prolonged planned exercise (cross-country running, long-distance hiking, skiing)
- eating disorders
- family disruption such as divorce or separation
- inadequate family motivation, support or understanding

Management at school

An individualized care plan should be developed by the parents, diabetes team, and the school to address the specific needs of the child.

General overview (periodic):

- Normal growth and pubertal development, avoiding obesity — measure height and weight and BMI and plot on growth chart at each visit
- Blood pressure check for hypertension yearly (age-specific centiles)
- Renal disease — screening for microalbuminuria, an early sign of nephropathy
- Circulation: — check pulses and sensation
- Eyes — retinopathy or cataracts are rare in children
- Feet — maintain good care, avoid tight shoes and obtain prompt treatment of infections – annually
- Screening for coeliac and thyroid disease at diagnosis
- Annual reminder to have flu vaccination

Knowledge and psychosocial aspects

- Good understanding of diabetes?
- Becoming self-reliant, but appropriate supervision?
- Taking exercise, sport? Diabetes not interfering with it?
- Leading as normal life as possible?
- Smoking, alcohol?
- Is 'hypo' treatment readily available?
- What are the main issues for the patient?

Puberty and adolescence

Diabetes in young people is influenced by biological, psychological, and social factors. Growth hormone, oestrogen and testosterone all antagonise insulin action and there is an increase in the insulin requirement. With increasing independence, the young person may explore behaviours such as smoking, use of alcohol, and sexual relationships. Conflict with parents is common. Some teenagers with diabetes, especially girls, have excessive weight gain and become obese. The weight gain not only affects their diabetes control, but may have a major impact on their body image. Eating disorders are more common in young people with diabetes. Successful long-term diabetes management depends on education to understand their condition, increasing self-reliance and responsibility.

The impact of diabetes in normal adolescence

Normal adolescence	How diabetes interferes
Biological factors	Insulin resistance secondary to growth and sex hormone secretion Growth and pubertal delay if diabetes control poor
Psychological factors	Reduced self-esteem e.g. related to impaired body image, difference from peers
Social factors	Different from peer group e.g. need for blood tests and injections Hypoglycaemic events — can be frightening and emphasize difference from friends
	Increased risk from alcohol, smoking, use of recreational drugs Vocational plans e.g. some restrictions in choices such as heavy goods vehicle licence, pilot Separation from parents more complex

The neurological sequelae include epilepsy, severe learning difficulties and microcephaly. This risk is greater in early childhood during the period of most rapid brain growth. Infants should never be starved for more than 4 hours. A blood glucose should be checked in any child who:
- becomes septicemic or appear seriously ill
- has a prolonged seizure
- develops an altered state of consciousness

Causes of hypoglycaemia beyond the immediate neonatal period
Fasting
- Insulin excess
- Excess exogenous insulin
- β-cell tumours/disorders
- Drug induced
- Autoimmune

- Beckwith syndrome
- Without hyperinsulinemia
- Liver disease
- Ketotic hypoglycaemia of childhood
- Inborn errors of metabolism
- Hormonal deficiency

Reactive/non fasting
- Galactosemia
- Leucine sensitivity
- Fructose intolerance
- Maternal diabetes
- Hormonal deficiency
- Aspirin/alcohol poisoning

Exercise 4
Study the following summary and then interpret basic information in English.

1. Regular assessment of the child with diabetes
Any episodes of hypoglycaemia, diabetic ketoacidosis, hospital admission?
Is there still awareness of hypoglycaemia?
Absence from school? School supportive of diabetes care?
Diary of blood glucose results or blood glucose read-out are appropriate actions to results being taken?
Insulin regimen appropriate?
Lipohypertrophy or lipoarthrophy at injection sites?
Diet – healthy diet, manipulating food intake and insulin to maintain good control?
2. Diabetes mellitus
Type 1 diabetes is usually managed by an intensive insulin regime, matching insulin to the carbohydrate eaten in a balanced diet. Exercise is encouraged.
Diabetic ketoacidosis is associated with a significant morbidity and mortality rate in children
3. Hypoglycaemia
Hypoglycaemia is a common problem in neonates during the first few days of life. Clinical features include:
sweating
pallor
central nervous system signs of irritability, headache, seizures, and coma.
Should be excluded in any child with septicaemia, who is seriously ill, has a prolonged seizure or altered state of consciousness

Low blood glucose on bedside testing must be confirmed by laboratory measurement
If the cause is unknown, diagnostic blood and urine samples should, if possible, be taken at the time

Exercise 5
Answer the following questions. Prepare short talks and/or dialogues on these topics

1. Describe problems in diabetes control.
2. Why is general overview important?
3. What are factors influencing diabetes in young people?
4. What is the impact of diabetes in normal adolescence?
5. Speak about hypoglycaemia in neonates.
6. What are causes of hypoglycaemia beyond the immediate neonatal period?

Translation 2

1. Good blood glucose control is particularly difficult in the following circumstances: eating too many sugary foods, infrequent or unreliable blood glucose testing, viral illnesses, vigorous exercise, eating disorders, divorce or separation, inadequate support or understanding. 2. General overview includes: measuring height and weight and BMI, checking blood pressure, screening for renal disease, checking pulses and sensation, maintaining good care of feet, screening for coeliac and thyroid disease. 3. Knowledge and psychosocial aspects include: good understanding of diabetes, becoming self-reliant, taking exercise, sport, and 'hypo' treatment. 4. Growth hormone, oestrogen and testosterone all antagonise insulin action and there is an increase in the insulin requirement.

Exercise 6
Study the following summary and then interpret basic information in English.

1. Eating disorders are more common in young people with diabetes. 2. Successful long-term diabetes management depends on education to understand their condition, increasing self-reliance and responsibility. 3. The impact of diabetes in normal adolescence includes: biological factors (insulin resistance, growth and pubertal delay), psychological factors (reduced self-esteem), and social factors (different from peer group, hypoglycaemic events, increased risk from alcohol, smoking, use of recreational drugs, vocational plans).

Exercise 7
Fill in the missing words. Choose the correct ones.

1. Clinical features of hypoglycaemia include: sweating, pallor, _____, headache, _____, and coma. The neurological _____ include epilepsy, severe learning difficulties and _____.	a microcephaly b seizures c sequelae d irritability
2. _____ should never ___ _____ for more than 4 hours.	a be starved b Infants
3. A blood glucose should ___ _____ in any child who: _____ seriously ill, has a prolonged seizure and develops an _____ _____ of consciousness.	a appears b altered state c be checked
4. Causes of _____ beyond the immediate _____ _____ are: fasting, reactive, ____-_____.	a neonatal period b hypoglycaemia c non-fasting

Text 3
Thyroid disorders
Congenital hypothyroidism
Detection of congenital hypothyroidism is important in neonatal screening, as it is:
- relatively common
- a preventable cause of severe learning difficulties

Causes of congenital hypothyroidism are:
- maldescent of the thyroid and athyrosis
- dishormonogenesis — an inborn error of thyroid hormone synthesis
- iodine deficiency
- hypothyroidism due to TSH deficiency

Most infants with congenital hypothyroidism are detected on routine neonatal biochemical screening performed on all newborn infants. Treatment with thyroxine should be started before 2 weeks to 3 weeks of age to reduce the risk of impaired neurodevelopment.

Clinical features of hypothyroidism

Congenital	Acquired
Usually asymptomatic and picked up on screening. Clinical features: • faltering growth • feeding problems • prolonged jaundice • constipation • pale, cold, mottled dry skin • coarse facies • large tongue • hoarse cry • goitre (occasionally) • umbilical hernia • delayed development	Females >males Short stature/poor growth • Cold intolerance • Dry skin • Cold peripheries • Bradycardia • Thin, dry hair • Pale, puffy eyes with loss of eyebrows • Goitre • Slow-relaxing reflexes • Constipation • Delayed puberty/amenorrhoea • Obesity • Slipped upper femoral epiphysis • Poor concentration • Deterioration in school work • Learning difficulties

Hyperthyroidism

This usually results from autoimmune thyroiditis (Graves disease) secondary to the production of thyroid-stimulating immunoglobulin (Tsis). Hyperthyroidism is less common in children than adults and can present with nonspecific symptoms.

Clinical features of hyperthyroidism

- Systemic
- Anxiety, restlessness
- Increased appetite
- Sweating
- Diarrhoea
- Weight loss
- Rapid growth in height

- Advanced bone maturity
- Tremor
- Tachycardia, wide pulse pressure
- Warm, vasodilated peripheries
- Goitre (bruit)
- Learning difficulties/behaviour problems
- Psychosis
- Eye signs (uncommon in children)
- Exophthalmos
- Ophthalmoplegia
- Lid retraction
- Lid lag

Parathyroid disorders

Parathyroid hormone (PTH) promotes bone formation via bone-forming cells (osteoblasts). Severe hypocalcaemia leads to muscle spasm, fits, stridor, and diarrhoea. Hypocalcaemia may also result in rickets. Associated abnormalities are short stature, obesity, subcutaneous nodules, short fourth metacarpals, and learning difficulties. Treatment of acute symptomatic hypocalcaemia is with an intravenous infusion of calcium gluconate. Chronic hypocalcaemia is treated with oral calcium and high doses of vitamin D analogues. Hyperparathyroidism results in a high calcium level, causing constipation, anorexia, lethargy and behavioural effects, polyuria, and polydipsia. Bony erosions of the phalanges may be seen on a hand radiograph.

Pituitary disorders
Causes of pituitary disorders
Congenital
Structural e.g. midline defects including septooptic dysplasia
Pituitary hypoplasia or aplasia

Acquired
Brain tumours affecting hypothalamus or pituitary gland e.g. craniopharyngioma
Cranial irradiation
Trauma e.g. affecting pituitary stalk
Infection e.g. post meningitis
Infiltration e.g. histiocytosis
Structural e.g. associated with cerebral malformation, hydrocephalus

Adrenal disorders
Congenital adrenal hyperplasia

- Autosomal recessive disorder of adrenal steroid biosynthesis.
- Females present with virilisation of the external genitalia.
- Males present with salt loss (80%) or tall stature and precocious puberty (20%).
- Long-term medical management with lifelong glucocorticoids, and mineralocorticoids/sodium chloride if salt loss.
- Additional corticosteroids must be given to cover illness or surgery.
- Salt-losing adrenal crisis needs urgent treatment with hydrocortisone, saline, and glucose given intravenously.
- Monitor growth, skeletal maturity, plasma androgens.
- Surgery for females.

Exercise 8
Study the following summary and then interpret basic information in English.

1. Congenital hypothyroidism
Is defined on routine neonatal biochemical screening
Although present antenatally, treatment started soon after birth results in satisfactory intellectual development
2. Acquired hypothyroidism
There is an increased risk in children with Down syndrome or Turner syndrome and of developing other autoimmune disorders, e.g. vitiligo, rheumatoid arthritis, diabetes mellitus.
Addison disease may also occur.
3. Adrenal insufficiency
May result in an adrenal crisis requiring urgent treatment.
Usually due to withdrawal from long-term corticosteroid therapy, congenital adrenal hyperplasia or, rarely, Adison disease.
4. Clinical features of Cushing syndrome
Growth failure/short stature
Face and trunk obesity
Red cheeks
Hirsutism
Striae
Hypertension
Bruising
Carbohydrate intolerance

| Muscle wasting and weakness |
| Osteopenia |
| Psychological problems. |

Exercise 9
Answer the following questions. Prepare short talks and/or dialogues on these topics

1. What are causes of congenital hypothyroidism?
2. What are clinical features of hypothyroidism?
3. What are clinical features of hyperthyroidism?
4. Describe parathyroid disorders.
5. What are causes of pituitary disorders (congenital, acquired)?
6. Speak about congenital adrenal hyperplasia.
7. What are clinical features of Cushing syndrome?

Exercise 10
Match the column A with the column B. Try to learn the expressions and/or sentences by heart.

A

1. Clinical features of congenital hypothyroidism are: ...
2. Clinical features of acquired hypothyroidism are: ...
3. Clinical features of hyperthyroidism are: ...
4. Clinical features of Cushing syndrome are: ...

B

a. ... *faltering growth, feeding problems, prolonged jaundice, constipation, pale, cold, mottled dry skin, coarse facies, large tongue, hoarse cry, goitre (occasionally), umbilical hernia, delayed development.*

b. ... *growth failure/short stature, face and trunk obesity, red cheeks, hirsutism, striae, hypertension, bruising, carbohydrate intolerance, muscle wasting and weakness, osteopenia, and psychological problems*

c. ... *anxiety, restlessness, increased appetite, sweating, diarrhoea, weight loss, rapid growth in height, advanced bone maturity, tremor, tachycardia, wide pulse pressure, warm, vasodilated peripheries, goitre (bruit), learning difficulties, behaviour problems, psychosis, eye signs, exophthalmos, ophthalmoplegia, lid retraction, lid lag.*

d. ... *short stature/poor growth, cold intolerance, dry skin, cold peripheries, bradycardia, thin, dry hair, pale, puffy eyes with loss of eyebrows, goitre, slow-relaxing reflexes, constipation, delayed*

puberty, amenorrhoea, obesity, slipped upper femoral epiphysis, poor
concentration, deterioration in school work, learning difficulties.

Translation 3

1. Detection of congenital hypothyroidism is important in neonatal screening. 2. Causes of congenital hypothyroidism are: maldescent of the thyroid, an inborn error of thyroid hormone synthesis, iodine deficiency, hypothyroidism due to TSH deficiency. 3. Treatment with thyroxine should be started before 2 weeks to 3 weeks of age to reduce the risk of impaired neurodevelopment. 4. Parathyroid hormone (PTH) promotes bone formation via bone-forming cells (osteoblasts). 5. Severe hypocalcaemia leads to muscle spasm, fits, stridor, and diarrhoea. 6. Treatment of acute symptomatic hypocalcaemia is with an intravenous infusion of calcium gluconate. 7. Hyperparathyroidism results in a high calcium level, causing constipation, anorexia, lethargy and behavioural effects, polyuria, and polydipsia.

Text 4
Musculoskeletal disorders
Variation of normal posture

Variations are common and may be noticed by parents or on routine developmental surveillance. Most resolve without any treatment but if severe, progressive, painful, functionally limiting or asymmetrical, they should be referred for a specialist opinion.

Clinical features of in-toeing in children
Metatarsus varus
- Occurs in infants
- Passively correctable
- Heel is held in the normal position
- No treatment required unless it persists beyond 5 years of age and is symptomatic

Medial tibial torsion
- Occurs in toddlers
- May be associated with bowing of the tibiae
- Self-corrects within about 5 years

Persistent anteversion of the femoral neck
- Presents in childhood
- Usually self-corrects by 8 years of age-specific

- May be associated with hypermobility of the joints
- Children sit between their feet with the hips fully internally rotated (W sitting)
- Most do not require treatment but femoral osteotomy may be required for persistent anteversion

Abnormal posture
Talipes equinovarus (club foot)

Positional talipes from intrauterine compression is common. The foot is normal size, the deformity is mild and can be corrected to the neutral position with passive manipulation. Talipes equinovarus is a complex abnormality. The entire foot is inverted and supinated, the forefoot adducted and the heel is located inwards and in plantar flexion. The position of the foot is fixed, often bilateral. Treatment is started promptly with plaster casting and bracing, which may be required for many months. It is usually successful.

The painful limb, knee, and back
Growing pains

Episodes of generalized pain in the lower limbs, referred as 'growing pains' are common in preschool and school-aged children. The pain often wakes the child from sleep and settles with massage of comforting. Features are:

- age range 3-12 years
- pain symmetrical in lower limbs and not limited to joints
- pain never present at the start of the day after waking
- physical activities not limited; no limp
- physical examination normal

Osteomyelitis

In osteomyelitis, there is infection of the metaphysis of long bone. The most common sites are the distal femur and proximal tibia. The skin is swollen directly over the affected site.

Presentation

This is usually with a markedly painful, immobile limb in a child with an acute febrile illness. Directly over the infected site there is swelling and exquisite tenderness, and it may be erythematous and warm. Moving a limb causes severe pain. Blood cultures are usually positive and the white blood count and acute-phase reactants are raised.

Treatment

Prompt treatment with parenteral antibiotics is required for several weeks to prevent bone necrosis, chronic infection, limb deformity and amyloidosis. Surgical drainage is performed if the condition does not respond rapidly to antibiotic therapy. The affected limb is initially rested in a splint and subsequently mobilized.

Back pain

Back pain is a symptom of concern in the very young and preadolescent ages as, in contrast to adults, a cause may often be identified.

- Mechanical causes — there may be muscle spasm or soft tissue pain from injury, often sport-related or from poor posture or abnormal loading (such as carrying heavy school bags on one shoulder).
- Tumours: benign or malignant. It may be the site of primary tumours or metastases.
- Vertebral osteomyelitis or discitis — there is localized tenderness. Treatment is with intravenous antibiotics.
- Spinal cord or nerve root entrapment — from tumour or prolapsed intervertebral disc – often associated with trauma or heavy lifting.
- Scheuermann disease — an osteochondritis of the vertebral body; may present with a fixed thoracic kyphosis with or without back pain. The diagnosis is usually made on X-ray.
- Spondylosis/spondylolisthesis — increased risks with certain sporting activities, e.g. bowling in cricket or gymnastics.
- Complex regional pain syndrome (CRPS) — diagnosed when no physical cause is found; may be exacerbated by psychological stress.

Red flag clinical features of back pain

- Young age — pathology more likely
- High fever — infection
- Night waking, persistent pain — osteoid osteoma or tumours
- Painful scoliosis — infection of malignancy
- Focal neurological signs including nerve root irritation, loss of bowel/bladder control — nerve root/spinal cord compression
- Associated weight loss, systemic malaise — malignancy.

Exercise 11

Answer the following questions. Prepare short talks and/or dialogues on these topics

1. Describe musculoskeletal disorders.

2.   What are clinical features of in-toeing in children?
3.   Give information about talipes equinovarus (club foot).
4.   What is meant by growing pains (the painful limb, knee, and back)?
5.   Speak about presentation and treatment of osteomyelitis.
6.   What can you say about back pain?

Translation 4

1. Variation of normal posture may be noticed by parents or on routine developmental surveillance. 2. If severe, progressive, painful, functionally limiting or asymmetrical, they should be referred for a specialist opinion. 3. Metatarsus varus occurs in infants, is passively correctable, heel is held in the normal position. 4. Medial tibial torsion occurs in toddlers, and may be associated with bowing of the tibiae, and persistent anteversion of the femoral neck. 5. It presents in childhood, and may be associated with hypermobility of the joints. 6. Children sit between their feet with the hips fully internally rotated (W sitting). 7. Talipes equinovarus (club foot) is a complex abnormality. 8. The entire foot is inverted and supinated, the forefoot adducted and the heel is located inwards and in plantar flexion. 9. Treatment is started promptly with plaster casting and bracing, which may be required for many months.

Exercise 12
Match the column A with the column B. Try to learn the expressions and/or sentences by heart.

A

1.   Episodes of generalized pain in the lower limbs, …
2.   Features are: pain symmetrical in lower limbs …
3.   In osteomyelitis, …
4.   The skin is swollen directly …
5.   Blood cultures are usually positive …
6.   Prompt treatment with parenteral antibiotics …
7.   The affected limb is initially rested …
8.   Back pain is a symptom of concern …
9.   There may be muscle spasm or soft tissue pain …

B

a.   … *in the very young and preadolescent ages.*
b.   … *referred as 'growing pains' are common in preschool and school-aged children.*

c.   ... *is required for several weeks to prevent bone necrosis, chronic infection, limb deformity and amyloidosis.*
d.   ... *there is infection of the metaphysis of long bone.*
e.   ... *pain is never present after waking, physical activities are not limited, and there is no limp.*
f.   ... *from injury or from poor posture or abnormal loading.*
g.   ... *and the white blood count and acute-phase reactants are raised.*
h.   ... *over the affected site.*
i.   ... *in a splint and subsequently mobilized.*

Exercise 13
Fill in the missing words. Choose the correct ones.

1. It may be the site of _____ tumours or _____.	a metastases b primary
2. Spinal cord or nerve root _____ from tumour or _____ _____ _____ is often associated with trauma or _____ _____.	a heavy lifting b prolapsed intervertebral disc c entrapment
3. _____ disease may present with a fixed _____ _____.	a thoracic kyphosis b Scheuermann
4. In _____/spondylolisthesis there is increased risks with certain sporting activities, e.g. _____.	a bowling b spondylosis
5. Complex _____ _____ syndrome (CRPS) is diagnosed when no physical cause __ _____, it may __ _____ by psychological stress.	a be exacerbated b is found c regional pain
6. _____ _____ of back pain are:_____ ___, high fever, night waking, _____ _____	a painful scoliosis b Clinical features c young age

7. _____ _____ _____ include nerve root irritation, loss of _____/_____ _____, nerve root/spinal cord _____, associated weight loss, systemic _____, malignancy.	a malaise
	b bowel/bladder control
	c Focal neurological signs
	d compression

Text 5
Limp

The limp can be divided into acute painful limp and chronic or intermittent limp, where pain may or may not be the presenting feature.

Causes of limp pain

Age 1-3 years

Acute painful limp	Chronic and intermittent limp
Infection — septic arthritis, osteomyelitis of hip or spine Transient synovitis Trauma — accidental/non-accidental Malignant disease — leukaemia, neuroblastoma	Developmental dysplasia of the hip (DDH), talipes Neuromuscular, e.g. cerebral palsy Juvenile idiopathic arthritis (JIA)

Age 3-10 years

Acute painful limp	Chronic and intermittent limp
Transient synovitis Septic arthritis/osteomyelitis Trauma and overuse injuries Perthes disease (acute) Juvenile idiopathic arthritis (JIA) Malignant disease, e.g. leukaemia Complex regional pain syndrome	Perthes disease (chronic) Neuromuscular disorder, e.g. Duchenne muscular dystrophy Juvenile idiopathic arthritis (JIA) Tarsal coalition

Age 11-16 years

Acute painful limp	Chronic and intermittent limp
Mechanical — trauma, overuse injuries, sport injuries Slipped capital femoral epiphysis (acute) Avascular necrosis of the femoral head Reactive arthritis Juvenile idiopathic arthritis (JIA) Septic arthritis/osteomyelitis Osteochondritis dissecans of the knee Bone tumours and malignancy Complex regional pain syndrome	Slipped capital femoral epiphysis (chronic) Juvenile idiopathic arthritis (JIA) Tarsal coalition

Contrast in clinical features of transient synovitis and septic arthritis of the hips

	Transient synovitis	Septic arthritis
Onset	Acute limp, non-weight bearing	Acute onset, non-weight bearing
Fever	Mild/absent	Moderate/high
Child's appearance	Child often looks well	Child looks ill
Hip movement	Comfortable at rest, limited internal rotation and pain on movement	Hip held flexed; severe pain **at rest** and worse on any attempt to move joint
White cell count	Normal	Normal/high
Acute-phase reactant/ESR	Slight increased/normal	Raised
Ultrasound	Fluid in joint	Fluid in joint
Radiograph	Normal	Normal/widened joint space
Management	Rest, analgesia	Joint aspiration, usually under ultrasound guidance Prolonged antibiotics, rest and analgesia
Course	Resolves<1 week, approx. 3% develops Perthes disease	Progressive and severe joint damage if not treated

Exercise 14
Study the following summary and then interpret basic information in English.

1. Variations of musculoskeletal normality and differential diagnosis Perceived disorder Bow legs Normal age range 1-3 years Differential diagnosis to consider Rickets, osteogenesis imperfecta, Blount disease
Perceived disorder Knock-knees 2 years Normal age range -7 years Differential diagnosis to consider Juvenile idiopathic arthritis (JIA)
Perceived disorder Flat feet Normal age range 1-2 years Differential diagnosis to consider congenital tarsal fusion, hypermobility
Perceived disorder In-toeing Normal age range 1-2 years Differential diagnosis to consider Tibial torsion, femoral anteversion

Perceived disorder Toe walking Normal age range 1-3 years Differential diagnosis to consider: Spastic diplegia, muscular dystrophy, JIA, mucopolysaccharidosis
2. Regarding talipes equinovarus: needs to be differentiated from positional talipes.
Check for neuromuscular disorder or spinal lesion and for developmental dysplasia of the hip (DDH)
Early plaster casting and bracing usually avoids the need for surgery, and is being adopted world-wide.
3. Osteomyelitis presents with fever, a painful, immobile limb, swelling and extreme tenderness, especially on moving the limb.
Blood cultures are usually positive.
Parenteral antibiotics must be given immediately.
Surgical drainage if unresponsive to antibiotic therapy.
4. Regarding hip disorders:
Developmental dysplasia of the hip (DDH) - identified on screening at birth or 8 weeks, detection of asymmetry of skinfolds around the hip. Limited abduction of the hip, shortening of the affected leg, or a limp or abnormal gait.
Transient synovitis – most common cause of acute hip pain or a limp; must be differentiated from septic arthritis.
Perthes disease – usually school-aged children with hip pain or limp.
Slipped capital femoral epiphysis – adolescent with a limp or hip pain.

Arthritis

Acute arthritis presents with pain, swelling, heat, redness and restricted movement in a joint. In a monoarthritis of acute onset, the child is also likely to be systemically unwell with fever; if septic arthritis or osteomyelitis is the cause, urgent diagnosis and treatment is required. With infection, more than one joint can be affected.

Causes of polyarthritis

Infection	Bacterial — septicaemia/septic arthritis, TB Viral — rubella, mumps, adenovirus, coxsackie B, herpes, hepatitis, parvovirus Other — Mycoplasma, Lyme disease, rickettsia Reactive — gastrointestinal infection, streptococcal infection Rheumatic fever
Inflammatory bowel disease	Henoch-Schönlein purpura, Kawasaki disease
Vasculitis	Crohn's disease, ulcerative colitis
Haematological disorders	Haemophilia, sickle cell disease

Malignant disorders	Leukaemia, neuroblastoma
Connective tissue disorders	Juvenile idiopathic arthritis (JIA), systemic lupus erythematosus (SLE), dermatomyositis, mixed connective tissue disease (MCDT), polyarteritis nodosa (PAN)
Other	Cystic fibrosa

Early treatment of septic arthritis is essential to prevent destruction of the articular cartilage and bone. If JIA is suspected, even if joint abnormality is not clear, referral to paediatric rheumatology is indicated as early treatment radically improves outcome.

Exercise 15
Study the following summary and then interpret basic information in English.

Diagnostic clues regarding musculoskeletal disorders
Genetic skeletal conditions

'Typical' symptom combinations	Pivotal clinical features	Possible diagnoses
Nocturnal wakening with leg pain	Normal child anaemia, bruising, irritability, infections	'Growing pains' Osteoid osteoma Leukaemia, lymphoma, neuroblastoma (young child)
'Clunk' on hip movement on neonatal and early infant screening, limp in an older infant	Older infant: asymmetrical upper leg skin folds, limited hip abduction	Developmental dysplasia of the hip (DDH)
Febrile, toxic-looking infant, irritability with nappy changing	Restricted joint range (especially hip) or limb movement	Septic arthritis Osteomyelitis
Sudden limp in an otherwise well young child	Unilateral restricted hip movement	Transient synovitis of the hip Perthes disease
Fever, erythematous rash, red eyes, irritability in infant or young child	Erythema/oedema of hands and feet, oral mucositis, cervical lymphadenopathy	Kawasaki disease
Irritability, fever, reluctance to move in an infant or young child	Stiff back, 'tripod' sitting	Discitis Vertebral osteomyelitis

Joint pain, stiffness, and restriction Loss of joint function	Persistent joint swelling Loss of joint range	Juvenile idiopathic arthritis
Hip pain in an obese adolescent boy	Unilateral hip restriction	Slipped capital femoral epiphysis
Lethargy, unwilling to do physical activities, irritability, rash	Eye lid erythema proximal muscle weakness	Juvenile dermatomyositis
Constitutional symptoms, lethargy, arthralgia in an adolescent female	Multisystem abnormalities, haematuria, facial erythema	Systemic lupus erythematosus

These are inherited abnormalities resulting in generalized developmental disorders of the bone, of which there are several hundred types. They usually result in reduced growth and abnormality of bone shape. The bones of the limbs and spine are often affected, resulting in short stature. Intelligence is usually normal.

Exercise 16
Answer the following questions. Prepare short talks and/or dialogues on these topics

1. What are causes of limp pain?
2. Characterize contrast in clinical features of transient synovitis and septic arthritis of the hips.
3. How does acute arthritis present?
4. What are causes of polyarthritis?
5. What can you say about genetic skeletal conditions?

Translation 5
1. The limp can be divided into acute painful limp and chronic or intermittent limp. 2. Causes of acute painful limp are: infection, transient synovitis, septic arthritis, osteomyelitis of hip or spine, trauma, malignant disease, transient synovitis, overuse injuries, Perthes disease, and juvenile idiopathic arthritis. 3. Complex regional pain syndrome includes: trauma, overuse injuries, sport injuries, slipped capital femoral epiphysis, avascular necrosis of the femoral head, reactive arthritis, juvenile idiopathic arthritis (JIA), osteochondritis, dissecans of the knee, bone tumours and malignancy, and complex regional pain syndrome. 4. Causes of chronic and intermittent limp are: developmental dysplasia of the hip (DDH), talipes, cerebral palsy, juvenile idiopathic arthritis (JIA), Perthes disease, Duchenne muscular dystrophy, tarsal coalition, slipped capital femoral epiphysis, tarsal coalition.

Exercise 17
Study the following summary and then interpret basic information in English.

1. Clinical features of transient synovitis are: acute limp, non-weight bearing, mild/absent fever, child often looks well, hip movement is comfortable at rest, with limited internal rotation and pain on movement, normal white cell count, acute-phase reactant/ESR slight, increased/normal, ultrasound shows fluid in joint, radiograph is normal, management includes rest, analgesia, disease resolves <1 week, approx. 3% develops Perthes disease.
2. Clinical features of septic arthritis of the hips are: acute onset, non-weight bearing, moderate/high fever, child looks ill, hip held flexed, severe pain at rest and worse on any attempt to move joint, white cell count is normal/high, raised acute-phase reactant/ESR, ultrasound shows fluid in joint, normal radiograph, widened joint space, management consists of joint aspiration, usually under ultrasound guidance and prolonged antibiotics, rest and analgesia, course is progressive and severe joint damage follows if not treated.

Exercise 18
Fill in the missing words. Choose the correct ones.

1. Acute arthritis presents with pain, _____, heat, _____ and _____ _____ in a joint.	a restricted movement b redness c swelling
2. In a monoarthritis of _____ _____, the child is also likely to be systemically _____ with fever.	a acute onset b unwell
3. If _____ _____ or _____ is the cause, _____ diagnosis and treatment is required.	a urgent b septic arthritis c osteomyelitis
4. Causes of polyarthritis are: infection, _____ _____ _____, vasculitis, _____ disorders, malignant disorders, and _____ _____ disorders.	a connective tissue b haematological c inflammatory bowel disease
5. Early treatment of _____ _____ is essential to prevent _____ _____ destruction of the and bone.	a septic arthritis b articular cartilage

6. Genetic _____ conditions are _____ _____ resulting in _____ developmental disorders of the bone.	a generalized b skeletal c inherited abnormalities
7. They usually result in _____ _____ and abnormality of _____ _____.	a bone shape b reduced growth
8. The bones of the _____ ___ _____ are often affected, resulting in _____ _____.	a limbs and spine b short stature

Key 9
Exercise 3
1 c, b, a; 2 c, b, a; 3 c, b, a; 4 c, a, b; 5 c, a, b; 6 c, b, a; 7 b, a, c

Exercise 7
1 d, b, c, a; 2 b, a; 3 c, a, b; 4 b, a, c

Exercise 10
1a; 2d; 3c; 4b

Exercise 12
1b; 2e; 3d; 4h; 5g; 6c; 7i; 8a; 9f

Exercise 13
1 b, a; 2 c, b, a; 3 b, a; 4 b, a; 5 c, b, a; 6 b, c, a; 7 c, b, d, a

Exercise 18
1 c, b, a; 2 a, b; 3 b, c, a; 4 c, b, a; 5 a, b; 6 b, c, a; 7 b, a; 8 a, b

VOCABULARY 9

abduction /æbˈdʌk.ʃən/
acetone /ˈæs.ɪ.təʊn/
adduct /ædˈdʌkt/
adenovirus /ˈæd.ɪ.nəʊˌvaɪə.rəs/
Adison disease /æd.ə.sən dɪˈziːz/
adjust /əˈdʒʌst/
adopt /əˈdɒpt/
amyloidosis /ˌa.məl.ɔːˌi.ˈdəʊ.sɪs/
analogue /ˈænəˌlɒg/
androgen /ænˈdrɒ.dʒən/
angle /ˈæŋgəl/
antagonise /ænˈtægəˌnaɪz/
anteversion /ænˈtɪ.vɜːˌʃən/
anticipate /ænˈtɪs.ɪ.peɪt/
Beckwith /ˈbek.wəth/ **syndrome** /ˈsɪn.drəʊm/
biosynthesis /ˌbaɪ.əʊ.ˈsɪn.θə.sɪs/
Blount /blunt/ **disease** /dɪˈziːz/
bowing /ˈbəʊɪŋ/
bowling /ˈbəʊlɪŋ/
bracing /ˈbreɪ.sɪŋ/
bruit /bruːt/
calcium /ˈkæl.si.əm/ **gluconate** /ˈgluː.kəˌneɪt/
capital /ˈkæpɪtəl/
cartilage /ˈkɑː.təl.ɪdʒ/
cartridge /ˈkɑː.trɪdʒ/
cast /kɑːst/
club foot /klʌb.fʊt/
clunk /klʌŋk/
coalition /ˌkəʊəˈlɪʃən/
coarse /kɔːs/
consciousness /ˈkɒnˌʃəs.nəs/
correctable /kəˈrekt.ə.bl̩/
cross-country /ˈkrɒsˌkʌntrɪ/ **running** /ˈrʌnɪŋ/
dermatomyositis /ˌdər.mə.təʊˌmaɪ.ə.ˈsaɪ.təs/
deterioration /dɪˌtɪə.ri.əˈreɪ.ʃən/
dip /dɪp/
discitis /dɪsˈkaɪ.tɪs/
dishormonogenesis /dɪs.hɔːˈməʊ.nəˈdʒen.ə.sɪs/
dysplasia /dɪsˈpleɪzɪə/
dizzy /ˈdɪzɪ/
drop /drɒp/
Duchenne /dɑːˌˈʃen/ **muscular** /ˈmə.skjə.lər/ **dystrophy** /ˈdi.strə.fiː/
entrapment /ɪnˈtræp.mənt/
epiphysis /əˈpɪf.ɪ.sɪs/
erosion /ɪˈrəʊ.ʒən/

error /ˈer.ər/
excitement /ɪkˈsaɪt.mənt/
exogenous /ekˈsɑdʒ.ə.nəs/
facies /ˈfeɪˌʃiˌiːz/
faint /feɪnt/
forefoot /ˈfɔːˌfʊt/
frightening /ˈfraɪtnɪŋ/
glucocorticoid /gluːkəˈkɔːtɪ.kɒ.ɪd/
glucose /ˈgluːkəʊz/ **meter** /ˈmiːtə/
haematuria /hiːˌməˈtjʊə.rɪ.ə/
hiking /ˈhaɪ.kɪŋ/
hirsutism /ˈhər.sə.ˌti.zəm/
hyperinsulinemia /ˌhaɪ.pə.ˌrin.sə.ləˈniː.miː.ə/
hypermobility /ˌhaɪ.pə.ˌməʊ.ˈbi.lə.tiː/
hyperparathyroidism /ˌhaɪ.pə.ˌpær.əˈθaɪ.rɔɪd.ɪsm/
hypothalamus /ˌhaɪ.pəʊˈθæl.ə.məs/
infrequent /ɪnˈfriː.kwənt/
interference /ˌɪn.təˈfɪə.rəns/
internally /ɪnˈtɜːnəlɪ/
intervertebral /ˌɪn.tɜːrˈvɜː.tɪ.brəl/ **disc** /dɪsk/
in-toeing /ˈin.ˈtəʊ.ɪŋ/
iodine /ˈaɪ.ə.diːn/
juvenile /ˈdʒuːvɪˌnaɪl/ **idiopathic** /ˌɪd.i.əˈpæθ.ɪk/ **arthritis** /ɑːˈθraɪ.tɪs/
ketotic /kiːˈtɑː.tik/ **hypoglycaemia** /ˌhaɪ.pəʊ.glaɪˈsiː.mi.ə/
Kussmaul /ˈkus.ˌmaul/ **breathing** /ˈbriːðɪŋ/
kyphosis /kaɪˈfəʊ.sɪs/
Legg-Calvé-Perthes /ˈleg.ˌkal.ˈveɪ.ˈpər.ˌtiːz/ **disease** /dɪˈziːz/
leucine /ˈlʊ.ˌsiːn/
licence /ˈlaɪ.sᵊns/
lid /lɪd/
limiting /ˈlɪm.ɪ.tɪŋ/
lipoatrophy /ˈlaɪ.ˌpəʊ.ˈa.trə.fiː/
lipohypertrophy /ˈlaɪ.ˌpəʊ.haɪˈpɜː.trə.fi/
load /ləʊd/
macrovascular /ˈmækrəʊ.væskjʊlə/
maldescent /mæl dɪˈsent/
maturity /məˈtjʊə.rɪ.ti/
measurement /ˈmeʒ.ə.mənt/
metacarpal /ˌmet.əˈkɑː.pəl/
metaphysis /ˌmə.ˈtaf.ə.səs/
metatarsus /ˌmet.əˈtɑː.səs/
microalbuminuria /ˈmaɪ.krəʊ.al.ˌbjʊ.mə.ˈnjʊər.ɪ.ə/
mineralocorticoids /ˌmɪn.ə.rəl.əˈkɔː.tɪ.kɒ.ɪdz/
monoarthritis /ˌmɒn.əʊ.ɑːˈθraɪ.tɪs/
muscular dystrophy /ˌmʌs.kjʊ.ləˈdɪs.trə.fi/
non-weight /ˌnɒnˈweɪt/
occur /əˈkɜː/

ophthalmoplegia /ˌɒf.θælˈmɒ ˈpliː.dʒiː..ə/
osteoblast /ˈɒstɪəʊˌblæst/
osteochondritis /ˌɒstɪ.əˌkɑːn.ˈdraɪt.əs/
osteogenesis /ˌɒstɪəˈdʒen.ə.sɪs/ **imperfecta** /ˌim.pər.ˈfek.tə/
osteoid /ˌɒstɪˌɔid/
osteoma /ˌɒstɪ.ˈəʊ.mə/
osteotomy /ˌɒstɪˈɒtəmɪ/
overuse /ˌəʊ.vəˈjuːz/
overview /ˈəʊ.və.vjuː/
Perthes /ˈper.ðez/ **disease** /dɪˈziːz/
phalanx /fælæŋks/ pl **phalanges**
pick /ˈpɪk/ **up** /ʌp/
pinch /pɪntʃ/
pituitary /pəˈtʊ.əˌter.i:/ **stalk** /ˈstɔːk/
pituitary gland /pɪˈtjuː.ɪ.tər.iˌglænd/
pivotal /ˈpɪvətəl/
plaster /ˈplɑː.stər/
precocious /prɪˈkəʊˌʃəs/
prolapsed /prəʊˈlæpst/
puffy /ˈpʌf.i/
radiograph /ˈreɪ.di.əˌgrɑːf/
read /riːd/ **out** /aʊt/
rest /rest/
restricted /rɪˈstrɪk.tɪd/
Rickettsiae /rɪˈkɛt.si.ə/
rotate /rəʊ ˈteɪt/
saline /ˈseɪ.laɪn/
Scheuermann /ʃojer.maen/ **disease** /dɪˈziːz/
self-reliant /ˌself rɪˈlaɪ.ənt/
septicaemia /ˌsep.tɪˈsiː.mi.ə/
septo-optic /ˌsep.təʊ.opˈtik/
shortening /ˈʃɔːtənɪŋ/
skinfold /ˈskinˌfəʊld/
slip /slɪp/
splint /splɪnt/
spondylolisthesis /spɒnˈdl.əʊ.lɪs.thiːˈ.sɪs/
spondylosis /ˌspɒn.dɪˈləʊ.sɪs/
supinate /ˈsuː.pɪn.eɪt/
sweatiness /ˈswe.tiː.nəs/
synovitis /saɪˈnəʊ.vaɪ.tɪs/
tarsus /ˈtɑː.səs/ pl **tarsi** /ˈtɑːr.ˌsaɪ/
tibia /ˈtɪb.i.ə/ pl **tibiae**
tibial /ˈtɪb.i.əl/
torsion /ˈtɔː.ʃən/
toxoplasma /ˌtɒksəʊˈplæzmə/
traction /ˈtrækˌʃən/
transglutaminase /tranzˈgluːtə.ˈmɪn.eɪs/

tripod /ˈtraɪ.pɒd/
tubular /ˈtjuː.bjʊ.lər/
ulceration /ˌʌl.sərˈeɪ.ʃən/
unreliable /ˌʌn.rɪˈlaɪə.bḷ/
unresponsive /ˌʌn.rɪˈspɒnt.sɪv/
unsteadiness /ʌnˈsted.i.nəs/
varus /ˈveə.rəs/
vasodilator /ˌveɪ.zəʊ.daɪˈleɪ.tər/
ventriculoperitoneal /venˌtrik.jə.ləʊ ˌper.ɪ.təˈni.əl/ **shunt** /ˈʃənt/
vertebral /ˈvɜː.tɪ.brə/
virilization /ˌvɪrɪlaɪˈzeɪʃən/
virology /vaɪˈrɒl.ə.dʒɪ/
vocational /vəʊˈkeɪ.ʃə.nəl/
volvulus /ˈvɒlvjʊləs/
weakness /ˈwiːk.nəs/
wheeze /wiːz/
whooping cough /ˈhuː.pɪŋ ˌkɒf/
widen /ˈwaɪ.dən/
wobbly /ˈwɒblɪ/
yeast /jiːst/

Neurological disorders; Causes of paroxysmal disorders; Motor disorders; The neurocutaneous syndromes; Adolescent medicine; Talking and listening with young people; Impact of chronic conditions; Health-risk behaviour

Text 1
Features of neurological disorders in children are:
- recurrent headaches caused by migraine and tension-type headaches
- febrile seizures
- epilepsy
- epilepsy syndromes, e.g. infantile spasms at 4-6 months, childhood absence epilepsy at 4-12 years
- motor disorders
- neural tube defects

The central nervous system comprises 100 000 million neurones and when it malfunctions it has the potential to operate a wide spectrum of clinical problems. These may involve impaired movement, vision, hearing, sensory perception, learning, memory, consciousness or sleep.

Headache
- Primary headaches: four main groups, comprising migraine, tension-type headache, cluster headache, and other primary headaches.
- Secondary headaches: underlying pathology e.g. from raised intracranial pressure or space-occupying lesions
- Trigeminal and other cranial neuralgias including root pain from herpes zoster

The classification of headache disorders
Primary headaches
- Migraine
- Tension-type headache
- Cluster headache and other trigeminal autonomic cephalalgias
- Other primary headaches

Secondary headaches
Headache attributed to:
- Medication overuse headache
- Head and/or neck trauma
- Cranial or cervical vascular disorder — vascular malformation or intracranial haemorrhage
- Non-vascular intracranial disorder — raised intracranial pressure, idiopathic intracranial hypertension
- A substance or its withdrawal — alcohol, solvent or drug abuse
- Infection — meningitis, encephalitis, abscess
- Disorder of homeostasis — hypercapnia or hypertension
- Disorder of facial or cranial structures — acute sinusitis
- Associated with emotional disorders
- Cranial neuralgias, central and primary facial pain, and other headaches
- Trigeminal and other cranial neuralgias and central causes of facial pain
- Other headaches

Headache type
- Tension-type headache — constriction band.
- Migraine without aura — bilateral or unilateral, pulsatile, gastrointestinal disturbance, e.g. nausea, vomiting, abdominal pain, photophobia. Lies in quiet, dark place. Relieved by sleep.
- Migraine with aura — preceded by aura (visual, sensory or motor), premonitory symptoms.
- Mixed-type headaches — common
- Red flag symptoms — space-occupying lesion
- Headache — worse lying down or with coughing and straining
- Headache — wakes up child (different from headache on awakening, not uncommon in migraine)
- Associated confusion, and/or morning or persistent nausea or vomiting
- Recent change in personality, behaviour or educational performance.

Red flag physical signs — space-occupying lesion
- Growth failure
- Visual field defects — craniopharyngioma
- Squint
- Cranial nerve abnormality

- Torticollis
- Abnormal coordination — for cerebellar lesions
- Gait — upper motor neurone or cerebellar signs
- Fundi-papilledema
- Bradycardia
- Cranial bruits — arteriovenous malformation

Other physical signs
- Visual acuity — for refractive errors
- Sinus tenderness — for sinusitis
- Pain on chewing — temporomandibular joint malocclusion
- Blood pressure — for hypertension

Seizures
A seizure is a paroxysmal abnormality of motor, sensory, autonomic, and/or cognitive function, due to transient brain dysfunction. The term includes epileptic, syncopal (anoxic), brainstem (hydrocephalic, coning), emotional or functional (psychogenic pseudo-seizures).

Causes of seizures
Epilepsies

Genetic (70-80%) — also called 'idiopathic', caused by alleles at several loci together rather than a single gene, so inheritance is 'complex'
- Structural, metabolic
- Cerebral dysgenesis/malformation
- Cerebral vascular occlusion
- Cerebral damage, e.g. congenital infection, hypoxic-ischaemic encephalopathy, intraventricular haemorrhage/ischaemia
- Cerebral tumour
- Neurodegenerative disorders
- Neurocutaneous syndromes
- Tuberous sclerosis

Acute symptomatic seizures
- Due to any **cortical** brain injury or insult, at the time of the trauma or illness
- Stroke, traumatic brain injury, intracranial infection
- Hypoglycaemia, hypocalcaemia, hypomagnesaemia, hyponatraemia/hypernatremia
- Poison/toxins
- Febrile seizures

- Non-epileptic seizures
- Convulsive syncope
- Cardiac syncope e.g. prolonged Q-T syndrome
- Neurally mediated syncope: cardio-inhibitory e.g. reflex asystolic syncope (reflex anoxic seizures); vasodepressor or mixed (vasovagal syncope)
- Expiratory apnoea syncope ('blue breath-holding spells')
- Hypovolaemic syncope e.g. with haemorrhage, dehydration or anaphylaxis
- Sudden rise in intracranial pressure e.g. hydrocephalic attack, haemorrhage
- Sleep disorders e.g. benign neonatal sleep myoclonus, hypnic jerks
- Functional/medically unexplained e.g. dissociative states

Exercise 1
Answer the following questions. Prepare short talks and/or dialogues on these topics

1. What do you know about features of neurological disorders in children?
2. Speak about the classification of headache disorders.
3. Characterize types of headache.
4. What are causes of seizures?
5. Describe acute symptomatic seizures.

Translation 1

1. Features of neurological disorders in children are: recurrent headaches, febrile seizures, epilepsy syndromes, motor disorders, and neural tube defects. 2. Clinical problems may involve: impaired movement, vision, hearing, sensory perception, learning, memory, consciousness or sleep. 3. Primary headaches include: migraine, tension-type headache, cluster headache, trigeminal, and autonomic cephalalgias. 4. Secondary headaches are attributed to: medication overuse, head and/or neck trauma, vascular malformation or intracranial haemorrhage, cranial or cervical vascular disorder, raised intracranial pressure, intracranial hypertension, alcohol, solvent or drug abuse, meningitis, encephalitis, abscess, hypercapnia or hypertension, acute sinusitis, cranial neuralgias, facial pain, trigeminal and other cranial neuralgias. 5. Types of headache are: tension-type, migraine, mixed-type. 6. Red flag symptoms are: headache, confusion, and/or morning or persistent nausea or vomiting, change in personality, behaviour or educational performance. 7. Red flag physical signs are: growth failure,

craniopharyngioma, squint, cranial nerve abnormality, torticollis, abnormal coordination, gait, fundi-papilledema, bradycardia, cranial bruits. 8. Other physical signs include: visual acuity, sinus tenderness, pain on chewing, blood pressure. 9. The term includes: epileptic, syncopal, brainstem, emotional or functional seizure.

Exercise 2
Study the following summary and then interpret basic information in English.

1. A seizure is a paroxysmal abnormality of motor, sensory, autonomic, and/or cognitive function, due to transient brain dysfunction.
2. Causes of seizures are: genetic, structural, metabolic, cerebral dysgenesis, malformation, cerebral vascular occlusion, cerebral damage, cerebral tumour, neurodegenerative disorders, neurocutaneous syndromes, tuberous sclerosis, congenital infection, hypoxic-ischaemic encephalopathy, intraventricular haemorrhage/ischaemia.
3. Acute symptomatic seizures appear due to any cortical brain injury or insult, stroke, hypoglycaemia, hypocalcaemia, hypomagnesaemia, hyponatraemia, hypernatremia, traumatic brain injury, intracranial infection, and poison, toxins.
4. Non-epileptic seizures include: convulsive syncope, cardiac syncope, neuronally mediated syncope, expiratory apnoea syncope, hypovolaemic syncope, sudden rise in intracranial pressure, and sleep disorders.

Text 2
Causes of paroxysmal disorders ('funny turns')
Temper
Blue 'breath-holding' spells ⇒

Occur in some toddlers when they are upset. The child cries, holds his breath in expiration and goes blue. Sometimes children will briefly lose consciousness but rapidly recover fully. Drug therapy is unhelpful. Attacks resolve spontaneously, but behaviour modification therapy with distraction may help.

Head trauma, cold food, fright, fever
Reflex asystolic syncope ⇒

Also called reflex anoxic seizures. Occur in infants or toddlers. Many have a first-degree relative with a history of faints. Commonest triggers are pain or discomfort, particularly from minor head trauma, cold food (such as ice-cream or cold drinks), fright or fever. Some children with febrile seizures may have experienced this phenomenon. After the triggering event, the child becomes very pale and falls to the floor. The hypoxia may induce a generalised tonic-clonic seizure. The episodes are due to cardiac asystole from vagal inhibition. The seizure is brief and the child rapidly recovers. Ocular compression under controlled conditions often leads to asystole and paroxysmal slow-wave discharge on the EEG.

Syncope (transient loss of consciousness) ⇒
Children may faint if in a hot and stuffy environment, on standing for long periods, or from fear. Clonic movements lasting a few seconds are common.

Migraine ⇒
May sometimes lead to paroxysmal headache involving unsteadiness or light-headedness as well as the more common visual or gastrointestinal disturbance. In some young people these episodes occur without headache.

Benign paroxysmal vertigo ⇒
This is characterised by recurrent episodes of vertigo, lasting from one to several minutes, associated with nystagmus, unsteadiness or even falling. It is a primary headache disorder of childhood occasionally due to a viral labyrinthitis.

Other causes ⇒
- Cardiac arrhythmia — prolonged QT interval may rarely cause collapse or cardiac syncope which may be related to exercise.
- Tics, daydreaming, night terrors
- Self-gratification — young children may stimulate their genitalia in order to achieve a feeling of comfort rather than sexual gratification.
- Non-epileptic attack disorder (NEAD)/functional seizures/medically unexplained seizures/dissociative states
- Pseudo-seizures — when children feign seizures
- Fabricated — seizures are fabricated by parents
- Induced illness (nonaccidental injury) — e.g. seizures from hypoglycaemia from an adult deliberately injecting insulin
- Paroxysmal movement disorders — well-circumscribed episodes. Genetically determined, no loss of consciousness.

Epilepsies of childhood
Epileptic seizure types
Generalised seizures
Onset in both hemisphere
In generalised seizures, there is:
- loss of consciousness if > 3 seconds duration

- no warning
- symmetrical seizure
- bilaterally synchronous seizure discharge on EEG

Absence seizures ⇒

Transient loss of consciousness, with an abrupt onset and termination, unaccompanied by motor phenomena except for some flickering of the eyelids and minor alteration in muscle tone. Absences can often be precipitated by hyperventilation

Myoclonic seizures ⇒

Brief, often repetitive, jerking movements of the limbs, neck or trunk

Non-epileptic myoclonic movements are also seen psychologically in hiccoughs (myoclonus of the diaphragm) or on passing through stage II sleep (sleep myoclonus)

Tonic seizures ⇒

Generalized increase in tone

Tonic-clonic seizures ⇒

Rhythmical contraction of muscle groups following the tonic phase.

In the rigid tonic phase, children may fall to the ground, sometimes injuring themselves. They do not breathe and become cyanosed. This is followed by the clonic phase, with jerking of the limbs. Breathing is irregular, cyanosis persists and saliva may accumulate in the mouth. There may be biting of the tongue and incontinence of urine. The seizure usually lasts from a few seconds to minutes, followed by unconsciousness or deep sleep for up to several hours.

Atonic seizures ⇒

Often combined with a myoclonic jerk, followed by transient loss of muscle tone causing a sudden fall to the floor or drop of the head.

Focal seizures

Onset in neural network limited to one cerebral hemisphere
Focal seizures:

- originate in a relatively small group of dysfunctional neurones in one of the cerebral hemispheres

- may be heralded by an aura (the sensory symptoms) which reflects the site of origin
- may or may not be associated with change of consciousness or evolve to generalized tonic-clonic seizure

Focal seizures ⇒
- Frontal seizures — motor phenomena
- Temporal lobe seizures — auditory or sensory (smell or taste) phenomena
- Occipital — positive or negative visual phenomena
- Parietal lobe seizures — contralateral altered sensation (dysesthesia)

Management

Management begins with diagnosis, but it is often uncertain initially. Once diagnosed, a clear explanation of the diagnosis and advice to help adjustment to the condition is needed. A specialist epilepsy nurse may assist families by providing education and continuing advice on lifestyle issues.

Exercise 3
Study the following summary and then interpret basic information in English.

1. Headaches
Headaches history
Premonitory symptoms, aura, character, position, radiation, frequency, duration, triggers, relieving and exacerbating factors?
Special consideration:
Triggers – stress, relaxation, food, menstruation?
Emotional or behavioural problems at home or school?
Vision checked – refractive error?
Head trauma?
Alcohol, solvent, or drug abuse?
Analgesia over-use?
2. Febrile seizures
Affect 3% of children; have a genetic predisposition.
Occur between 6 months and 6 years of age.
Are usually brief, generalized tonic-clonic seizures occurring with a rapid rise in fever.
If a bacterial infection, especially meningitis is present, it needs to be identified and treated.
Advise family about management of seizures, consider rescue therapy.

| If simple – does not affect intellectual performance. |
| If complex, 4-12% risk of subsequent epilepsy. |
| **3. Epilepsy** |
| Affects 1 in 200 children. |
| Classified according to seizure type, epilepsy type, and underlying aetiology. |
| An inter-ictal EEG is performed whenever an epilepsy is diagnosed to help categorize the epilepsy type |
| Antiepileptic drug therapy should be considered where the seizures are intrusive, and selected according to seizure and epilepsy type. |
| Requires liaison with the school about how to manage seizure and avoiding situations which could lead to injury |

Exercise 4

Answer the following questions. Prepare short talks and/or dialogues on these topics

1. Describe causes of paroxysmal disorders (temper, head trauma, cold food, fright, fever, syncope, migraine, benign paroxysmal vertigo).
2. Characterize epilepsies of childhood.
3. Speak about absence seizures, myoclonic seizures, tonic seizures, tonic-clonic seizures, atonic seizures and focal seizures.

Translation 2

1. Blue 'breath-holding' spells occur in some toddlers when they are upset. 2. The child cries, holds his breath in expiration and goes blue. 3. Reflex asystolic syncope occur in infants or toddlers. 4. Commonest triggers are pain or discomfort, particularly from minor head trauma, cold food (such as ice-cream or cold drinks), fright or fever. 5. After the triggering event, the child becomes very pale and falls to the floor. 6. The episodes are due to cardiac asystole from vagal inhibition. 7. Children may faint if in a hot and stuffy environment, on standing for long periods, or from fear. 8. Migraine may sometimes lead to paroxysmal headache involving unsteadiness or light-headedness as well as the more common visual or gastrointestinal disturbance. 9. Benign paroxysmal vertigo is characterised by recurrent episodes of vertigo. 10. In generalised seizures there is: loss of consciousness, no warning, symmetrical seizure bilaterally, synchronous seizure. 11. Absence seizures are characterized by transient loss of consciousness with an abrupt onset and termination. 12. Myoclonic seizures contain brief, often repetitive, jerking movements of the limbs, neck or trunk. 13. Tonic seizures mean generalized increase in tone. 14. Tonic-clonic seizures include rhythmical contraction of muscle groups following the tonic phase.

Exercise 5
Fill in the missing words. Choose the correct ones.

1. Children ____ ____ to the ground, they __ ___ _____ and become _____.	a cyanosed b do not breathe c may fall
2. This __ _____ by the clonic phase, with _____ __ ___ _____.	a is followed b jerking of the limbs
3. Breathing is _____, cyanosis persists, saliva may _____ in the mouth and there may be _____ of the tongue and _____ of urine.	a accumulate b biting c incontinence d irregular
4. Atonic seizures are often _____ ____ a myoclonic jerk, followed by _____ loss of _____ ____ causing a sudden fall to the floor or ____ of the head.	a muscle tone b drop c transient d combined with
5. _____ _____ originate in a relatively small group of _____ neurones, may __ _____ by an aura and may or may not be associated with change of _____.	a be heralded b consciousness c dysfunctional d Focal seizures

Text 3
Motor disorders

Movement is governed by three main cerebral control centres. Patterns of information, modulated by afferent sensory information (joint position, crude touch, visual, auditory and vestibular), pass down the brainstem spinal cord, through synapse in the anterior horns and along peripheral nerves to the target muscles. The first question to ask when seeing a child with a motor disorder is whether this is a central or a peripheral nervous system disorder.

Causes of movement disorders

Corticospinal (pyramidal) tract disorders	Basal ganglia disorders	Cerebellar disorders
Cerebral dysgenesis, e.g. neuronal migration disorder Global hypoxia-ischaemia Antenatal ischemic stroke Cerebral tumour Acute disseminated encephalomyelitis	Acquired brain injury: Acute and profound hypoxia-ischaemia Carbon monoxide poisoning Post-cardiopulmonary bypass chorea Post-streptococcal chorea (rheumatic fever)	Acute – medication and drugs, including alcohol and solvent abuse Postviral – particularly varicella infection
Postictal paresis Hemiplegic migraine	Mitochondrial cytopathies Wilson disease Huntington disease Vitamin E deficiency Pontocerebellar hypoplasia	Posterior fossa lesions or tumours e.g. medulloblastoma Genetic and degenerative disorders, e.g. Friedrich ataxia and ataxia telangiectasia

Neuromuscular disorder

Disorders of the anterior horn cell	Spinal muscular atrophy Poliomyelitis
Disorders of the peripheral nerve	Hereditary motor sensory neuropathies Acute post-infectious polyneuropathy Bell palsy
Disorders of neuromuscular transmission	Myasthenia gravis
Muscle disorders	Muscle dystrophies Inflammatory myopathies Benign acute myositis Polymyositis/dermatomyositis Myotonic disorders Dystrophia myotonica Metabolic myopathies Congenital myopathies

Causes of a hypotonic 'floppy' infant

Central	Hypoxic-ischaemic encephalopathy Intracranial haemorrhage Cerebral malformations Chromosome/genetic Congenital infections: toxoplasma, rubella, cytomegalovirus, herpes Acquired infections Peroxisomal disorders Drug effects (e.g. benzodiazepines)

Spinal cord	Birth trauma (especially breech delivery) Syringomyelia
Anterior horn cell	Spinal muscular atrophy
Neuromuscular junction	Myasthenia gravis (transient/congenital) Infantile botulism
Muscle	Muscular dystrophies (e.g. congenital myotonic dystrophy) Congenital myopathies (e.g. central core disease)
Peripheral nerve	Hereditary motor and sensory neuropathies Inborn errors of metabolism
Metabolic myopathies	Carnitine deficiency

Causes of ataxia

- Friedrich ataxia
- Ataxia telangiectasia
- Cerebellar agenesis/dysgenesis
- Postinfectious cerebellitis – varicella
- Posterior fossa tumours
- Other hereditary cerebellar ataxia
- Miller Fisher syndrome (a variant of Guillain-Barré syndrome)
- Mitochondrial disease
- Drugs
- Toxins e.g. ethanol

Exercise 6
Study the following summary and then interpret basic information in English.

1. Intracranial haemorrhage
History of significant head injury — remember that an extradural haemorrhage may be present even if lucid afterwards.
Subdural haematoma and retinal haemorrhages in an infant — consider non-accidental injury caused by shaking or direct trauma
2. Strokes
Occur in infants and children
In infants, occur in the perinatal period, and may present in late infancy with a hemiplegia or with seizures.
In children, are seen in association with cardiac or sickle cell disease, following varicella infection or neck trauma. However, often no cause is evident.
3. Neural tube defects
Include anencephaly, encephalocele, spina bifida occulta, meningocele, and myelomeningocele.

| The birth prevalence has fallen owing to antenatal screening. |
| The birth prevalence is reduced by periconceptual folic acid. |
| Myelomeningoceles can cause paralysis of the legs, dislocation of the hip and talipes, sensory loss, neuropathic bladder and bowel, scoliosis and hydrocephalus. |

Hydrocephalus

In hydrocephalus, there is an accumulation of cerebrospinal fluid in the brain. In babies and children this can be congenital, associated with cerebral malformations, or obstruction to the flow of cerebrospinal fluid leading to dilatation of the ventricular system proximal to the site of obstruction

Causes of hydrocephalus

Non-communicating (obstruction in the ventricular system)
- Congenital malformation:
- Aqueduct stenosis
- Atresia of the outflow foramina of the fourth ventricle
- Chiari malformation (cerebellar tonsils herniation through foramen magnum)
- Posterior fossa neoplasm or vascular malformation
- Intraventricular haemorrhage in preterm infant

Communicating (failure to reabsorb CSF)
- Subarachnoid haemorrhage
- Meningitis, e.g. pneumococcal, tuberculous

Hydrocephalus
- In infants, presents with excessive increase in head circumference, separation of skull sutures, bulging of the anterior fontanelle, distension of scalp veins and sun setting of the eyes.
- Older children present with symptoms of raised intracranial pressure.

Treatment is usually with a ventriculoperitoneal shunt.

Exercise 7
Answer the following questions. Prepare short talks and/or dialogues on these topics

1. Characterize motor disorders.
2. What are causes of movement disorders?
3. What is meant by neuromuscular disorders?

4.   What causes a hypotonic 'floppy' infant?
5.   What causes ataxia?
6.   Describe causes of hydrocephalus.

Translation 3

1. The first question to ask when seeing a child with a motor disorder is whether this is a central or a peripheral nervous system disorder. 2. Corticospinal (pyramidal) tract disorders are: cerebral dysgenesis, global hypoxia-ischaemia, antenatal ischemic stroke, cerebral tumour, acute disseminated encephalomyelitis, postictal paresis, or hemiplegic migraine. 3. Basal ganglia disorders include: acquired brain injury, acute and profound hypoxia-ischaemia, carbon monoxide poisoning, post-cardiopulmonary bypass chorea, post-streptococcal chorea (rheumatic fever), mitochondrial cytopathies, Wilson disease, Huntington disease, vitamin E deficiency, or pontocerebellar hypoplasia. 4. Cerebellar disorders are: acute (medication and drugs, including alcohol and solvent abuse), postviral (varicella infection), posterior fossa lesions or tumours, and genetic and degenerative disorders. 5. Neuromuscular disorders are divided into: disorders of the anterior horn cell, disorders of the peripheral nerve, disorders of neuromuscular transmission, muscle disorders. 6. Causes of a hypotonic 'floppy' infant can be: central spinal cord, anterior horn cell, neuromuscular junction, muscle peripheral nerve, metabolic myopathies. 7. We distinguish: Friedrich ataxia, ataxia telangiectasia, cerebellar agenesis/dysgenesis, postinfectious cerebellitis, Miller Fisher syndrome, mitochondrial disease. 8. In hydrocephalus, there is an accumulation of cerebrospinal fluid in the brain. 9. In babies and children this can be congenital, associated with cerebral malformations, or obstruction to the flow of cerebrospinal fluid. 10. Causes of hydrocephalus can be: congenital malformation, aqueduct stenosis, atresia of the outflow foramina of the four ventricle, Chiari malformation, intraventricular haemorrhage, failure to reabsorb CSF.

Text 4
The neurocutaneous syndromes

The nervous system and the skin have a common ectodermal origin. Embryological disruption causes syndromes involving abnormalities to both systems — the neurocutaneous syndromes.

Neurofibromatosis

Neurofibromata appear in the course of any peripheral nerve, including cranial nerves. In order to make the diagnosis, two or more of these criteria need to be present:

- six or more café-au-lait spots
- more than one neurofibroma
- axillary freckling
- optic glioma which may cause visual impairment
- one Lisch nodule: a hamartoma of the iris seen on slit-lamp examination
- bony lesions from sphenoid dysplasia, which can cause eye protrusion
- a first-degree relative with NF-1.

Tuberous sclerosis

Many people who carry the gene have no stigmata other than cutaneous features and no associated neurological features.

The cutaneous features consist of:

- depigmented 'as leaf' shaped patches
- roughened patches of skin usually over the lumbar spine
- angiofibromata in a butterfly distribution over the bridge of the nose and cheeks

Neurological features are seen in 50%, including:

- infantile spasms and developmental delay
- epilepsy — often local
- intellectual disability, often with autism

Other features include:

- fibromata beneath the nails (subungual fibromata)
- dense white areas on the retina
- rhabdomyomata of the heart
- angiomyolipomas and polycystic kidneys
- cysts in the lungs

Neurodegenerative disorders

These are disorders that cause a deterioration in motor and intellectual function. Abnormal neurological features develop, including seizures, spasticity, abnormal head circumference (macrocephaly or microcephaly), involuntary movement disorders, visual and hearing loss, and behaviour change.

Some examples of neurodegenerative disorders seen in children

Age 0-2 years	Presentation	Diagnostic investigations
Infantile neuronal ceroid lipofuscinosis (NCL)	Developmental arrest by end of first year, seizures and blindness	Skin biopsy, blood enzyme analysis, DNA testing
Krabbe leukodystrophy	Irritability, hypertonia, myoclonus	White cell enzymes
Rett syndrome		DNA testing
Tay Sachs	Regression by 6-18 months, with characteristic hand wringing	White cell enzymes
	Hypotonia, seizures, and blindness	

Age 2-5 years	Presentation	Diagnostic investigations
Mucopolysaccharidosis type III	Developmental delay, behavioural disturbances, dysmorphism	Urinary glycosaminoglycans and blood white cell enzymes
NCL – late infantile	Myoclonus, motor difficulties, blindness	Skin biopsy, enzymes analysis, DNA testing
Alpers		Genetic tests
	Seizures, developmental regression, hypotonia and hepatic derangement	

Age 5-12 years	Presentation	Diagnostic investigations
Juvenile NCL	Cognitive and motor decline. Visual deterioration. Seizures later	Vacuolated lymphocytes on light microscopy, fingerprinting on electron microscopy, DNA testing
Adrenoleukodystrophy Niemann-Pick disease type C Friedreich ataxia	Cognitive development slowed, visual impairment, seizures	Very Long Chain Fatty Acids (VLCFA), DNA testing
	Seizures, vertical gaze, palsy	Sea blue histiocytes on bone marrow aspiration, DNA testing
	Ataxia, pyramidal signs, and peripheral neuropathy	

Age 12+ years	Presentation	Diagnostic investigations
Wilson disease	Psychiatric, extrapyramidal	Plasma copper and caeruloplasmin, penicillamine challenge
Juvenile Huntington	Progressive dystonia, dementia, seizures, corticospinal tract signs	DNA testing

Exercise 8
Answer the following questions.

1. Characterize the neurocutaneous syndromes (neurofibromatosis, tuberous sclerosis neurodegenerative disorders).
2. Give some examples of neurodegenerative disorders seen in children (age 0-2 years, age 2-5 years, age 5-12 years, age 12+ years)

Translation 4

1. The nervous system and the skin have a common ectodermal origin. 2. Embryological disruption causes syndromes involving abnormalities to both systems – the neurocutaneous syndromes. 3. In order to make the diagnosis of neurofibromatosis, two or more of these criteria need to be present: café-au-lait spots, neurofibroma, axillary optic glioma, freckling, Lisch nodule, bony lesions. 4. Many people who carry the gene of tuberous sclerosis have no stigmata other than cutaneous features and no associated neurological features. 5. The cutaneous features consist of: depigmented patches, roughened patches, or angiofibromata. 6. Neurological features include: infantile spasms epilepsy, intellectual disability, autism. 7. Other features include: subungual fibromata, dense white areas on the retina, rhabdomyomata of the heart, angiomyolipomas and polycystic kidneys, cysts in the lungs. 8. Neurodegenerative disorders cause a deterioration in motor and intellectual function. 9. Abnormal neurological features develop, including seizures, spasticity, macrocephaly or microcephaly, involuntary movement disorders, visual and hearing loss, and behaviour change. 10. Some examples of neurodegenerative disorders seen in children are: ataxia, behavioural disturbances, blindness, cognitive and motor decline, cognitive development slowed, corticospinal tract signs, dementia, developmental delay, developmental arrest, dysmorphism, hepatic derangement, hypertonia, hypotonia, irritability, motor difficulties, myoclonus, palsy, peripheral neuropathy, progressive dystonia, psychiatric problems, pyramidal signs, regression, vertical gaze, visual deterioration, visual impairment.

Text 5
Adolescent medicine
Features of adolescent medicine are:
- the adolescent consultation differs from the paediatric consultation
- the HEADS acronym assists in taking a psychosocial history
- mortality of adolescents aged 15-19 years is now greater than that of young children
- chronic illness may impact on adolescent development, which in turn may impact on the chronic illness, e.g. adherence
- prominent mental health problems are eating disorders and self-harm.

The transition from being a child to an adult involves many biological, psychological, and social changes with adolescent brain developmental continuing into the third decade. Difficulties may arise when obtaining specialist medical care. Paediatric facilities e.g. children's wards, are often geared to the needs of young children rather than adolescents, whilst older adolescents may be overwhelmed by the medical conditions encountered on adult wards and the independence expected of them.

HEADS acronym for psychosocial history taking in adolescents

H ⇒
Home life
   Relationships, social support, household chores

E ⇒
Education
   School, exams, work experience, career, university, financial issues

A ⇒
Activities
Exercise, sport, other leisure activities
   Social relationships, friends, peers, who can they rely on? Bullying?

D ⇒
Driving
- Drugs — drug use, cigarettes, alcohol. How much? How often?
- Diet — weight, caffeine (diet drinks), binges/vomits

S ⇒

- **Sexual health** — Concerns, periods, contraception (and in relation to medication)
- **Sleep** — How much? Hard to get to sleep? Wake often?
- **Suicide**/affect — Early waking? Depression, self-harm, body image
- **Safety** — Safety issues around substance use, sexual activity, Internet use, etc.

Communicating with adolescents

The adolescent has a greater active role in the consultation. An integral component of adolescent healthcare if offering young persons the opportunity to be seen independently of their parents for at least part of the visit. Some practical points about communication and working with adolescents are:

- make the adolescent the central person in the consultation
- engage the adolescent by talking about his/her interests
- is the mother or father answering for the adolescent? Does the adolescent seem to want this or resent being interrupted?
- avoid being judgemental or lecturing
- an authoritarian approach is likely to result in a rebellious stance
- frame difficult questions so they are less threatening and judgemental. (How much alcohol do you drink in comparison with your friends? Lots of young people smoke – do you?)
- confidentiality must be respected. Explain that you will keep everything you are told confidential, unless they or somebody else is at risk of serious harm.
- Bear in mind proxy presentations, e.g. abdominal pain, when the real reason is anxiety about the possibility of pregnancy, or sexually transmitted infection (STI) or the result of recreational drug use
- a full adolescent psychosocial history is useful as well as identifying protective or resilient factors
- communicate and explain concepts appropriate to their cognitive development
- history taking should avoid making the assumption of heterosexuality with questions about sexual partners asked in a gender-neutral way

Young people have the right to a chaperone. Also, find out if they would prefer a doctor of the same sex.

Development changes in adolescence
Early adolescence

Biological	Psychological	Social
Early puberty: Females — breast bud, pubic hair development, start of growth spurt Males — testicular enlargement, start of genital growth	Concrete thinking, but begin to develop moral concepts and awareness of their sexual identity	The early emotional separation from parents, start of strong peer identification, early exploratory behaviours, e.g. may start smoking

Mid-adolescence

Biological	Psychological	Social
Females — end of growth spurt, menarche, changes in body shape Males — sperm production, voice breaks, start of growth spurt Acne Blushing Need for more sleep	Abstract thinking, but still seen as ‚bulletproof‘, increasing verbal dexterity, may develop a fervent ideology (religious, political)	Continuing emotional separation from parents, strong peer group identification, development of sexual identity and orientation, early vocational plans

Late adolescence

Biological	Psychological	Social
Males — end of puberty, continued growth in height, strength, and body hair	Complex abstract thinking, identification of difference between law and morality, increased impulse control, further development of personal identity, further development of rejection of ideologies.	Social autonomy, may develop intimate relationships, further education or employment, may begin or develop financial independence

Exercise 9
Answer the following questions. Prepare short talks and/or dialogues on these topics

1. What are the features of adolescent medicine?
2. What does HEADS acronym for psychosocial history taking in adolescents stand for?

3. Name the rules of communicating with adolescents.
4. What are development changes in adolescence?

Translation 5

1. Features of adolescent medicine are: the adolescent consultation differs from the paediatric consultation, mortality of adolescents is now greater than that of young children, chronic illness may impact on adolescent development, prominent mental health problems are eating disorders and self-harm. 2. The transition from being a child to an adult involves many biological, psychological, and social changes. 3. HEADS acronym for psychosocial history taking in adolescents stands for: home life, education, activities, driving, drugs, diet, sexual health, sleep, suicide, safety. 4. Some practical points about communication and working with adolescents are: engage the adolescent by talking about his/her interests, avoid being judgemental or lecturing. 5. Explain that you will keep everything you are told confidential, unless they or somebody else is at risk of serious harm. 5. A full adolescent psychosocial history is useful as well as identifying protective or resilient factors. 6. Biological development changes in early adolescence are: in females – breast bud, pubic hair development, start of growth spurt, in males – testicular enlargement, start of genital growth. 7. Psychological development changes in early adolescence are: concrete thinking, begin to develop moral concepts and awareness of their sexual identity.

Exercise 10
Match the column A with the column B. Try to learn the expressions and/or sentences by heart.

A

1. Social development changes in early adolescence are: ...
2. Biological development changes in mid-adolescence are: ...
3. Psychological development changes in mid-adolescence are: ...
4. Social development changes in mid-adolescence are: ...
5. Biological development changes in late adolescence are: ...
6. Psychological development changes in late adolescence are: ...
7. Social development changes in late adolescence are: ...

B

a.   *... in males – end of puberty, continued growth in height, strength, and body hair.*

b. *... abstract thinking, increasing verbal dexterity, may develop a fervent ideology (religious, political).*

c. *... social autonomy, may develop intimate relationships, further education or employment, may begin or develop financial independence.*

d. *... complex abstract thinking, identification of difference between law and morality, increased impulse control, further development of personal identity, further development of rejection of ideologies.*

e. *... in females – end of growth spurt, menarche, changes in body shape, in males – sperm production, voice breaks, start of growth spurt, acne, blushing, need for more sleep.*

f. *... the early emotional separation from parents, start of strong peer identification, early exploratory behaviours.*

g. *... continuing emotional separation from parents, strong peer group identification, development of sexual identity and orientation, early vocational plans.*

Text 6
Summary
Talking and listening with young people

- Always give them the opportunity to be seen independently of their parents.
- Explain and assure confidentiality.
- Psychological screening is useful to:
- engage young people
- assess risk
- identify protective/resilient factors: they assist formulation of interventions.

Consent and confidentiality
Consent

Conflict rarely arises about a treatment, as usually the adolescent, his/her parents and doctors agree that it is necessary.

Confidentiality

Adolescents want to know that information they have disclosed to their doctor is not revealed to others, whether parents, school or police, without their permission. Confidentiality should be kept unless there is a risk of serious harm, from physical or sexual abuse, from suicidal thoughts or to others from homicidal intent. Difficulties relating to confidentiality are usually about contraception, abortion, STIs, substance abuse, or mental health. It is usually desirable for the parents to be informed. The adolescent should be encouraged to tell them or allow the doctor to do so.

Range of health problems

Adolescence is considered a healthy stage of life compared with early childhood or old age. The range of health problems affecting adolescents include:

- common acute illnesses: respiratory disorders, skin conditions, musculoskeletal problems including sport injuries, and somatic complaints.
- chronic illness and disability: e.g. asthma, epilepsy, diabetes, cerebral palsy, juvenile idiopathic arthritis, sickle cell disease. There is also a range of uncommon disorders such as malignant disease and connective tissue disorders. Children with many congenital disorders which often used to be fatal in childhood now survive into adolescence or adult life.
- high prevalence of somatic symptoms: e.g. fatigue, headaches, backache
- mental health problems including suicide and deliberate self-harm
- eating disorders and weight problems
- those associated with health-risk behaviours, such as smoking, drinking, drug abuse and sexual health, contraception, and teenage pregnancy.

Mortality

Although deaths in adolescents from communicable diseases have declined markedly, this has not been matched by mortality from road traffic accidents, other injuries and suicide. Alcohol is thought to be a contributing factor in one-third of these deaths.

Some of the ways in which chronic illness and development interact with each other
Biological

Effect of chronic illness on development	Effect of development on chronic illness
Delayed puberty Short stature Reduced bone mass accretion Malnutrition secondary to inadequate intake due to	Pubertal hormones may impact on disease, e.g. growth hormone worsens diabetes and increases insulin requirements; females with cystic fibrosis may have deterioration in

| increased caloric requirement of disease or anorexia
Localized growth abnormalities in inflammatory joint disease, e.g. premature fusion of epiphyses | lung function; corticosteroid toxicity worse in the peripubertal phase
Increased caloric requirement may worsen disease control or result in undernutrition — may need dietary supplements or overnight feeding with nasogastric tube or gastrostomy
Growth may cause scoliosis |

Psychological

Effect of chronic illness on development	Effect of development on chronic illness
Regression to less mature behaviour Adopt sick role Impaired development of sense of attractive/sexual self Parental stress, depression, financial problems in providing care; siblings may suffer	Deny that their health may suffer from their actions Poor adherence and disease control Reject medics like parents

Social

Effect of chronic illness on development	Effect of development on chronic illness
Reduced independence when should be separating Failure of peer relationships Social isolation — unable to participate in sports or social events School absence and decline in school performance, may lower self-esteem Vocational failure	Risk behaviour may adversely affect disease, e.g. smoking and asthma or cystic fibrosis, alcohol and diabetic control, sleep deprivation and epilepsy Chaotic eating habits lead to malnutrition or obesity

Exercise 11
Answer the following questions. Prepare short talks and/or dialogues on these topics

1. How to talk and listen to young people (consent and confidentiality)?
2. What can you say about range of health problems and mortality?
3. Give examples of some of the ways in which chronic illness and development interact with each other (biological, psychological, social).

Translation 6

1. Always give young people the opportunity to be seen independently of their parents. 2. Adolescents want to know that information they have disclosed to their doctor is not revealed to others, whether parents,

school or police, without their permission. 3. Confidentiality should be kept unless there is a risk of serious harm from physical or sexual abuse, from suicidal thoughts or to others from homicidal intent. 4. Difficulties relating to confidentiality are usually about contraception, abortion, STIs, substance abuse, or mental health. 5. Common acute illnesses include: respiratory disorders, skin conditions, musculoskeletal problems and somatic complaints. 6. Chronic illness and disability are e.g. asthma, epilepsy, diabetes, cerebral palsy, juvenile idiopathic arthritis, or sickle cell disease. 7. There is high prevalence of somatic symptoms: fatigue, headaches, backache.

Exercise 12
Match the column A with the column B. Try to learn the expressions and/or sentences by heart.

A

1. Problems can also be associated with health-risk behaviours, …
2. Biological ways in which chronic illness and development interact with each other are: …
3. Pubertal hormones may impact on disease, e.g. …
4. Psychological ways in which chronic illness and development interact with each other are: …
5. Social ways in which chronic illness and development interact with each other are:

B

a. … *reduced independence, failure of peer relationships, social isolation, school absence and decline in school performance, vocational failure, smoking, alcohol, sleep deprivation, chaotic eating habits.*
b. … *growth hormone, cystic fibrosis, corticosteroid toxicity, or increased caloric requirement.*
c. … *regression to less mature behaviour, adopt sick role, impaired development of sense of attractive/sexual self, parental stress, depression, financial problems, poor adherence and disease control, reject medics like parents.*
d. … *delayed puberty, short stature, reduced bone mass accretion, malnutrition, and localized growth abnormalities.*
e. … *such as smoking, drinking, drug abuse and sexual health, contraception, and teenage pregnancy.*

Text 7
Impact of chronic conditions
Chronic illness may disrupt biological, psychological, and social development.

Adherence
Poor adherence is a problem for many people. Adolescents wish to avoid parental supervision, and may give the management of their illness a lower priority than social and recreational activities. They may not believe that taking the medication really matters. Peer relationships and self-image are very important when considering adherence. Side-effects are also important, particularly those that affect well-being or appearance. Adherence may be influenced by lack of knowledge and/or poor recall of previous disease education. If the communication has not been updated with increasing age, the adolescent's knowledge may be poor, with little understanding about his/her illness, what medications he/she is taking and why. The implications of their condition on the rest of their health and their life needs to be considered. This may include sexual health, or future vocational development. Similarly, the implications of other health-risk behaviours, such as substance use, tattoos, and piercing may need to be discussed.

Ways to maximize adherence

Assess the size of the problem and be non-judgemental	Ask: Some people have trouble taking their medication. When was the last time you forgot?
Take time to explore practicalities	Try to put yourself in the adolescent's shoes and think through the detail of their regimen with them. 'Which is the most difficult dose to remember?' 'How do you fit in taking your tablets into your daily routine?' Make regimen as simple as possible. Do not forget practical issues — poor adherence may be as simple as not having any private space at school to take the treatment
Explore beliefs	May harbour strange or incorrect beliefs about medications, e.g. falsely attribute a side-effect, and therefore refuse to take the medication
Use daily routines to 'anchor' adherence	Find daily activities to anchor taking the medication, e.g. brushing teeth or 'with breakfast and dinner' instead of 'twice a day'. Find the least chaotic time of day: may be morning or evening! Let the suggestions come from the adolescent
Motivation	Negotiate short term treatment goals. Search for factors that motivate the young person

Involve and contract	Plan the regimen with the adolescent. Some may respond to a written contract that both sides agree to stick to.
Written instructions	Most of what is said has been shown to be forgotten once they leave the room!
Take time to explain	Check level of knowledge on each occasion
Solution-focused approach	Find out what has been going well and why. Use this information e.g. ‚How have you managed to remain out of hospital for 3 weeks this month?'

Fatigue, headache, and other somatic symptoms

Fatigue, headache, abdominal pain, backache, and dizziness are common in adolescence. Organic disease must be excluded by history, examination, and occasionally, investigation. The symptoms may be a physical manifestation of psychological problems, and are precipitated by factors such as bullying or parental discord. Occasionally the symptoms are so severe that they affect quality of life, with impairment of school attendance, academic result, and peer relationship. Further investigation and assessment will be required.

Mental health problems

Main mental health problems and disorders in adolescents

Problem or disorder	Prevalence
Depression	3-5 %
Anxiety	4-6 %
Attention deficit hyperactivity disorder	2-4 %
Eating disorders	1-2 %
Conduct disorder	4-6 %
Substance misuse disorder	2-3 %

Exercise 13
Answer the following questions. Prepare short talks and/or dialogues on these topics

1. Describe adherence and ways to maximize adherence.
2. What may be impact of chronic conditions?
3. What are ways to maximize adherence?
4. Characterize fatigue, headache, and other somatic symptoms.
5. What can you say about mental health problems?

Translation 7

1. Chronic illness may disrupt biological, psychological, and social development. 2. Adherence may be influenced by lack of knowledge and/or poor recall of previous disease education. 3. The adolescent's knowledge may be poor, with little understanding about his/her illness, what medications he/she is taking and why. 4. Similarly, the implications of other health-risk behaviours, such as substance use, tattoos, and piercing may need to be discussed. 5. Ways to maximize adherence include: assess the size of the problem, be non-judgemental, take time to explore practicalities, explore beliefs, use daily routines to 'anchor' adherence and motivation, involve and contract written instructions, take time to explain. 6. Fatigue, headache, abdominal pain, backache, and dizziness are common in adolescence. 7. The symptoms may be a physical manifestation of psychological problems, and are precipitated by factors such as bullying or parental discord. 8. Main mental health problems and disorders in adolescents are: depression, anxiety, attention deficit, hyperactivity disorder, eating disorders, conduct disorder, and substance misuse disorder.

Text 8
Health-risk behaviour

During adolescence, young people begin to explore 'adult' behaviours, including smoking, drinking, drug use and sex. These behaviours, are often referred to as 'risk-taking' behaviours.

Sexual health

Having sexual intercourse at an early age is often associated with unsafe sex. This may be because of a lack of knowledge, lack of access to contraception, being drunk or high on drugs, or unable to rest being pressurized by his/her partner. Risk-taking behaviour in adolescents can result in STIs or unplanned pregnancy. STIs may present with urethral or vaginal discharge, urinary symptoms, pain on micturition, abdominal or loin pain, or postcoital vaginal bleeding. Chlamydia can lead to later infertility. In young teenagers, it is more likely to present with a vaginal discharge.

Management of sexually transmitted infections

Relevant questions include those related to the risk of STIs: number of partners; any partners during travel abroad; contraception used; whether vaginal, oral, or anal sex; any discharge, lower abdominal pain, urinary symptoms; and last menstrual period. However, many STIs are asymptomatic. If indicated, swabs should be taken for virology and microbiology (to look for human papilloma virus, herpes simplex virus, chlamydia, and gonorrhoea). HIV testing may be indicated.

Contraception

Condoms, followed by the oral contraceptive pill, are the most of contraception used. Emergency contraception can provide significant protection from pregnancy for up to 72 hours after unprotected intercourse. Side-effects include nausea and lethargy.

Teenage parenthood

Teenage girls may present with complaints such as abdominal pain, fatigue, breast tenderness, or appetite changes rather than late or missed menstrual period. Children of teenaged mothers have a higher infant mortality, a higher rate of childhood accidents, illness, and admissions to hospital. Deprivation from the mother's lack of financial and emotional support and the paucity of her own education and life experience, is the strongest risk factor.

Health promotion

The reasons to undertake health promotion in adolescents are:
- health-risk behaviours (smoking, alcohol, drug misuse, unsafe sexual activity) as well as health-promoting behaviours (regular physical exercise, nutrition)
- health-risk behaviours often continue into adult life
- health-risk behaviours may have a direct effect on their lives, e.g. teenage pregnancy, road traffic accidents
- increasing obesity and diabetes
- The main areas for **health-promotion** are:
- health-risk behaviours
- mental health
- violent behaviour
- physical activity, nutrition, and obesity
- parent-adolescent communication

There are a number of **approaches** to health promotion for adolescents:
- provide suitable information
- banning cigarette advertising, making emergency contraception available in pharmacies,
- programme to reduce bullying, and reducing drug misuse in a whole school
- training programmes to reject certain courses of behaviour

• health promotion by professionals

Exercise 14
Study the following summary and then interpret basic information in English.

1. Chronic conditions during adolescence
Chronic illness and/or disability may disrupt adolescent development. Consideration should be made of the impact of the chronic condition on the rest of health as well as education and leisure.
2. Transition to adult services
Transitional care aims to address medical, psychosocial, and educational/vocational issues as young people move from child- to adult-centred services.
3. The main health problems of adolescents
Common acute illness: respiratory disorders, skin conditions, musculoskeletal problems Chronic illness and disability, including previously fatal congenital disorders Somatic symptoms: fatigue, headache, backache and abdominal pain Mental health problems Health-risk behaviours: smoking, drinking, drug abuse, road traffic accidents Sexual health: sexually transmitted infections, contraception, teenage pregnancy Eating disorders and obesity

Exercise 15
Answer the following questions. Prepare short talks and/or dialogues on these topics

1. What is meant by health-risk behaviour?
2. Speak about sexual health and management of sexually transmitted infections.
3. What should the adolescents know about contraception and teenage parenthood?
4. What are the reasons to undertake health promotion in adolescents?

Translation 8

1. During adolescence, young people begin to explore 'adult' behaviours, including smoking, drinking, drug use and sex. 2. Having sexual intercourse at an early age may be because of a lack of knowledge, lack of access to contraception, being drunk or high on drugs. 3. STIs may present with urethral or vaginal discharge, urinary symptoms, pain on micturition, abdominal or loin pain, or postcoital vaginal bleeding. 4. Relevant questions include those related to the risk of STIs: number of partners, any partners during travel abroad, contraception used, whether vaginal, oral, or anal sex. 5. If indicated, swabs should be taken for virology and microbiology (to look for human papilloma virus, herpes simplex virus, chlamydia, and

gonorrhoea). 6. Condoms, followed by the oral contraceptive pill, are the most of contraception used. 7. Children of teenaged mothers have a higher infant mortality, a higher rate of childhood accidents, illnesses, and admissions to hospital. 8. The main areas for health-promotion are: health-risk behaviours, mental health, violent behaviour, physical activity, nutrition and obesity, and parent-adolescent communication.

Key 10
Exercise 5
1 c, b, a; 2 a, b; 3 d, a, b, c; 4 d, c, a, b; 5 d, c, a, b

Exercise 10
1f; 2e; 3b; 4g; 5a; 6d; 7c

Exercise 12
1e; 2d; 3b; 4c; 5a

VOCABULARY 10

abortion /əˈbɔː.ʃən/
abrupt /əˈbrʌpt/
accretion /əˈkriːʃən/
accumulate /əˈkjuː.mjʊ.leɪt/
acquired /əˌkwaɪ.əd/
adherence /ədˈhɪə.rənt s/
adjustment /əˈdʒʌst.mənt/
adopt /əˈdɒpt/
adrenoleukodystrophy /əˌdriːnəʊˈluːkəʊˈdɪstrəfɪ/
advise /ədˈvaɪz/
agenesis /eɪˈdʒenɪsɪs/
allele /əˈliːl/
Alpers disease /alˈperz dɪˈziːz /
alteration /ˌɒl.təˈreɪ.ʃən/
altered /ˈɒl.tərd/
anchor /ˈæŋ.kər/
anencephaly /æn.en.ˈse.fə.liː/
angiofibroma /anˈdʒiː..əʊ.faɪ.brəʊˈmæ/
angiomyolipoma /anˈdʒiː..əʊ.lɪmˈfəʊmə/
anoxia /ænˈɒk.si.ə/
apnoea /ˈæp.ni.ə/
appearance /əˈpɪə.rənt s/
aqueduct /ˈækwɪˌdʌkt/
arteriovenous /ɑː.tɪə.ri.əʊˈviː.nəs/
assumption /əˈsʌmp.ʃən/
assure /əˈʃɔːr/
asystolic /ˌæsɪsˈtɒlɪk/
ataxia /əˈtæk.si.ə/
atonic /ˌeɪ.ˈtɒ.nik/
atresia /əˈtriː.ʃə/
atrophy /ˈæt.rə.fi/
attribute /ˈæt.rɪ.bjuːt/
auditory /ˈɔː.dɪtərɪ/
authoritarian /ɔːˌθɒrɪˈteərɪən/
awaken /əˈweɪ.kən/
awareness /əˈweə.nəs/
axillary /æˈksɪl.ər.i/
ban / bæn/
band /bænd/
Bell palsy /ˈpɔːl.zi/
benign /bɪˈnaɪn/
binge /bɪndʒ/
biting /ˈbaɪ.tɪŋ/
blush /blʌʃ/
botulism /ˈbɒt.jʊ.lɪ.zəm/

brainstem /ˈbreɪn.stem/
breech /briːtʃ/
bridge /brɪdʒ/
bruit /bruːt/
bud /bʌd/
bulging /ˈbʌl.dʒɪŋ/
bulletproof /ˈbʊl.ɪt.pruːf/
butterfly /ˈbʌt.ə.flaɪ/
bypass /ˈbaɪ.pɑːs/
carbon monoxide /ˌkɑː.bən.məˈnɒk.saɪd/
carnitine /karˈni.tiːn/
central /ˈsen.trəl/
cephalalgia /ˌsefəˈlældʒɪə/
cerebellar /ˌser.ə.ˈbe.lər/
cerebellitis /serˈe.bel.aɪˈtɪs/
cerebral /ˈser.ɪ.brəl/
cerebrospinal /ˌser.əbrəˈspaɪ.nəl/
ceroid /sɪərəɪd/
ceruloplasmin /se.ruˈləʊ.plazˈmin/
chaperone /ˈʃæp.ə.rəʊn/
Chiari /kiːahrˈiː/ syndrome /ˈsɪndrəʊm/
chlamydia /kləm.iˈde.ə/ pl chlamydiae
chorea /koˈrɪə/
chores /tʃɔːz/
chromosome /ˈkrəʊməˌsəʊm/
circumference /səˈkʌm.fər.əns/
circumscribe /ˌsɜːkəmˈskraɪb/
cluster headache /ˈklʌs.tərˌhed.eɪk/
cognitive /ˈkɒg.nɪ.tɪv/
comparison /kəmˈpær.ɪ.sən/
comprise /kəmˈpraɪz/
concept /ˈkɒn.sept/
conception /kənˈsepʃən/
confidential /ˌkɒn.fɪˈden.tʃəl/
confidentiality /ˌkɒn.fɪ.den.tʃiˈæl.ɪ.ti/
confusion /kənˈfjuː.ʒən/
congenital /kənˈdʒen.ɪ.təl/
conization /kəʊnɪ.zəɪˈʃən /
constriction /kənˈstrɪkˌʃən/
contraception /ˌkɒntrəˈsepʃən/
contralateral /ˌkɒn.trə.ˈlæt.ər.əl/
convulsive /kənˈvʌl.sɪv/
copper /ˈkɒp.ər/
core /kɔːr/
corticospinal /ˌkɔːtɪkəʊˈspaɪnᵊl/
craniopharyngioma /ˈkreɪ.ni.əʊ.fəˌrin.dʒiː.ˈəʊ.mə/
crude /kruːd/

cytomegalovirus /ˌsaɪ.təʊ.ˌmeg.ə.lə.ˈvaɪ.rəs/
cytopathy /ˌsaɪtɒpəθɪ/
daydream /ˈdeɪ.driːm/
deficiency /dɪˈfɪʃ.ən.si/
deliberate /dɪˈlɪb.ər.ət/
deliberately /dɪˈlɪb.ər.ət.li/
dense /dens/
deny /dɪˈnaɪ/
depigmented /deˈpɪg.mənt.ɪd/
derangement /dɪˈreɪndʒd.mənt/
dermatomyositis /ˌdər.mə.təʊ.ˌmaɪ.ə.ˈsaɪ.təs/
desirable /dɪˈzaɪə.rə.bl̩/
dexterity /dekˈster.ə.ti/
diaphragm /ˈdaɪ.ə.fræm/
discharge /dɪsˈtʃɑːdʒ/
disclose /dɪsˈkləʊz/
discord /ˈdɪs.kɔːd/
dislocation /ˌdɪs.lə.ˈkeɪ.ʃən/
disrupt /dɪsˈrʌpt/
disseminated /dɪˈsem.ɪ.neɪt.ɪd/
dissociative /dɪˈsəʊ.ʃi.eɪt.ɪv/
distension /dɪˈsten.ʃən/
dizziness / ˈdɪz.ɪ.nəs/
dreaming /driːmɪŋ/
dysesthesia /dɪsəsˈθiːzɪə/
dysgenesis /ˌdis.ˈdʒe.nə.səs/
dysmorphia /dɪsˈmɔːfɪə/
dystonia /dɪsˈtəʊnɪə/
dystrophia /dɪˈstrəʊfɪə/
ectodermal /ˌektəʊˈdɜːməl/
encephalocele /in.ˈsef.ə.ləʊ.ˌsiː.l/
encephalomyelitis /enˌsefələʊˌmaɪəˈlaɪtɪs/
encephalopathy /enˌsef.əˈlɒp.ə.θi/
engage /ɪnˈgeɪdʒ/
epiphysis /əˈpɪf.ɪ.sɪs/
ethanol /ˈeθ.ə.nɒl/
evident /ˈev.ɪ.dənt/
expiratory /ˌɪk.spɪr.ə.tər.i/
exploratory /ɪkˈsplɒrətərɪ/
extradural /ˈek.strə.ˈdjʊr.əl/
extrapyramidal /ˌek.strə.pə.ˈra.mə.dᵊl/
fabricate /ˈfæbrɪˌkeɪt/
faint /feɪnt/
falsely /ˈfɒl.sli/
feign /feɪn/
fervent /ˈfɜːvənt/
fibroma /faɪˈbrəʊmə/

fit in /fɪt ɪn/
flicker /ˈflɪkə/
floppy /ˈflɒp.i/
folic /ˈfəʊ.lik/ **acid** /ˈæs.ɪd/
foramen /fəˈreɪ.mən/ pl **foramina**
fossa /ˈfɒs.ə/ pl **fossae**
frame /freɪm/
freckle /ˈfrekəl/
Friedreich ataxia /əˈtæk.si.ə/
frontal /ˈfrʌn.təl/
fundus /ˈfʌn.dəs/ pl **fundi**
fusion /ˈfjuː.ʒən/
ganglion pl **ganglia** /ˈgæŋ.gli.ə/
gaze /geɪz/
gear /gɪə/
gene /dʒiːn/
generalized /ˈdʒenrəˌlaɪzd/
glioma /glaɪˈəʊmə/
glycosaminoglycan /glaɪkəʊs.ə.mi.ˈnəʊ.glaɪˈkæn/
gonorrhoea /ˌgɒn.əˈriː.ə/
govern /ˈgʌv.ən/
Guillain-Barré /giˈjæn bəˈrei/ **syndrome** /ˈsɪndrəʊm/
hamartoma /hæmˈærˈtəʊˈmə/
harbour /ˈhɑːbə/
hemiplegia /ˌhæm.ɪˈpliː.dʒi.ə/
hemiplegic /ˌhe.mi.ˈpliː.dʒik/
herald /ˈher.əld/
hereditary /həˈred.ɪ.tər.i/
herniation /ˌhɜː.niˈeɪ.ʃən/
herpes /ˈhɜː.piːz/ **simplex** /ˈsɪm.pleks/
hiccough /ˈhɪk.ʌp/
histiocyte /ˈhɪstɪəˌsaɪt/
homicidal /ˌhɒm.ɪˈsaɪ.dəl/
horn /hɔːn/
human /ˈhjuː.mən/ **papilloma virus** /ˌpa.pə.ˈləʊ.məˈvaɪə.rəs/
Huntington's disease /ˈhʌn.tɪŋ.tənz dɪˌziːz/
hydrocephalic /ˌhaɪdrəʊseˈfælɪk/
hydrocephalus /ˌhaɪ.drəˈsef.ə.ləs/
hypernatremia /ˌhaɪ.pə.neɪ.ˈtriː.miː.ə/
hypertonia /ˌhaɪ.pəˈtəʊ.niə/
hypnic /ˈhɪpnɪk/
hypomagnesaemia /ˌhaɪ.pəʊˌmæg.nəˈsiː.mi.ə/
hyponatraemia /ˌhaɪ.pəʊ.næˈtriː.mɪ.ə/
hypoplasia /ˌhaɪ.pəʊ.ˈpleɪ.ʒə/
hypotonia /ˌhaɪpəʊˈtəʊ.niə/
hypoxic-ischaemic /haɪˈpɒk.sɪk ɪsˈkiː.mɪk/ **IgA** /ˌaɪ.dʒiː.ˈeɪ/
ictal /ɪktəl/

impact /ˈɪm.pækt/
implication /ˌɪm.plɪˈkeɪ.ʃən/
inborn /ˈɪnˈbɔːn/
infantile /ˈɪn.fən.taɪl/
infertility /ˌɪn.fəˈtɪl.ɪ.ti/
inheritance /ɪnˈherɪtəns/
inhibition /ˌɪn.hɪˈbɪʃ.ən/
inhibitory /ɪnˈhɪb.ɪ.tər.i/
intent /ɪnˈtent/
inter- /ɪnˈtɜːr/
intercourse /ˈɪntəˌkɔːs/
intervention /ˌɪn.təˈven.ʃən/
intraventricular /ɪn.trə.venˈtrɪk.jə.lər/
intrusive /ɪnˈtruː.sɪv/
involuntary /ɪnˈvɒləntərɪ/
iris /ˈaɪrɪs/
jerk /dʒɜːk/
judgemental /dʒʌdʒˈmen.təl/
juvenile /ˈdʒuːvɪˌnaɪl/
Krabbe leukodystrophy /krabˈiːˌluːkəʊˈdɪstrəfɪ/
labyrinthitis /ˌlæbərɪnˈθaɪtɪs/
lecture /ˈlek.tʃə/
leukodystrophy /ˌluːkəʊˈdɪstrəfɪ/
liaison /liˈeɪ.zɒn/
light-headedness /ˌlaɪtˈhed.ɪd.nəs/
lipofuscinosis /ˌlɪpəʊfʌskɪˈnəʊsɪs/
Lisch nodule /lishˈnɒdjuːl/
locus pl **loci** /ˈləʊkəs/
loin /lɔɪn/
lucid /ˈluː.sɪd/
lumbar /ˈlʌm.bər/
lymphocyte /ˈlim.fə.saɪt/
macrocephaly /ˌmækrəʊ.ˈsef.ə.li/
magnum /ˈmægnəm/
malformation /ˌmæl.fəˈmeɪ.ʃən/
matter /ˈmæt.ər/
medulloblastoma /mɪˌdʌləʊbæsˈtəʊmə/
menarche /menˈɑː.ki/
meningocele /meˈnɪŋgəʊˌsiːl/
microbiology /ˌmaɪkrəʊbaɪˈɒlədʒɪ/
microcephaly /ˌmaɪ.krəʊ.ˈsef.ə.li/
micturition /ˌmɪktjʊˈrɪ.ʃən/
Miller Fisher syndrome /miler fishˈer sɪndrəʊm/
mitochondrial /ˌmaɪtəʊˈkɒndrɪəl/
motor /ˈməʊ.tər/
mucopolysaccharidosis /ˌmjuːkəʊˌpɒlɪˈsækəˌraɪd əʊsɪs/
myasthenia /ˌmaɪəsˈθiː.nɪ.ə/ **gravis** /græv.ɪs/

myelomeningocele /ˌmaɪ.ə.ləʊ.menˈɪŋ.gə.siːl/
myoclonic /ˌmaɪəʊˈklɒn.ɪk/
myoclonus /ˌmaɪ.əˈkləʊ.nəs/
myopathy /ˌmɑɪ.oʊˈpə.θi/
myositis /ˌmaɪəʊˈsaɪtɪs/
myotonic /ˌmaɪəˈtɒnɪk/
negotiate /nɪˈɡəʊʃiˌeɪt/
neural tube /ˈnjʊə.rəl tjuːb/
neurocutaneous /ˌnjʊə.rəʊˈkjuˈteɪ.ni.əs/
neurofibroma /ˌnjʊərəʊˈfaɪ.brəʊmə/
Niemann-Pick disease /niːˈmən pik dɪˈziːz/
nystagmus /nɪˈstæg.məs/
occipital /ɒkˈsɪp.ɪ.təl/
occult /ˈɒkʌlt/
overnight /ˌəʊ.vəˈnaɪt/
palsy /ˈpɔːl.zi/
papilledema /pəˈpɪl.ə.ɪˈdiː.mə/
paralysis /pəˈræl.ə.sɪs/
parenthood /ˈpeərənthʊd/
parietal /pəˈraɪə.təl/
paroxysmal /ˈpær.ɒk.sɪz.məl/
patch /pætʃ/
paucity /ˈpɔː.sə.ti/
perception /pəˈsep.ʃən/
peri- /ˌperi/
permission /pəˈmɪʃ.ən/
peroxisomal /pəˌrɒksɪˈsəʊməl/
persistent /pəˈsɪs.tənt/
personality /ˌpɜː.sənˈæl.ə.ti/
phenomenon /fəˈnɒm.ɪ.nən/ pl **phenomena**
pierce /ˈpɪə.s/
pneumococcal /ˌnjuː.məˈkɒkəl/
poliomyelitis /poʊ.li.oʊ.maɪ.ə.laɪ.tɪs/
polycystic disease /pɒl.iˌsɪs.tɪk dɪˌziːz/
polymyositis /ˌpɒlɪˈmaɪəs aɪtɪs/
polyneuropathy /ˈpɒlɪnjʊˈrɒpəθɪ/
pontocerebellar /pɒnˈto.ser.e.belˈar/
postcoital /ˌpəʊstˈkəʊɪtᵊl/
posterior /pɒsˈtɪə.ri.ər/
postictal /ˈpəʊstˈɪkt.əl/
practicality /ˌpræktɪˈkælɪtɪ/
pre monitoring /priːˈmɒnɪtərɪŋ/
precipitate /prɪˈsɪp.ɪ.teɪt/
predisposition /ˌpriːdɪs.pəˈzɪʃ.ən/
profound /prəˈfaʊnd/
protective /prəˈtek.tɪv/
protrusion /prəˈtruː.ʒən/

310

proxy /ˈprɒksɪ/
pseudoseizure /ˌsjuːdəʊˈsiːʒə/
psychogenic /ˌsaɪ.kəʊˈdʒɛ.nɪk/
pulsatile /ˈpʌlsəˌtaɪl/ **mass** /mæs/
pyramidal /pɪˈræm.ɪ.dəl/
recall / rɪˈkɔːl/
refractive /rɪˈfræk.tɪv/
regimen /ˈredʒ.ɪ.mən/
regression /rɪˈgreʃ.ən/
reject /rɪˈdʒekt/
rejection /rɪˈdʒek.ʃən/
religious /rɪˈlɪdʒəs/
repetitive /rɪˈpet.ə.tɪv/
rescue /ˈreskjuː/
resilient /rɪˈzɪl.i.ənt/
retinal /ˈret.ɪ.nəl/
Rett syndrome /ˈret sɪndrəʊm/
reveal /rɪˈviːl/
rhabdomyoma /ˌræbdəʊmaɪˈəʊmə/
rigid /ˈrɪdʒɪd/
roughen /ˈrʌfən/
scoliosis /ˌskɒl.iˈəʊ.sɪs/
self-gratification /selfˌgræt.ɪ.fɪˈkeɪ.ʃən/
sensory / ˈsent.sər.i/
setting /ˈsetɪŋ/
shunt /ʃʌnt/
side /saɪd/ **effect** /ɪˈfekt/
sinusitis /ˌsaɪ.nəˈsaɪ.tɪs/
slit-lamp /slɪt læmp/
spasm /ˈspæz.əm/
spasticity /spæsˈtɪs.ə.ti/
sperm /spɜːm/
sphenoid /sfiːn.ɒ.ɪd/
spina bifida /ˌspaɪ.nəˈbɪf.ɪ.də/
spurt /spɜːt/
squint /skwɪnt/
stance /stɑːns/
stenosis /steˈnəʊ.sɪs/
stick /stɪk/ **(stuck, stuck)**
straining /streɪn.ɪŋ/
stuffy /ˈstʌfɪ/
subdural /sʌbˈdjʊ.ə.rəl/
subungual /sʌbˈʌŋgwəl/
suture /ˈsuː.tʃər/
swab /swɒb/
synchronous /ˈsɪŋ.krə.nəs/
syncope /ˈsɪŋ.kə.pi/

syringomyelia /sə.rɪngˈɡəʊ.maɪ.iːˈliː.ə/
tattoo /təˈtuː/
Tay Sachs /ˌteɪˈsæks/ **hypertonia** /ˌhaɪpəˈtəʊnɪə/
telangiectasia /tɪˌlændʒiekˈteɪ.zɪə/
temper /ˈtem.pər/
temporal /ˈtem.pər.əl/
temporomandibular /ˌtem.pər.ə.mænˈdɪ.bjʊ.lə/
termination /ˌtɜːˈmɪˈneɪ.ʃən/
terror /ˈterə/
testicular /tesˈtɪk.jə.lər/
tonsil /ˈtɒnt.səl/
torticollis /tɔːˈtɪˈkɒl.ɪs/
toxoplasma /ˌtɒksəʊˈplæzmə/
traction /ˈtræk.ʃən/
transglutaminase /tranzˈɡluːtəˈmɪn.eɪs/
trigeminal /traɪˈdʒem.ɪ.nəl/
tuberculous /ˌtjʊˌbɜːkjʊˈləs/
tuberous /ˈtʃuː.bə.rəs/ **sclerosis** /skləˈrəʊ.sɪs/
tubular /ˈtjuː.bjʊ.lər/
ulceration /ˌʌl.sərˈeɪˌʃən/
unsafe /ʌnˈseɪf/
unsteadiness /ʌnˈsted.i.nəs/
urethral /jʊəˈriː.θrəl/
vacuole /ˈvækjʊˌəʊl/
vagal /ˈveɪ ɡəl/
variant /ˈveərɪənt/
vasodepressor /ˌvəɪzəʊ dɪˈprəsə/
vasovagal /ˌveɪ.zəʊˈvæg.əl/
ventriculoperitoneal /ven.ˌtrik.jə.ləʊ ˌper.ɪ.təˈniːˈel/ **shunt** /ˈʃənt/
vertical /ˈvɜː.tɪ.kəl/
vertigo /ˈvɜː.tɪ.ɡəʊ/
vestibular /vesˈtɪb.jə.lər/
virology /vaɪˈrɒl.ə.dʒɪ/
virus /ˈvaɪ.rəs/
vocational /vəʊˈkeɪ.ʃə.nəl/
volvulus /ˈvɒlvjʊləs/
wheeze /wiːz/
whooping cough /ˈhuː.pɪŋ ˌkɒf/
Wilson /ˈwilˈsɒn/ **disease** /dɪˈziːz/
wring /rɪŋ/
yeast /jiːst/

Perspectives of paediatric nursing; Documentation of nursing care; Childhood injuries: risk factors; Key elements of family - centred care; Using defining characteristics to select an appropriate nursing diagnosis; Social, cultural, and religious influences on child health promotion.

Text 1
United Nations' Declaration of the Rights of the Child
All children need:
- to be free from discrimination
- to develop physically and mentally in freedom and dignity
- to have a name and nationality
- to have adequate nutrition, housing, recreation, and medical services
- to receive special treatment if handicapped
- to receive love, understanding, and material security
- to receive an education and develop his or her abilities
- to be the first to receive protection in disaster
- to be protected from neglect, cruelty, and exploitation
- to be brought up in a spirit of friendship among people

Health promotion objectives
- increase physical activity and fitness
- improve nutrition
- reduce tobacco use
- reduce alcohol and other drugs abuse
- improve family planning
- improve mental health and reduce mental disorder
- reduce violent and abusive behaviour
- enhance and expand community-based health promotion programs

Health protection objectives
- reduce unintentional injuries
- improve occupational safety and health
- improve environmental health and reduce human exposure to hazardous substances (i.e., lead)

- ensure safety of food and drugs
- improve oral health

Preventive services objectives
- improve nutritional and infant health
- reduce heart disease, stroke, and end-stage renal disease
- prevent and control cancer
- reduce and control human immunodeficiency virus (HIV) infection
- prevent sexually transmitted disease
- increase immunization and prevent infectious diseases
- improve clinical preventive services by reducing barriers to health care

Surveillance and data systems
- improve surveillance and data systems to track progress toward the objectives

American Nurses' Association Standards of Maternal and Child Health Nursing Practice

Standard I:	The nurse helps children and parents attain and maintain optimum health.
Standard II:	The nurse assists families to achieve and maintain a balance between the personal growth needs of individual family members and optimum family functioning.
Standard III:	The nurse intervenes with vulnerable clients and families at risk to prevent potential developmental and health problems.
Standard IV:	The nurse promotes an environment free of hazards to reproduction, growth and development, wellness, and recovery from illness
Standard V:	The nurse detects changes in health status and deviations from optimum development.
Standard VI:	The nurse carries out appropriate interventions and treatment to facilitate survival and recovery from illness.
Standard VII:	The nurse assists clients and families to understand and cope with developmental and traumatic situations during illness, childbearing, childrearing, and childhood.
Standard VIII	The nurse actively pursues strategies to enhance access to and utilization of adequate health care services.
Standard IX:	The nurse improves maternal and child health nursing practice through evaluation of practice, education, and research.

Exercise 1
Answer the following questions. Prepare short talks and/or dialogues on these topics

1. What can you say about United Nations' Declaration of the Rights of the Child (health promotion objectives, preventive services objectives)?
2. What do you know about American Nurses' Association Standards of Maternal and Child Health Nursing Practice (standard I: - standard IX)?

Translation 1

1. All children need: to be free from discrimination, to develop physically and mentally in freedom and dignity, to have adequate nutrition, housing, recreation, and medical services, to be the first to receive protection in disaster, and to be protected from neglect, cruelty, and exploitation. 2. Health promotion objectives are: increase physical activity and fitness, improve mental health and reduce mental disorder, reduce violent and abusive behaviour. 3. Health protection objectives include: improving environmental health and reducing human exposure to hazardous substances (i.e., lead), reducing unintentional injuries. 3. Preventive services objectives mean: improve nutritional and infant health, reduce heart disease, stroke, and end-stage renal disease, reduce and control human immunodeficiency virus (HIV) infection, increase immunization and prevent infectious diseases. 4. The nurse helps children and parents attain and maintain optimum health. 5. The nurse intervenes with vulnerable clients and families at risk to prevent potential developmental and health problems. 6. The nurse detects changes in health status and deviations from optimum development. 7. The nurse carries out appropriate interventions and treatment to facilitate survival and recovery from illness. 8. The nurse assists clients and families to understand and cope with developmental and traumatic situations during illness, childbearing, childrearing, and childhood.

Text 2
Documentation of nursing care
Initial assessments and reassessments
Nursing diagnoses and/or patient care needs
Interventions identified to meet the patient's nursing care
Nursing care provided
Patient's response to, and the outcomes of, the care provided

Abilities of patient and/or, as appropriate, significant other(s) to manage continuing care needs after discharge

Classification systems for nursing diagnoses
Human response patterns

- **Exchanging** — involves mutual giving and receiving
- **Communicating** — involves sending messages
- **Relating** — involves establishing bonds
- **Valuing** — involves the assigning of relative worth
- **Choosing** — involves the selection of alternatives
- **Moving** — involves activity
- **Perceiving** — involves the reception of information
- **Knowing** — involves the meaning associated with information
- **Feeling** — involves the subjective awareness of sensation or affect

Functional health patterns

- **Health perception — health management pattern** – perceptions related to general health management and preventive practices
- **Nutritional-metabolic pattern** — intake of food and fluids related to metabolic requirements
- **Elimination pattern** — regularity and control of excretory functions, bowel, bladder, skin, and wastes
- **Activity-exercise pattern** — activity patterns that require energy expenditure and provide for rest
- **Sleep-rest pattern** — effectiveness of sleep and rest periods
- **Cognitive-perceptual pattern** — adequacy of language, cognitive skills, and perception related to required or desired activities; includes pain perception
- **Self-perception – self-concept pattern** — beliefs and evaluation of self-worth
- **Role-relationship pattern** — family and social roles, especially parent-child relationships
- **Sexuality-reproductive pattern** — problems or potential problems with sexuality or reproduction
- **Coping-stress tolerance pattern** — stress tolerance level and coping patterns, including support systems
- **Value-belief pattern** — values, goals, or beliefs that influence health-related decisions and actions

AHCPR clinical practice guidelines relevant to paediatric practice

- Acute pain management: operative or medical procedures and trauma
- Urinary incontinence in adults
- Pressure ulcers in adults: prediction and intervention
- Treatment of pressure ulcers in adults
- Diagnosis and treatment of depressed outpatients in primary care settings
- Diagnosis and treatment of sickle cell disease
- Initial evaluation and early treatment of the HIV-infected individual
- Management of cancer-related pain
- Diagnosis and treatment of heart failure
- Otitis media in children

Exercise 2
Answer the following questions. Prepare short talks and/or dialogues on these topics

1. What does Documentation of nursing care include?
2. Describe Classification systems for nursing diagnoses.
3. What are human response patterns and functional health patterns?
4. What can you say about health perception and health management?

Translation 2

1. Documentation of nursing care consists of: initial assessments, nursing diagnoses, interventions identified, nursing care provided, outcomes of the care provided, abilities to manage continuing care needs after discharge. 2. Classification systems for nursing diagnoses are: human response patterns (communicating, choosing, moving, perceiving, knowing, feeling) and functional health patterns (nutritional-metabolic pattern, elimination pattern, activity-exercise pattern, sleep-rest pattern, cognitive-perceptual pattern, self-concept pattern, role-relationship pattern, sexuality-reproductive pattern, coping-stress tolerance pattern, value-belief pattern).

Text 3
Childhood injuries: risk factors

Sex	• preponderance of males; difference mainly due to behavioural characteristics; especially aggression
Temperament	• children with difficult temperament profile, especially persistence, high activity and negative reactions to new situations
Stress	• predisposes to increased risk taking and self-destructive behaviour; general lack of self-protection
Alcohol and drug use	• associated with higher incidence of motor vehicle injuries, drownings, homicides, and suicides
Previous history of injury	• associated with increased likelihood of another injury, especially if initial injury required hospitalization
Developmental characteristics	• mismatch between child's developmental level and skill required for activity (e. g., all-terrain vehicles); • natural curiosity to explore environment; • desire to assert self and challenge rules • in older child, desire for peer approval and acceptance
Cognitive characteristic **Infancy** **Young child:** **School-age child** **Adolescent**	(age specific) • sensorimotor: explores environment through taste and touch • object permanence: actively searches for attractive object; • cause and effect: unaware of consequential dangers; • transductive reasoning: may fail to learn from experiences; for example, falling from a step is not perceived as same type of danger as climbing a tree; • magical and egocentric thinking: cannot comprehend danger to self or others; cannot take place of others to realize danger; if thinking something is safe, believes it to be so • transitional cognitive processes; unable to fully comprehend causal relationships; attempts dangerous acts without detailed planning regarding consequences
	• formal operations: preoccupied with abstract thinking and loses sight of reality; may lead to feeling of invulnerability
Anatomic characteristics (especially in young children):	• large head — predisposes to cranial injury; • large spleen and liver with wide costal arch — predispose to direct trauma to these organs; • small and light body — may be thrown easily, especially inside a moving vehicle
Other factors	• poverty, family stress (i.e., maternal illness, recent environmental change), substandard alternative child care, young maternal age, low maternal education, multiple siblings

Exercise 3
Answer the following questions. Prepare short talks and/or dialogues on these topics

1. Which are risk factors of childhood injuries (in infancy, young child, school-age child, adolescent)?
2. What factors may influence injuries (sex, temperament, stress, alcohol and drug use, previous history of injury, developmental characteristics, cognitive characteristic, anatomic characteristics)?

Translation 3

1. Risk factors of childhood injuries are: aggression, high activity and negative reactions to new situations, risk taking and self-destructive behaviour. 2. Other risks are: incidence of motor vehicle injuries, small and light body may be thrown easily, especially inside a moving vehicle. 3. Drownings, homicides, and suicides are all emergency situations. 4. Mismatch between child's developmental level and skill required for activity, as well as desire for peer approval and acceptance may also be dangerous. 4. Children are often unaware of consequential dangers, cannot comprehend danger to self or others, are unable to fully comprehend causal relationships, lose sight of reality and may lead to feeling of invulnerability. 5. Poverty, family stress, young maternal age, low maternal education are important risks, too.

Text 4
Key elements of family — centred care

- Recognizing that the family is the constant in a child's life, whereas the service systems and personnel within those systems fluctuate
- Facilitating parent/professional collaboration at all levels of health care: care of an individual child; program development, implementation, and evaluation; policy information
- Honouring the racial, ethnic, cultural, and socioeconomic diversity of families
- Recognizing family strengths and individuality and respecting different methods of coping
- Sharing with parents, on a continuing basis and in a supportive manner, complete and unbiased information
- Encouraging and facilitating family-to-family support and networking

- Understanding and incorporating the developmental needs of infants, children, and adolescents and their families into health care systems
- Implementing comprehensive policies and programs that provide emotional and financial support to meet the needs of families
- Designing accessible health care systems that are flexible, culturally competent, and responsive to family-identified needs

Exploring your relationships with children and families

To foster therapeutic relationships with children and families, you must first become aware of your caregiving style, including how effectively you can take care of yourself. The following questions should help you understand the therapeutic quality of your professional relationships.

Negative actions

- Are you overinvolved with children and their families?
- Do you work overtime to care for the family?
- Do you spend off-duty time with children's families either in or out of the hospital?
- Do you call frequently (either the hospital or home) to see how the family is doing?
- Do you show favouritism toward certain patients?
- Do you buy clothes, toys, food, or other items for the child and family?
- Do you compete with other staff members for the affection of certain patients and families?
- Do other staff members comment to you about your closeness to the family?
- Do you attempt to influence families' decisions rather than facilitate their own decision making?
- Are you under-involved with children and families?
- Do you restrict parent or visitor to access to children, using excuses such as the unit is too busy?
- Do you focus on the technical aspects of care and lose sight of the person who is the patient?
- Are you overinvolved with children and under-involved with their parents?
- Do you become critical when parents don't visit their children?
- Do you compete with parents for their children's affection?

Positive actions

- Do you strive to empower families?
- Do you explore families' strength and needs in an effort to increase family involvement?
- Have you developed teaching skills to instruct families rather than doing everything for them?
- Do you work with families to find ways to decrease their dependence on health care providers?
- Can you separate families' needs from your own needs?
- Do you strive to empower yourself?
- Are you aware of your emotional responses to different people and situations?
- Do you seek to understand how your own family experiences influence reactions to patients and families, especially as they affect tendencies toward overinvolvement or under-involvement?
- Do you have a calming influence, not one that will amplify emotionality?
- Have you developed interpersonal skills in addition to technical skills?
- Have you learned about ethnic and religious family patterns?
- Do you communicate directly with persons with whom you are upset or take issue?
- Are you able to "step back" and withdraw emotionally, if not physically, when emotional overload occurs, yet remain committed?
- Do you take care of yourself and your needs?
- Do you maintain clear, open communication?
- Do you periodically interview family members to determine their current issues (e. g., feelings, attitudes, responses, wishes), communicate these findings to peers, and update records?
- Do you avoid relying on initial interview data, assumptions, or gossip regarding families?
- Do you ask questions if families are not participating in care?
- Do you assess families for feelings of anxiety, fear, intimidation, worry about making a mistake, a perceived lack of competence to care for their child, or fear of health care professionals' overstepping their boundaries into family territory or vice versa?
- Do you explore these issues with family members and provide encouragement and support to enable families to help themselves?
- Do you keep communication channels open among self, family, physicians, and other care providers?

- Do you resolve conflicts and misunderstandings directly with those who are involved?
- Do you clarify information for families or seek appropriate person to do so?
- Do you recognize that from time to time a therapeutic relationship can change to a social relationship or an intimate friendship?
- Are you able to acknowledge the fact when it occurs and understand why it happened?
- Can you ensure that there is someone else who is more objective and take your place in the therapeutic relationship?

Exercise 4
Answer the following questions. Prepare short talks and/or dialogues on these topics

1. Characterize key elements of family - centred care.
2. What to do to foster therapeutic relationships with children and families?
3. What can you say about negative actions?
4. What can you say about positive actions?

Translation 4

1. Key elements of family - centred care are: facilitating parent/ professional collaboration at all levels of health care; honouring the racial, ethnic, cultural, and socioeconomic diversity of families; understanding and incorporating the developmental needs of infants, children, and adolescents and their families into health care systems; designing accessible health care systems that are flexible, culturally competent, and responsive to family-identified needs. 2. The following questions should help you understand the therapeutic quality of your professional relationships: Do you work overtime to care for the family?; Do you buy clothes, toys, food, or other items for the child and family?; Do you attempt to influence families' decisions?; Do you restrict parent or visitor to access to children?; Do you compete with parents for their children's affection? (negative actions). 3. Questions about positive actions may include: Have you developed teaching skills to instruct families rather than doing everything for them?; Do you work with families to find ways to decrease their dependence on health care providers?; Are you aware of your emotional responses to different people and situations?; Do you take care of yourself and your needs?; Do you avoid relying on initial interview data, assumptions, or gossip regarding families?; Do you keep communication channels open among self, family, physicians, and

other care providers?; Do you recognize that from time to time a therapeutic relationship can change to a social relationship or an intimate friendship?; Can you ensure that there is someone else who is more objective and take your place in the therapeutic relationship?

Text 5
Using defining characteristics to select an appropriate nursing diagnosis

An 18-months-old child is admitted with respiratory distress and a presumptive diagnosis of epiglottitis. Initial nursing actions are focused on the physiologic status of the child. As the condition stabilizes, family assessment data are gathered. The child's immunizations are current, he is clean and well nourished, and his developmental age is appropriate. The parents are present at admission. Both are employed, and the child is cared for by the maternal grandparents. The mother is distraught about the sudden onset of the respiratory distress. She states that earlier just a "runny nose" was present. She asks appropriate questions and seems to understand that epiglottitis is a sudden illness that typically follows symptoms of a cold. She asks what she can do to make her child more comfortable and less fearful, and she is able to implement the suggestions. The father supports both the child and the mother but assumes a more passive, "listening" role. At least three nursing diagnoses that relate to family/parent situations can be considered. The first step is to review the definition and defining characteristics for each and decide which is most appropriate for this family:

Altered parenting — inability to nurturing figure to create an environment that promotes optimum growth and development of another human being.
- **Selected defining characteristics:** inattentive to infant/child needs; inappropriate caretaking behaviours

Family coping: potential for growth — family member has effectively managed adaptive tasks involved with client's health challenge and is exhibiting desire and readiness for enhanced health and growth in regard to self and in relation to client.
- **Selected defining characteristics**: family member attempts to describe growth impact or crisis on own values, priorities, goals, or relationships

Altered family process — inability of family system (household members) to meet needs of members, carry out family functions, or maintain communication for mutual growth and maturation

- **Selected defining characteristics:** inability of family members to relate to each other for mutual growth and maturation; failure to send and receive clear messages; inability to accept and receive help

Among these choices, the most appropriate nursing diagnosis is "family coping: potential for growth." The parents are attentive to the child's needs and appear to have appropriate caregiving skills. The sudden illness of the child has disrupted the family's pattern, but the mother demonstrates effective coping and the ability to learn and implement new comforting skills. The other two diagnoses require some maladaptive feature, which is not found in this situation.

Exercise 5
Answer the following questions. Prepare short talks and/or dialogues on these topics

1. Sum up defining characteristics of the casualty.
2. What is the first step is to review the definition and defining characteristics?
3. Speak about altered parenting, family coping, and altered family process.

Exercise 6
Study the following summary and then interpret basic information in English.

1. Low birth weight, which is closely related to early gestational age, is considered the leading cause of neonatal death.
2. Injuries are the leading cause of death in children over age 1 year, with the majority of injuries being due to motor vehicle injuries.
3. Childhood morbidity encompasses acute illness, chronic disease, and disability.
4. Eighty percent of childhood illnesses are attributable to infections, with respiratory infections occurring two to three times as often as all other illnesses combined.
5. The "new morbidity" refers to behavioural, social, and educational problems that can significantly alter a child's health.
6. Children's developmental stage and their environment are important determinants in the prevalence of injuries at a given age and thus help to direct preventive measures.
7. Two strategies for injury prevention in children are (1) **passive**, which provides automatic protection by product and environmental design; and (2) **active**, which persuades people to change their behaviours for increased self-protection.

Exercise 7
Fill in the missing words. Choose the correct ones.

1. During the first half of the 1900s, public health initiatives, such as environmental strategies to _____ _____ and the development of _____, were the major advances leading to _____ childhood deaths.	a decreased b antibiotics c control infection
2. During the latter half of the 1900s, the advancement and medical __ _____ __ knowledge and technology, specifically in care of ____-____ and ___-_____-_____ newborns, lowered the number of deaths in children, especially the neonatal _____ ____.	a mortality rate b low-birth-weight c high-risk d application of
3. _____ _____ involves care and accountability by one nurse for a small patient population. Associate nurses making up the primary care share patient _____ _____ in the _____ __ the primary nurse.	a absence of b care responsibilities c Primary nursing
4. The paediatric nurse's roles include a _____ _____, family advocacy, disease prevention/ health promotion, health teaching, support - _____, _____, collaboration, ethical decision making, research, and health care _____.	a counselling, coordination b planning c therapeutic relationship
5. With the shift in focus from _____ __ _____ to promotion of health, nurses' roles are expanding outside traditional _____ ____ _____, such as in _____ ____ centres, schools, and the family's home.	a ambulatory care b treatment of disease c health care facilities
6. The process of nursing children and families includes accurate and comprehensive assessment, analysis and synthesis of _____ ____ to arrive at a _____ _____, planning of care, implementation of the plan, and _____ __ _____.	a evaluation of interventions b nursing diagnosis c assessment data

Translation 5

1. An 18-months-old child is admitted with respiratory distress and a presumptive diagnosis of epiglottitis. 2. As the condition stabilizes, family assessment data are gathered. 3. The child's immunizations are current, he is clean and well nourished, and his developmental age is appropriate. 4. The child is cared for by the maternal grandparents. 5. The mother is distraught about the sudden onset of the respiratory distress. 6. She asks appropriate questions and seems to understand that epiglottitis is a sudden

illness that typically follows symptoms of a cold. 7. The first step is to review the definition and decide which is most appropriate for this family: altered parenting, family coping, altered family process. 8. Low birth weight, which is closely related to early gestational age, is considered the leading cause of neonatal death. 9. Childhood morbidity encompasses acute illness, chronic disease, and disability. 10. Eighty percent of childhood illnesses are attributable to infections, especially respiratory infections.

Exercise 8
Fill in the missing words. Choose the correct ones.

1. Children's _____ _____ and their _____ are important determinants in the _____ __ _____.	a prevalence of injuries b developmental stage c environment
2. The paediatric nurse's roles include a therapeutic relationship, family advocacy, _____ _____/health promotion, _____ _____ , support-counselling, coordination, collaboration, _____ _____ _____, research, and health care planning.	a ethical decision making b health teaching c disease prevention
3. The _____ __ _____ children and families includes accurate and comprehensive assessment, of _____ ____ _____ assessment data to arrive at a nursing diagnosis, planning of care, _____ __ the plan, and evaluation of interventions.	a implementation of b analysis and synthesis c process of nursing

Text 6
Social, cultural, and religious influences on child health promotion
- Nurses have a responsibility to understand the influence of culture, race, and ethnicity on the development of social and emotional relationships, childrearing practices, and attitudes toward health.
- Culture is the sum total of mores, traditions, and beliefs about how people function and encompasses other products of human works and thoughts specific to members of an intergenerational group, community, or population.
- A child's self-concept evolves from ideas about his of her social roles.
- Primary groups are characterized by intimate contact, mutual support, and behaviour constraint among members.
- Secondary groups have limited intermittent contact, little mutual support, and no pressure for conformity.

- Guilt and shame are two behaviours commonly conditioned in children to control social behaviour.
- Important subcultural influences on children include ethnicity, social class, occupation, poverty, affluence, religion, schools, peers, and biculture.
- Membership in a minority group presents special challenges for children, although changes in societal attitudes are slowly taking place.
- A child's physical characteristics and susceptibility to health problems are strongly related to ethnic and cultural variations of hereditary and socioeconomic forces.
- Hereditary and socioeconomic forces play an important role in a child's susceptibility to health problems.
- Groups of children suffering from greater physical and mental problems are those living in poverty who are homeless or have migrant families.
- Drug response, food sensitivity, disease resistance, physical characteristics, and disease states may demonstrate ethnic or cultural variations.
- Because of verbal and nonverbal communication is an important culture consideration, nurses need to acknowledge and respect their patient's practices in order to productive interaction to occur.
- Cultural beliefs related to cause of illness and maintenance of health may focus on natural forces, supernatural forces, or imbalance of forces.
- In planning and implementing patient care, nurses need to strive to adapt ethnic practices to the family's health needs rather than attempt to change long-standing beliefs.
- No cultural group is homogeneous; every racial and ethnic group contains great diversity.

Exercise 9
Answer the following questions. Prepare short talks and/or dialogues on these topics

1. Characterize responsibilities of nurses.
2. What is meant by the term culture?
3. What are primary and secondary groups?
4. Explain important subcultural influences on children.
5. What can you say about membership in a minority group?
6. What do you know about hereditary and socioeconomic forces?

7. Speak about problems of those living in poverty who are homeless or have migrant families.
8. Why do the nurses need to acknowledge and respect their patient's practices?

Translation 6

1. Nurses have a responsibility to understand the influence of culture, race, and ethnicity on the development of social and emotional relationships, childrearing practices, and attitudes toward health. 2. A child's self-concept evolves from ideas about his or her social roles. 3. Primary groups are characterized by intimate contact, mutual support, and behaviour constraint among members. 4. Secondary groups have limited intermittent contact, little mutual support, and no pressure for conformity. 5. Important subcultural influences on children include ethnicity, social class, occupation, poverty, affluence, religion, schools, peers, and biculture. 6. Hereditary and socioeconomic forces play an important role in a child's susceptibility to health problems. 7. Groups of children suffering from greater physical and mental problems are those living in poverty who are homeless or have migrant families. 8. Nurses need to acknowledge and respect their patient's practices in order to productive interaction to occur.

Key 11
Exercise 7
1 c, b, a; 2 d, c, b, a; 3 c, b, a; 4 c, a, b; 5 b, c, a; 6 c, b, a

Exercise 8
1 b, c, a; 2 c, b, a; 3 c, b, a

VOCABULARY 11

abusive /əˈbjuː.sɪv/
acceptance /əkˈsep.təns/
accountability /əˌkaʊn.təˈbɪl.ɪ.tɪ/
accurate /ˈæk.jʊ.rət/
addition /əˈdɪʃ.ən/
adequacy /ˈæd.ə.kwə.si/
advance /ədˈvɑːnt s/
advancement /ədˈvɑːnsmənt/
advocacy /ˈæd.və.kə.sɪ/
affect /əˈfekt/
affection /əˈfek.ʃən/
affluence /ˈæfluəns/
alternative /ɒlˈtɜː.nə.tɪv/
ambulatory /ˌæm.bjəˈleɪ.tər.i/
amplify /ˈæm.plɪ.faɪ/
appropriate / əˈprəʊ.pri.ət/
approval /əˈpruː.vəl/
arch /ɑːtʃ/
assert /əˈsɜːt/
assign /əˈsaɪn/
assumption /əˈsʌmp.ʃən/
attain /əˈteɪn/
attitude /ˈæt.ɪ.tjuːd/
attributable /əˈtrɪ.bjʊt.ə.bəl/
awareness /əˈweə.nəs/
belief /bɪˈliːf/
bond /bɒnd/
boundary /ˈbaʊn.dər.i/
bring /brɪŋ/ up /ʌp/
calming /kɑːm.ɪŋ/
caregiving /ˈkeəˌgɪvɪŋ/
causal /ˈkɔːzəl/
challenge /ˈtʃæl.ɪndʒ/
childbearing /ˈtʃaɪldˌbeə.rɪŋ/
clarify /ˈklær.ɪ.faɪ/
closeness /kləʊsnɪs/
cognitive /ˈkɒg.nɪ.tɪv/
collaboration /kəˌlæb.əˈreɪʃən/
comforting /ˈkʌm.fə.tɪŋ/
comment /ˈkɒm.ent/
committed /kəˈmɪ.tɪd/
compete /kəmˈpiːt/
competence /ˈkɒm.pɪ.tənt s/
comprehend /ˌkɒm.prɪˈhend/
comprehensive /ˌkɒm.prɪˈhen.sɪv/

conformity /kənˈfɔːm.ɪ.tɪ/
consequential /ˌkɒnsɪˈkwen.ʃəl/
constraint /kənˈstreɪnt/
continue /kənˈtɪn.juː/
coping /ˈkəʊp.ɪŋ/
costal /ˈkɒs.təl/
counselling /ˈkaʊnt.səl.ɪŋ/
cruelty /ˈkruː.əltɪ/
curiosity /ˌkjʊərɪˈɒsɪtɪ/
decrease /dɪˈkriːs/
dependence /dɪˈpen.dənt s/
desire /dɪˈzaɪər/
detect /dɪˈtekt/
determinant /dɪˈtɜː.mɪ.nənt/
determine /dɪˈtɜː.mɪn/
deviation /ˌdiː.vɪˈeɪʃən/
dignity /ˈdɪg.nɪ.ti/
disaster /dɪˈzɑː.stər/
discharge /dɪsˈtʃɑːdʒ/
disorder /dɪˈsɔː.dər/
distraught /dɪˈstrɔːt/
diversity /daɪˈvɜː.sɪ.ti/
drowning /ˈdraʊn.ɪŋ/
elimination /ɪˌlɪm.ɪˈneɪ.ʃən/
empower /ɪmˈpaʊər/
encompass /ɪnˈkʌm.pəs/
encouragement /ɪnˈkʌr.ɪdʒ.mənt/
ensure /ɪnˈʃɔːr/
environmental /ɪnˌvaɪə.rən.ˈmen.təl/
epiglottitis /ˌep.ɪ.gləˈtaɪ.tɪs/
establish /ɪˈstæb.lɪʃ/
evolve /ɪˈvɒlv/
excretory /ˈek.skrə.ˌtɔː.r.iː/
excuse /ɪkˈskjuːz/
expand /ɪkˈspænd/
expenditure /ɪkˈspendɪtʃə/
experience /ɪkˈspɪə.ri.ənts/
exploitation /ˌek.splɔɪˈteɪ.ʃən/
explore /ɪkˈsplɔːr/
exposure /ɪkˈspəʊ.ʒə/
facilitate /fəˈsɪl.ɪ.teɪt/
favouritism /ˈfeɪvərɪˌtɪzəm/
fluctuate /ˈflʌk.tju.eɪt/
foster /ˈfɒstə/
gather /ˈgæð.ər/
gestational /dʒesˈteɪ.ʃən.əl/
gossip /ˈgɒsɪp/

guilt /gɪlt/
hereditary /həˈred.ɪ.tər.i/
homicide /ˈhɒm.ɪ.saɪd/
homogeneous /ˌhəʊməˈdʒiːnɪəs/
housing /ˈhaʊ.zɪŋ/
imbalance /ˌɪmˈbæl.ənt s/
immunodeficiency /ˌɪm.jʊ.nəʊ .dɪˈfɪʃ.ənt .si/
implement /ˈɪm.plɪ.ment/
implementation /ˌɪm.plɪ.menˈteɪ.ʃən/
improve /imˈpruːv/
incidence /ˈɪn.sɪ.dəns/
influence /ˈɪn.flʊ.əns/
initial /ɪˈnɪʃəl/
initiative /ɪˈnɪʃ.ə.tɪv/
instruct /ɪnˈstrʌkt/
intermittent /ˌɪn.təˈmɪt.ənt/
intervene /ˌɪn.təˈviːn/
intervention /ˌɪn.təˈven.ʃən/
intimidation /ɪnˌtɪm.ɪˈdeɪ.ʃən/
invulnerability /ɪnˌvʌl.nºr.əˈbɪl.ə.ti/
lead /led/
lose /luːs/ **sight** /saɪt/ **of** /ɒv/
maintain /meɪnˈteɪn/
maladaptive /mæl.əˈdæp.tɪv/
mismatch /ˌmɪsˈmætʃ/
mores /ˈmɔːreɪz/
mutual /ˈmjuː.tʃu.əl/
neglect /nɪˈglekt/
objective /əbˈdʒek.tɪv/
occupational /ˌɒk.jʊˈpeɪ.ʃən.əl/
off-duty /ˌɒfˈdʒuː.ti/
otitis /əʊˈtaɪ.tɪs/ **media** /ˈmiːdɪə/
outpatient /ˈaʊt.peɪ.ʃənt/
overinvolved /ˌəʊ.və.ɪnˈvɒlvd/
overstepping /ˌəʊ.vəstep.ɪŋ/
participate /pɑːˈtɪs.ɪ.peɪt/
pattern /ˈpæt.ən/
perceive /pəˈsiːv/
perceptual /pəˈseptjʊəl/
permanence /ˈpɜːmənəns/
persuade /pəˈsweɪd/
poverty /ˈpɒv.ə.ti/
prediction /prɪˈdɪkʃən/
predispose /ˌpriː.dɪˈspəʊz/
preoccupied /ˌpriːˈɒk.jʊ.paɪd/
preponderance /prɪˈpɒndərəns/
pressure /ˈpreʃ.ə/ **ulcer** /ˈʌl.sər/

presumptive /prɪˈzʌmptɪv/
prevalence /ˈprevələns/
pursue /pəˈsjuː/
realize /ˈrɪə.laɪz/
reassessment /ˌriː.əˈses.mənt/
recovery /rɪˈkʌv.ər.i/
religious /rɪˈlɪdʒəs/
requirement /rɪˈkwaɪə.mənt/
rest /rest/
restrict /rɪˈstrɪkt/
runny /ˈrʌn.i/ **nose** /nəʊz/
security /sɪˈkjʊə.rɪ.ti/
self-concept /self ˈkɒn.sept/
self-destructive /ˌself dɪˈstrʌk.tɪv/
self-perception /ˌself pəˈsep.ʃən/
self-protection /ˌself prəˈtek.ʃən/
self-worth /ˌselfˈwɜːθ/
sensation /senˈseɪ.ʃən/
separate /ˈsep.ər.ət/
shame /ʃeɪm/
share /ʃeə/
spirit /ˈspɪr.ɪt/
status /ˈsteɪ.təs/
stress /stres/
strive /straɪv/
substandard /sʌbˈstændəd/
supernatural /ˌsuːpəˈnætʃrəl/
surveillance /səˈveɪ.ləns/
susceptibility /səˌsep.tɪˈbɪl.ɪ.ti/
tolerance /ˈtɒl.ər.əns/
transduction /trænzˈdʌk.ʃən/
transmitted /trænzˈmɪt.ɪd/
treatment /ˈtriː.mənt/
unaware /ˌʌn.əˈweər/
unbiased /ʌnˈbaɪəst/
under-involved /ˌʌn.də.ɪnˈvɒlvd/
understanding /ˌʌn.dəˈstæn.dɪŋ/
unintentional /ˌʌnɪnˈtenʃənəl/
upset /ʌpˈset/
utilization /ˌjuːtɪlɪˈzeɪʃən/
value /ˈvæl.juː/
vice versa /ˈvaɪsɪ ˈvɜːsə/
violent /ˈvaɪə.lənt/
vulnerable /ˈvʌl.nər.ə.bl̩/
waste /weɪst/
withdraw /wɪðˈdrɔː/

Family home care; Stages in development of language; Toy Safety; Childhood stress

Text 1
Feelings and behaviours of children related to divorce

Infancy	• effects of reduced mothering or lack of mothering • increased irritability • disturbance in eating, sleeping, and elimination • interference with attachment process
Early preschool children (ages 2-3 years)	• frightened and confused • blame themselves for the divorce • fear of abandonment • increased irritability, whining, tantrums • regressive behaviours (e. g., thumb-sucking, loss of elimination control) • separation anxiety
Later preschool children (ages 3-5 years)	• fear of abandonment • blame themselves for the divorce; decreased self-esteem • bewilderment regarding all human relationships • become more aggressive in relationships with others (e. g., siblings, peers) • engage in fantasy to seek understanding of the divorce
Early school-age children (ages 5-6 years)	• depression and immature behaviour • loss of appetite and sleep disorders • may be able to verbalize some feelings and understand some divorce — related changes • increased anxiety and aggression • feel abandonment by departing parent
Middle school-age children (ages 6-8 years)	• panic reactions • feelings of deprivation — loss of parent, attention, money, and secure future • profound sadness, depression, fear, and insecurity • feelings of abandonment and rejection • fear regarding the future • difficulty expressing anger at parents • intense desire for reconciliation of parents • impaired capacity to play and enjoy outside activities • decline in school performance • altered peer relationships — become bossy, irritable, demanding, and manipulative

	• frequent crying, loss of appetite, sleep disorders • disturbed routine, forgetfulness
Later school age children (ages 9-12 years)	• more realistic understanding of divorce • intense anger directed at one or both parents • divided loyalties • able to express feelings of anger • ashamed of parental behaviour • feel the need for revenge; may wish to punish the parent they hold responsible • feel lonely, rejected, and abandoned • altered peer relationships • decline in school performance • may develop somatic complaints • may engage in aberrant behaviour such as lying, stealing • temper tantrums • dictatorial attitude
Adolescents (ages 12-18 years)	• able to disengage themselves from parental conflict • feel a profound sense of loss — of family, childhood • feelings of anxiety • worry about themselves, parents, siblings • express anger, sadness, shame, embarrassment • may withdraw from family and friends • disturbed concept of sexuality • may engage in acting-out behaviours

Psychologic tasks for children after divorce
Task 1: Understanding the divorce

Young children: understand the immediate changes and differentiate fantasy from reality; manage concerns regarding abandonment, placement in foster care, not seeing departed parent again.

Adolescents/young adults: understand what led to marital failure, evaluate parents' actions; draw useful conclusions or their own lives.

Task 2: Strategic withdrawal

Acknowledge concern and provide appropriate help to parents and siblings; remove divorce from being their total focus and get back to their own interests, pleasures, activities, peer relationships, etc. Parents must help children to remain children to complete this task.

Task 3: Dealing with loss

Deal with loss of intact family and loss of presence of one parent, usually the father. May be most difficult task. Deal with feelings of rejection and blame for making one parent leave. Task is easier if child has good relationship with both parents.

Task 4: Dealing with anger

Manage anger at parents for deciding to divorce, yet are aware of parents' needs, anxiety, and loneliness. Diminished anger and forgiveness come about together.

Task 5: Working out guilt

Deal with sense of guilt for causing marital difficulties and driving wedge between parents. Need to separate guilty ties and get on with their lives.

Task 6: Accepting permanence of divorce

Overcome early denial and fantasies of parents getting back together. Task may not be completed until parent remarries or child separates from parents and leaves.

Task 7: Taking a chance on love

Most important task for growing children-adolescents and young adults. Remain open to love, commitment, marriage, fidelity. Able to turn away from parents' model.

Exercise 1
Answer the following questions. Prepare short talks and/or dialogues on these topics

1. What can you say about feelings and behaviours of children related to divorce?
2. Characterize psychologic tasks for children after divorce (understanding the divorce, dealing with loss, dealing with anger, accepting permanence of divorce).

Exercise 2
Study the following summary and then interpret basic information in English.

1. Since there is no agreement about the definition of family, family is what the client considers it to be.
2. Three theories that have significant relevance and application to paediatric nursing are family systems theory, family stress theory, and developmental theory.

3. Although the traditional family structure has been nuclear or extended, in recent years other forms such as the single-parent family have emerged.	
4. Family size and positioning within the family structure have a strong impact on a child's development.	

Exercise 3
Fill in the missing words. Choose the correct ones.

1. _____ _____ and a basic understanding of childhood _____ and development are two _____ ____ of focus for parents.	a growth b essential areas c Interpersonal skills
2. Parental control tends to be predominantly one of three types: _____, _____, or _____.	a authoritarian, b permissive, c authoritative
3. Three areas of special concern to adoptive families include the initial _____ process, the task of telling the children they ___ _____ and identify formation during _____	a are adopted, b adolescence c attachment
4. Marital factors within the home _____ _____ a child's development. The _____ __ _____ on a child depends on the child's age and sex, the outcome, and the quality of ___ _____-_____ relationship and parental care following the divorce.	a the parent-child b impact of divorce c significantly influence
5. Single-parenting and stepparenting create adjustment difficulties and ___ _____ to the already-demanding parental role. Significant numbers of children will live in a _____-_____ or _____ family at some point.	a single-parent b reconstituted c add stress

Translation 1

1. Feelings and behaviours of children related to divorce are e.g.: disturbance in eating, sleeping, and elimination, somatic complaints; profound sadness, separation anxiety, frequent crying, feelings of anxiety, depression and immature behaviour, increased irritability, decreased self-esteem, fear, and insecurity deprivation, altered peer relationships; feeling frightened and confused, lonely, rejected; children express anger, sadness, shame, embarrassment, forgetfulness, aberrant behaviour such as lying, stealing, they become bossy, irritable, demanding, and manipulative. 2.

Psychologic tasks for children after divorce are: understanding the divorce (manage concerns regarding abandonment); strategic withdrawal (get back to their own interests, pleasures, activities, peer relationships, etc.); dealing with loss (deal with feelings of rejection and blame for making one parent leave); dealing with anger (manage anger at parents for deciding to divorce); working out guilt (guilt for causing marital difficulties); accepting permanence of divorce (overcome early denial and fantasies of parents getting back together); taking a chance on love (able to turn away from parents' model). 3. Family is what the client considers it to be. 4. Three theories are family systems theory, family stress theory, and developmental theory. 5. Family size and positioning within the family structure have a strong impact on a child's development. 6. Parental control tends to be predominantly one of three types: authoritarian, permissive, or authoritative. 7. The impact of divorce on a child depends on the child's age and sex, the outcome, and the quality of the parent-child relationship. 8. Significant numbers of children will live in a single-parent or reconstituted family at some point.

Text 2
Growth and development of children. Developmental age periods
Prenatal period: Conception to birth
- **germinal**: Conception to approximately 2 weeks
- **embryonic**: 2 to 8 weeks
- **foetal**: 8 to 40 weeks (birth)

A rapid growth rate and total dependency make this one of the most crucial periods in the developmental process. The relationship between maternal health and certain manifestations in the newborn emphasizes the importance of adequate prenatal care to the health and well-being of the infant.

Infancy period: Birth to 12 or 18 months
- **neonatal**: Birth to 28 days
- **infancy**: 1 to approximately 12 months

The infancy period is one of rapid motor, cognitive, and social development. Through mutuality with the caregiver (parent), the infant establishes basic trust in the world and the foundation for future interpersonal relationships. The critical first month of life, although part of the infancy period, is often differentiated from the remainder because of the major physical adjustments to extrauterine existence and the psychological adjustment to the parent.

Early childhood: 1 to 6 years
- **toddler**: 1 to 3 years
- **preschool**: 3 to 6 years

This period, which extends from the time the children attain upright locomotion until they enter school, is characterized by intense activity and discovery. It is a time of marked physical and personality development. Motor development advances steadily. Children at this age acquire language and wider social relationships, learn role standards, gain self-control and mastery, develop increasing awareness of dependence and independence, and begin to develop a self-concept.

Middle childhood: 6 to 11 or 12 years
Frequently referred to as the "school age," this period of development is one in which the child is directed away from the family group and is centred around the wider world of peer relationships. There is steady advancement in physical, mental, and social development with emphasis on developing skill competencies. Social cooperation and early moral development take on more importance with relevance for later life stages. This is a critical period in the development of a self-concept.

Later childhood: 11 to 19 years
- **prepubertal**: 10 to 13 years
- **adolescence**: 13 to approximately 18 years

The period of rapid maturation and change known as adolescence is considered to be a transitional period that begins at the onset of puberty and extends to the point of entry into the adult world – usually high school graduation. Biologic and personality maturation are accompanied by physical and emotional turmoil, and there is redefining of the self-concept. In the late adolescent period, the child begins to internalize all previously learned values to focus on an individual, rather than a group, identity.

Attributes of temperament

Activity	Level of physical motion during activity, such as sleep, eating, play, dressing and bathing.

Rhythmicity	Regularity in the timing of physiologic functions, such as hunger, sleep, and elimination.
Approach-withdrawal	Nature of initial responses to a new stimulus, such as people, situations, places, foods, toys, and procedures. **Approach** responses are positive, displayed by activity or expression; **withdrawal** responses are negative expressions or behaviours.
Adaptability	Ease or difficulty with which the child adapts or adjusts to new or altered situations.
Threshold of responsiveness (sensory threshold)	Amount of stimulation, such as sounds or light, required to evoke a response in the child.
Intensity of reaction	Energy level of the child's reactions regardless of quality or direction.
Mood	Amount of pleasant, happy, friendly behaviour, compared with unpleasant, unhappy, crying, unfriendly behaviour exhibited by the child in various situations.
Distractibility	Ease with which a child's attention or direction of behaviour can be diverted by external stimuli.
Attention span and persistence	Length of time a child pursues a given activity (**attention**) and the continuation of an activity in spite of obstacles (**persistence**).

Exercise 4
Answer the following questions. Prepare short talks and/or dialogues on these topics

1. Characterize developmental age periods (prenatal period, infancy, early childhood).
2. Characterize developmental age periods (middle childhood, later childhood).
3. What are attributes of temperament (activity, rhythmicity, approach-withdrawal, threshold of responsiveness, intensity of reaction, mood, distractibility, attention span and persistence)?

Translation 2
1. Prenatal period consists of: germinal, embryonic, and foetal period. 2. Infancy period consists of: neonatal and infancy period. 3. Early childhood contains: toddler and preschool period. 4. In middle childhood there is steady advancement in physical, mental, and social development. 5. Later childhood contains prepubertal period and adolescence. 6. Attributes of temperament are: activity (level of physical motion during sleep, eating, play, dressing and bathing); rhythmicity (regularity in the timing of hunger,

sleep, and elimination); approach-withdrawal (nature of initial responses to people, situations, places, foods, toys, and procedures); adaptability (ease or difficulty with which the child adjusts to new or altered situations); threshold of responsiveness (amount of stimulation to evoke a response in the child); intensity of reaction (energy level of the child's reactions); mood (amount of pleasant behaviour, compared with unpleasant behaviour); attention span and persistence (length of attention in spite of obstacles); distractibility (ease with which a child's attention can be diverted).

Text 3
Stages in development of language

Prelinguistic stage	the period before children utter their first meaningful words; develops in step-like fashion over first 10 to 12 months from crying through cooing to babbling
Holophrastic stage	the period when children's speech consists of one-word utterances, some of which are thought to be holophrases (single-word utterances that represent the meaning of an entire sentence); begins at about 1 year of age
Telegraphic stage	the period when children's speech consists solely of context words, omitting the less meaningful parts of speech (such as articles, prepositions, and auxiliary verbs); begins at about 18 to 24 months of age
Preschool period	the period when children begin to produce some very lengthy sentences and speech increases in complexity (ages 30 months to 5 years)
Middle childhood period	the period when children refine their language skills and increase linguistic competence (ages 6 to 14 years). They use bigger words, produce longer and more complex utterances, and learn subtle exceptions to grammatical rules. They begin to understand even the most complex syntactic structures of their native language

Stages of role taking
Egocentric or undifferentiated perspective (approximately 3 to 6 years). Children are unaware of any perspective other than their own — whatever is right for them is agreeable to others.

- **Social-informational role taking** (approximately 6 to 8 years). Children recognize that people can have perspectives that differ from their own but only because these persons have received different information. Children are unable to think about the thinking of others and imagine how others will react to an event.

- **Self-reflective role taking** (approximately 8 to 10 years). Children know that their own and others' viewpoints may conflict even when they receive the same information. They are able to consider another's point of view and recognize that others can place themselves in their shoes. Consequently, children are able to anticipate another's reactions to their behaviour but are unable to consider their own and another's perspective at the same time.
- **Mutual role taking** (approximately 10 to 12 years). Children can consider their own and another's point of view simultaneously and realize that others are able to do the same. They can also assume the perspective of a disinterested child and anticipate the way the active participants (self and other) will react to the viewpoint of either participant.
- **Social and conventional system role taking** (approximately 12 to 15 years). Young people now attempt to understand the perspective of another by comparing it with that of the social system in which they operate. They expect others to consider and assume perspectives on events congruent with most persons in their social group.

Age characteristics of play

Exploratory stage	**Age**: approximately 3 to 12 months **Activities**: grasping, holding, and examining articles; exploration via creeping or crawling
Toy stage	**Age**: 1 to 7 or 8 years **Activities**: imitating adult behaviour with replicas of adult tools
Play stage	**Age**: 8 to 12 years **Activities**: interest in toys diminishes; interest in games, sports, and hobbies increases
Daydreaming stage	**Age**: characteristic of older children and pubescents **Activities**: Playing the martyr misunderstood and mistreated by everyone or the hero or beauty admired by everyone

Exercise 5
Answer the following questions. Prepare short talks and/or dialogues on these topics

1. Give the characteristics of stages in development of language (prelinguistic stage, holophrastic stage, telegraphic stage, preschool period, middle childhood period).

2. What is meant by stages of role taking (egocentric, social-informational role taking, self-reflective role taking, mutual role taking, social and conventional system role taking)?

3. What do you know about age characteristics of play (exploratory stage, toy stage, play stage, daydreaming stage)?

Translation 3

1. Prelinguistic stage is the period before children utter their first meaningful words. 2. Holophrastic stage is the period when children's speech consists of one-word utterances. 3. Telegraphic stage is the period when children's speech consists solely of context words. 4. Preschool period is the period when children begin to produce lengthy sentences. 5. Middle childhood is the period when children produce longer and more complex utterances and they begin to understand complex syntactic structures. 6. In egocentric perspective (3 to 6 years) children think that whatever is right for them is agreeable. 7. Social-informational role taking (6 to 8 years) - children are unable to think about the thinking of others.

Exercise 6
Match the column A with the column B. Try to learn the expressions and/or sentences by heart.

A

1. Self-reflective role taking (8 to 10 years) -
2. Mutual role taking (10 to 12 years) -
3. Social and conventional system role taking (12 to 15 years) -
4. Exploratory stage of play includes
5. Toy stage activities
6. During play stage
7. Activities in daydreaming stage

B

a. ... *young people now attempt to understand the perspective of another.*
b. ... *children are able to consider another's point of view and they are able to anticipate another's reactions.*
c. ... *are playing the martyr misunderstood and mistreated by everyone or the hero or beauty admired by everyone.*
d. ... *interest in games, sports, and hobbies increases.*
e. ... *grasping, holding, and examining articles and exploration via creeping or crawling.*

f.   ... *children can consider their own and another's point of view simultaneously.*

g.   ... *include imitating adult behaviour.*

Text 4
Family home care
Toy Safety
Selection

Select toys that suit the skills, abilities, and interests of children. Select toys that are safe for the specific child; look for a label that indicates the intended age-group. Toys that are safe for one age may not be safe for another.

- For infants, toddlers, and all children who still mouth objects, avoid toys with small parts that may pose a fatal choking hazard or aspiration hazard. Toys in this category are usually labelled: "Not recommended for children under 3 years".
- For infants avoid toys with strings or cords that are 7 inches or longer, since they may cause strangulation.
- For all children under 8 years, avoid electric toys with heating elements.
- For children under 5 years, avoid arrows and darts.
- Check for safety labels, such as "flame retardant" or "flame resistant".
- Select toys durable enough to survive rough play; look for sturdy construction such as tightly secured eyes, nose, or any small parts.
- Select toys light enough that they will not cause harm if one falls on a child.
- Look for toys with smooth, rounded edges. Avoid toys with sharp edges that can cut or have sharp points.
- Points on the inside of the toy can puncture if the toy is broken.
- Avoid toys with any shooting or throwing objects that can injure eyes.
- This includes toys into which other missiles, such as sticks or pebbles, might be used as substitutes for the intended projectiles.
- Arrows and darts used by children should have blunt tips and be manufactured from resilient materials; make certain tips are securely attached.
- Make certain that materials in toys are nontoxic.
- Avoid toys that make loud noises that might be damaging to a child's hearing. Even some squeaking toys are too loud when held close to the ear.

- Make certain that arrows or darts have soft tips, rubber suction cups, or other protective tips. Check to be certain that tips are secure.
- If selecting a toy gun, be certain that the barrel of the entire gun is brightly coloured to avoid being mistaken as a real gun.
- Check toy instructions for clarity. They should be clear to an adult and, when appropriate, to the child.

Supervision

Maintain a safe play environment.

- Remove and discard plastic wrappings on toys immediately; they could suffocate a child.
- Remove large toys, bumper pads, and boxes from playpens; an adventuresome child can use such items as a means of climbing or falling out.
- Set "ground rules" for play. Supervise young children closely during play. Teach children how to use toys properly and safely. Instruct older children to keep their toys away from younger brothers, sisters, and friends. Keep children who are playing with riding toys away from stairs, hills, traffic, and swimming pools. Establish and enforce rules regarding protective gear.
- Insist that children wear helmets when using bicycles, skate boards, or in-line skates.
- Insist that children wear gloves and wrist, elbow, and knee pads when using skateboards or in-line skates.
- Instruct children on electrical safety.
- Teach children the proper way to unplug an electric toy – pull on the plug, not the cord.
- Teach children to beware of electrical appliances and even electrically operated playthings; frequently children are unfamiliar with the hazards of electricity in association with water.
- Teach children the safe use of utensils that under certain circumstances can cause injury — scissors, knives, needles, heating elements, or loops, long string, or cord.

Maintenance

Inspect old and new toys regularly for breakage, loose parts, and other potential hazards.

- Look for jagged or sharp edges or broken parts that might constitute a choking hazard.

- Check movable parts to make certain they are attached securely to the toys; sometimes pieces that are safe when attached to the toy become a danger when detached.
- Examine all outdoor toys regularly for rust and weak or sharp parts that could become a danger to a child.
- Check electrical cords and plugs for cracked or fraying parts.
- Maintain toys in good repair, without signs of possible hazards, such as sharp edges, splinters, weak seems, or rust.
- Make repairs immediately, or discard out of reach of children.
- Sand sharp wooden toys or splintered surfaces smooth.
- Use only paint labelled "nontoxic" to repaint toys, toy boxes, or children's furniture.

Storage

Provide a safe place for children to store toys. Select a toy chest or toy box that is ventilated, is free of self-locking devices that could trap a child inside, and has a lid designed not to pinch a child's fingers or fall on a child's head. If containers other than toy chest are used for storage purposes, they should be fitted with spring loaded support devices if they have a hinged lid to avoid entrapment and suffocation. Teach children to store toys safely in order to prevent accidental injury from stepping, tripping, or falling on a toy. Playthings meant for older children and adults should be safely stowed away on high shelves, in locked closets, or in other areas unavailable to younger children.

Exercise 7
Answer the following questions. Prepare short talks and/or dialogues on these topics

1. How to select toys?
2. How to maintain a safe play environment?
3. Why is inspecting old and new toys for breakage, loose parts, and other potential hazards important?
4. What can you say about providing a safe place for children to store toys?

Translation 4

1. Select toys that suit the skills, abilities, and interests of children. 2. For infants, toddlers, and all children who still mouth objects, avoid toys with small parts that may pose a fatal choking hazard or aspiration hazard. 3. Check for safety labels, such as "flame retardant" or "flame resistant" 4.

Select toys durable enough to survive rough play. 5. Select toys light enough that they will not cause harm if one falls on a child. 6. Look for toys with smooth, rounded edges. 7. Avoid toys with any shooting or throwing objects that can injure eyes. 8. Avoid toys that make loud noises that might be damaging to a child's hearing. 9. Make certain that arrows or darts have soft tips. 10. If selecting a toy gun, be certain that the barrel of the entire gun is brightly coloured to avoid being mistaken as a real gun. 11. Remove and discard plastic wrappings on toys immediately; they could suffocate a child. 12. Instruct older children to keep their toys away from younger brothers, sisters, and friends. 13. Keep children who are playing with riding toys away from stairs, hills, traffic, and swimming pools. 14. Insist that children wear helmets when using bicycles, skate boards, or in-line skates.

Exercise 8
Match the column A with the column B. Try to learn the expressions and/or sentences by heart.

A

1. Insist that children wear gloves and wrist, elbow, and knee pads ...
2. Teach children to beware of electrical appliances ...
3. Teach children the safe use of utensils that can cause injury – ...
4. Inspect old and new toys regularly ...
5. Check movable parts ...
6. Maintain toys in good repair, ...
7. Use only paint labelled "nontoxic" ...
8. Select a toy chest or toy box that is ventilated, ...
9. Teach children to store toys safely ...

B

a. ... *scissors, knives, needles, heating elements, or loops, long string, or cord.*
b. ... *for breakage, loose parts, and other potential hazards.*
c. ... *to make certain they are attached securely to the toys.*
d. ... *in order to prevent accidental injury from stepping, tripping, or falling on a toy.*
e. ... *to repaint toys, toy boxes, or children's furniture*
f. ... *without signs of possible hazards, such as sharp edges, splinters, weak seems, or rust.*
g. ... *is free of self-locking devices that could trap a child inside, and has a lid designed not to pinch a child's fingers or fall on a child's head.*

h.   ... *and even electrically operated playthings; frequently children are unfamiliar with the hazards of electricity in association with water.*

i.   ... *when using skateboards or in-line skates.*

Text 5
Childhood stress
Warning signs:
- bed-wetting
- boasts of superiority
- complaints of feeling afraid or upset without being able to identify the source
- complaints of neck or back pains
- complaints of pounding heart
- complaints of stomach upset, queasiness, or vomiting
- compulsive cleanliness
- compulsive ear tugging, hair pulling, or eyebrow plucking
- cruel behaviour toward people or pets
- decline in school achievement
- defiance
- demand for constant perfection
- depression
- dirtying pants
- dislike of school
- downgrading of self
- easily startled by unexpected sounds
- explosive crying
- extreme nervousness
- frequent daydreaming and retreats from reality
- frequent urination or diarrhoea
- headaches
- stress scale for children
- hyperactivity, or increased tension or alertness
- increased number of minor spills, falls, and other accidents
- irritability
- listlessness or lack of enthusiasm
- loss of interest in activities usually approached with vigor
- lying
- nightmares or night terror
- nervous laughter
- nervous ticks, twitches, or muscle spasms
- obvious attention-seeking

- overeating
- poor concentration
- poor eating
- poor sleep
- psychosomatic illness
- stealing
- stuttering
- teeth grinding (sometimes during sleep)
- thumb-sucking
- uncomfortable urge to run and hide
- unusual difficulty in getting along with friends
- unusual jealousy of close friends and siblings
- unusual sexual behavioural, such as spying or exhibitionism
- unusual shyness
- use of alcohol, drugs, or cigarettes
- withdrawal from usual social activities

Stress scale for children

Life event	Value
• Death of a parent	100
• Divorce of parents	73
• Separation of parents	65
• Parent's jail term	63
• Death of a close family member (e. g., grandparent)	63
• Personal injury or illness	53
• Parent's remarriage	50
• Suspension or expulsion from school	47
• Parent's reconciliation	45
• Long vacation (summer etc.)	45
• Parent or sibling illness	44
• Mother's pregnancy	40
• Anxiety over sex	39
• Birth or adoption of a new baby	39
• New school or classroom or new teacher	39
• Money problems at home	38
• Death or moving away of close friend	37
• Changes in studies	36
• More quarrels with parents (or parents quarrelling more)	35

• Change in school responsibilities	29
• Sibling going away to school	29
• Family arguments with grandparents	29
• Winning school or community awards	28
• Mother or father going to work or stopping work	26
• School beginning or ending	26
• Family's living standard changing	25
• Change in personal habits (e. g., bedtime, homework, etc.)	24
• Trouble with parents (e. g., lack of communication, hostility, etc.)	23
• Change in school hours, schedule of courses.	23
• Family's moving	20
• New sports, hobbies, family recreation activities	20
• Change in church activities (more involvement or less)	19
• Change in social activities (e. g., new friends, loss of old ones, peer pressures)	18
• Change in sleeping habits, giving up naps, etc.	16
• Change in number of family get-togethers	15
• Change in eating habits (e. g., going on or off diet, new way of family cooking)	13
• Vacation	13
• Christmas	12
• Breaking home, school, or community rules	11

Add up the points for items that have touched the child's life in the last 12 months. Score below 150, the child is carrying an average stress load. Score between 150 and 300, the child has a better-than-average chance of showing some symptoms of stress. Score over 300, the child's stress load is heavy and there is a strong likelihood for experiencing a serious change in health and/or behaviour.

Exercise 9
Answer the following questions. Prepare short talks and/or dialogues on these topics

1. What are warning signs of childhood stress?
2. Describe stress scale for children.

Exercise 10
Study the following summary and then interpret basic information in English.

1. Growth and development of children are strongly influenced by both genetic and environmental factors.
2. The major development phases are prenatal, infancy, early childhood, middle childhood, or adolescent phases.
3. Information about normal growth and development is derived from both cross-sectional and longitudinal studies.
4. Growth and development follow predictable patterns in direction, sequence, and pace.
5. Biologic growth is determined by height, weight, bone age, and dentition.

Exercise 11
Fill in the missing words. Choose the correct ones.

1. External proportions and _____ _____ change with _____ ___.	a advancing age b organ systems
2. _____ _____ in development are those times when the child is more sensitive to _____ stimulation or more susceptible to _____ influences.	a beneficial b Critical periods c detrimental
3. Temperament is a way of _____, _____, ___ _____ to people and situations.	a thinking, b behaving, c and reacting
4. _____ attributes of children can be described as easy, difficult, or _____-__-_____-__.	a slow-to-warm-up b Temperamental
5. According to Freud's _____ _____, during childhood certain regions of the body assume a prominent psychological _____ as the source of new _____.	a pleasures b psychosexual theory c significance
6. Erikson's psychosocial theory emphasizes the concept of _____ _____ in personality development when children _____ __ _____ core conflicts; each successive stage is built on _____ _____ of _____ _____.	a strive to master b successful completion c early stages d critical periods

7. Piaget's theory of _____ _____ describes children's progress through stages of _____ _____ in an orderly _____ _____ that enables them to _____ _____ to the environment.	a make adaptations b mental activity c cognitive development d sequential manner
8. _____ ___ _____ development are accomplished __ _ _____ with _____ _____.	a cognitive development b Moral and spiritual c in conjunction
9. Children are born with the capacity for _____ ___ _____ and _____ rules of language by the time they _____ _____.	a enter school b master c speech and language

Exercise 12
Match the column A with the column B. Try to learn the expressions and/or sentences by heart.

A
1. According to social learning theory, …
2. In the context of the family children learn to apply appropriate …
3. To develop a positive self-concept, children need …
4. Through play children learn about their world …
5. Play provides a means of development in the areas of …
6. Growth and development are affected by …
7. Children's vulnerability and reaction to stress …
8. The mass media can be influential …

B
a. … *depend to a large extent on their age, coping behaviours, and support systems.*
b. … *in children's learning and behaviour.*
c. … *recognition for their achievements and the approval of others.*
d. … *a variety of conditions and circumstances, including heredity, physiologic function, gender of the child, disease, physical environment, nutrition, and interpersonal relationships.*

e.   ... *sensorimotor and intellectual progress, socialization, creativity, self-awareness, and moral behaviour; it serves as a means for release of tension and expression of emotions.*
f.   ... *and how to relate to things, people, and situations.*
g.   ... *children learn appropriate behaviour through conditioning and observation of role models.*
h.   ... *sex labels to themselves, acquire sex-appropriate behaviours, develop a preference to their biologic sex, and identify with the parent of the same sex.*

Translation 5

1. Warning signs of childhood stress are: bed-wetting, explosive crying, extreme nervousness, compulsive ear tugging, hair pulling, or eyebrow plucking, teeth grinding, thumb-sucking, nervous ticks, twitches, or muscle spasms, complaints of neck or back pains, complaints of pounding heart, complaints of stomach upset, queasiness, or vomiting, hyperactivity, or increased tension or alertness, overeating, poor eating, poor sleep, nightmares or night terror, frequent daydreaming and retreats from reality, increased number of minor spills, falls, and other accidents, use of alcohol, drugs, or cigarettes, cruel behaviour toward people or pets. 2. Stress scale for children includes: divorce of parents, separation of parents, parent's remarriage, birth or adoption of a new baby, new school or classroom or new teacher, money problems at home, more quarrels with parents, family arguments with grandparents, change in social activities, change in sleeping habits, giving up naps, change in eating habits, breaking home, school, or community rules. 3. Growth and development of children are strongly influenced by both genetic and environmental factors. 4. The major development phases are prenatal, infancy, early childhood, middle childhood, or adolescent phases. 5. Growth and development follow predictable patterns in direction, sequence, and pace. 6. Biologic growth is determined by height, weight, bone age, and dentition. 7. Temperament is a way of thinking, behaving, and reacting to people and situations.

Exercise 13
Match the column A with the column B. Try to learn the expressions and/or sentences by heart.

A

1.   According to Freud's psychosexual theory, during childhood ...
2.   Erikson's psychosocial theory emphasizes the concept of critical periods ...

3. Piaget's theory of cognitive development describes…
4. According to social learning theory, …
5. In the context of the family children …
6. To develop a positive self-concept, …
7. Play provides a means of development in the areas …
8. Children's vulnerability and reaction to stress depend …

B

a. …*of sensorimotor and intellectual progress, socialization, creativity, self-awareness, and moral behaviour*

b. … *to a large extent on their age, coping behaviours, and support systems.*

c. … *children's progress through stages of mental activity in an orderly sequential manner.*

d. … *children learn appropriate behaviour through conditioning and observation of role models.*

e. … *children need recognition for their achievements and the approval of others.*

f. … *certain regions of the body assume a prominent psychological significance.*

g. … *in personality development when children strive to master core conflicts.*

h. … *learn to apply appropriate sex labels to themselves.*

Key 12
Exercise 3
1 c, a, b; 2 c, b, a; 3 c, a, b; 4 c, b, a; 5 c, a, b

Exercise 6
1b; 2f; 3a; 4e; 5g; 6d; 7c

Exercise 8
1i; 2h; 3a; 4b; 5c; 6f; 7e; 8g; 9d

Exercise 11
1 b, a; 2 b, a, c; 3 a, b, c; 4 b, a; 5 b, c, a; 6 d, a, b, c; 7 c, b, d, a; 8 b, c, a; 9 c, b, a

Exercise 12
1g; 2h; 3c; 4f; 5e; 6d; 7a; 8b

Exercise 13
1f; 2g; 3c; 4d; 5h; 6e; 7a; 8b

VOCABULARY 12

abandonment /əˈbæn.dən.mənt/
aberrant /æˈber.ənt/
acquire /əˈkwaɪər/
adaptability /əˌdæp.təˈbɪl.ɪ.tɪ/
adaptation /ˌæd.əpˈteɪ.ʃən/
adjustment /əˈdʒʌst.mənt/
admired /ədˈmaɪ.əd/
adopt /əˈdɒpt/
advance /ədˈvɑːnt s/
adventuresome /ədˈventʃəsəm/
agreeable /əˈgrɪəbəl/
agreement /əˈgriː.mənt/
alertness /əˈlɜːt.nəs/
altered /ˈɒl.təd/
anger /ˈæŋ.gər/
anticipate /ænˈtɪs.ɪ.peɪt/
anxiety /æŋˈzaɪ.ə.ti/
arrow /ˈær.əʊ/
ashamed /əˈʃeɪmd/
aspiration /ˌæspɪˈreɪʃən/
assume /əˈsjuːm/
attachment /əˈtætʃ.mənt/
authoritarian /ɔːˌθɒrɪˈteərɪən/
authoritative /ɔːˈθɒrɪtətɪv/
away /əˈweɪ/
babble /ˈbæbəl/
barrel /ˈbær.əl/
bewilderment /bɪˈwɪldəmənt/
blame /bleɪm/
blunt / blʌnt/
boast /bəʊst/
bossy /ˈbɒsɪ/
breakage /ˈbreɪ.kɪdʒ/
bumper /ˈbʌm.pər/
chest /tʃest/
choke /tʃəʊk/
closet /ˈklɒzɪt/
commitment /kəˈmɪt.mənt/
compare /kəmˈpeər/
complaint /kəmˈpleɪnt/
conception /kənˈsep.ʃən/
conclusion /kənˈkluː.ʒən/
confused /kənˈfjuːzd/
congruent /ˈkɒŋgrʊənt/
conjunction /kənˈdʒʌŋk.ʃən/

continuation /kənˌtɪnjʊˈeɪʃən/
conventional /kənˈventˌʃən.əl/
coo /kuː/
cord /kɔːd/
core /kɔːr/
cracked /krækt/
crawl /krɔːl/
create /kriːˈeɪt/
creep /kriːp/
cross-section /krɒs.ˈsek.ʃən/
crucial /ˈkruː.ʃəl/
cruel /ˈkruː.əl/
cup /kʌp/
dart /dɑːt/
daydream /ˈdeɪ.driːm/
deal /dɪəl/ with /wɪð/
decline /dɪˈklaɪn/
defiance /dɪˈfaɪəns/
demanding /dɪˈmɑːn.dɪŋ/
dentition /denˈtɪʃ.ən/
depart /dɪˈpɑːt/
deprivation /ˌdep.rɪˈveɪʃən/
detached /dɪˈtætʃt/
detrimental /ˌdet.rɪˈmen.təl/
dictatorial /ˌdɪktəˈtɔːrɪəl/
differ /ˈdɪf.ər/
differentiate /ˌdɪfəˈrenʃieɪt/
discard /dɪˈskɑːd/
discovery /dɪˈskʌvərɪ/
disengage /ˌdɪsɪnˈgeɪdʒ/
disturbance /dɪˈstɜːbəns/
downgrade /ˈdaʊn.ˌgreɪd/
durable /ˈdjʊərəbəl/
ease /iːz/
edge /edʒ/
egocentric /ˌiːgəʊˈsentrɪk/
embarrassment /ɪmˈbær.əs.mənt/
embryonic /ˌembrɪˈɒnɪk/
emerge /ɪˈmɜːdʒ/
engage /ɪnˈgeɪdʒ/
enthusiasm /ɪnˈθjuː.zi.æz.ᵊm/
entrapment /ɪnˈtræpmənt/
evoke /ɪˈvəʊk/
exception /ɪkˈsepˌʃən/
exhibitionism /ˌeksɪˈbɪʃəˌnɪzəm/
exploratory /ɪkˈsplɒrətərɪ/
explosive /ɪkˈspləʊ.sɪv/

express /ɪkˈspres/
expulsion /ɪkˈspʌl.ʃən/
extended /ɪkˈsten.dɪd/
extrauterine /ˌek.strə.ˈjʊ.tə.rən/
fall /ˈfɔːl/ **out** /aʊt/
fidelity /fɪˈdel.ə.ti/
flame /fleɪm/
foetal /ˈfiː.təl/
forgetfulness /fəˈget.fʊl.nɪs/
forgiveness /fəˈgɪvnɪs/
foundation /faʊnˈdeɪ.ʃən/
fray /freɪ/
frightened /ˈfraɪ.tənd/
gear /gɪə/
germinal /ˈdʒɜː.mə.nəl/
give /gɪv/ **up** /ʌp/
graduation /ˌgrædjʊˈeɪʃən/
grasp /grɑːsp/
grind /graɪnd/ (**ground, ground**)
gun /gʌn/
habit /ˈhæb.ɪt/
hinged /ˈhɪndʒd/
holding /ˈhoʊl.dɪŋ/
holophrastic /ˌhoʊ.lə.ˈfra.stik/
imagine /ɪˈmædʒ.ɪn/
imitate /ˈɪm.ɪ.teɪt/
immature /ˌɪm.əˈtʃʊər/
impact /ˈɪm.pækt/
infancy /ˈɪn.fənt.si/
insecurity /ˌɪn.sɪˈkjʊə.rɪ.ti/
intended /ɪnˈten.dɪd/
intense /ɪnˈtens/
interference /ˌɪn.təˈfɪə.rəns/
internalize /ɪnˈtɜː.nə.laɪz/
irritability /ˌɪr.ɪ.təˈbɪl.ɪ.ti/
jagged /ˈdʒæg.ɪd/
jail /dʒeɪl/
jealousy /ˈdʒel.ə.si/
laughter /ˈlɑː.ftə/
light /laɪt/
listlessness /ˈlɪstlɪsnɪs/
loaded /ˈləʊdɪd/
locked /lɒkt/
locomotion /ˌləʊkəˈməʊʃən/
loneliness /ˈləʊn.li.nəs/
lonely /ˈləʊnlɪ/
longitudinal /ˌlɒn.dʒɪˈtjuː.dɪ.nəl/

loop /luːp/
loyalty /ˈlɔɪ.əl.ti/
manage /ˈmæn.ɪdʒ/
manipulative /məˈnɪpjʊlətɪv/
marital /ˈmær.ɪ.təl/
marriage /ˈmær.ɪdʒ/
martyr /ˈmɑːtə/
master /ˈmɑː.stər/
mastery /ˈmɑː.stər.i/
meaningful /ˈmiː.nɪŋ.fəl/
missile /ˈmɪs.aɪl/
mistreat /ˌmɪsˈtriːt/
misunderstood /ˌmɪsʌndəˈstʊd/
mothering /ˈmʌðərɪŋ/
movable /ˈmuː.vəbəl/
mutuality /ˌmjuː.tʃuˈæləti/
nap /næp/
nightmare /ˈnaɪt.meər/
nuclear /ˈnjuː.klɪər/
obstacle /ˈɒbstəkəl/
omit /əʊˈmɪt/
orderly /ˈɔː.dəl.i/
outcome /ˈaʊt.kʌm/
overcome /ˌəʊ.vəˈkʌm/
pad /pæd/
pebble /ˈpebəl/
perfection /pəˈfekʃən/
permissive /pəˈmɪsɪv/
persistence /pəˈsɪstəns/
pinch /pɪntʃ/
playpen /ˈpleɪˌpen/
pluck /plʌk/
plug /plʌg/
point /pɔɪnt/
pounding /ˈpaʊn.dɪŋ/
predictable /prɪˈdɪk.tə.bl̩/
predominantly /prɪˈdɒmɪnəntlɪ/
prelinguistic /ˌpriː.lɪŋˈgwɪs.tɪk/
profound /prəˈfaʊnd/
projectile /prəˈdʒek.taɪl/
pulling /ˈpʊl.ɪŋ/
puncture / ˈpʌŋk.tʃə/
punish /ˈpʌnɪʃ/
quarrel /ˈkwɒrəl/
queasiness /ˈkwiːzɪnɪs/
recent /ˈriː.sənt/
recognition /ˌrek.əgˈnɪʃ.ən/

reconciliation /ˌɹek.ənˌsɪl.iˈeɪ.ʃən/
reconstitute /ˌɹiːˈkɒn.stɪ.tjuːt/
refine /ɹɪˈfaɪn/
regarding /ɹɪˈgɑː.dɪŋ/
regressive /ɹɪˈgɹesɪv/
regularity /ˌɹeg.jʊˈlær.ə.ti/
reject /ɹɪˈdʒekt/
rejection /ɹɪˈdʒek.ʃən/
remarriage /ˌɹiːˈmærɪdʒ/
resilient /ɹɪˈzɪl.i.ənt/
resistant /ɹɪˈzɪs.tənt/
retardant /ɹɪˈtɑː.dᵊnt/
retreat /ɹɪˈtriːt/
revenge /ɹɪˈvendʒ/
rhythmicity /ˈɹɪðmɪsə.tiː/
role /ɹəʊl/ **taking** /teɪk.ɪŋ/
rough /ɹʌf/
rounded /ˈɹaʊn.dɪd/
rust /ɹʌst/
sand /sænd/ **sharp** /ˈʃɑːrp/
scale /skeɪl/
score /skɔː/
secure /sɪˈkjʊə/
seem /siːm/
self-control /ˌself.kənˈtɹəʊl/
self-esteem /ˌself.ɪˈstiːm/
self-locking /ˌself lɒk.ɪŋ/
self-reflective /ˌself ɹɪˈflek.tɪv/
sensorimotor /sensɒ.re.məʊ.tər/
separation /ˌsep.əˈreɪ.ʃən/
sequential /sɪˈkwen.ʃəl/
sharp /ʃɑːp/
shooting /ˈʃuː.tɪŋ/ **pain** /peɪn/
shyness /ʃaɪnɪs/
simultaneously /ˌsɪm.əlˈteɪ.ni.əs.li/
single-parenting /ˈsɪŋgəl.ˈpeərəntɪŋ/
smooth /smuːð/
somatic /səˈmæt.ɪk/
splinter /ˈsplɪn.tər/
spring /spɹɪŋ/
spying /spaɪ.ɪŋ/
squeak /skwiːk/
stage /steɪdʒ/
steadily /ˈsted.ɪ.li/
steplike /ˈstep.laɪk/
stepparent /ˈstepˌpeərənt/
stepping /step.ɪŋ/

stick /stɪk/
stick /stɪk/ (stuck, stuck)
stow /stəʊ/
strangulation /ˌstræŋ.gjʊˈleɪ.ʃən/
string /strɪŋ/
strive /straɪv/
sturdy /ˈstɜːdɪ/
stuttering /ˈstʌtərɪŋ/
subtle /ˈsʌt.əl/
successive /səkˈsesɪv/
suction /ˈsʌk.ʃən/
suffocate /ˈsʌf.ə.keɪt/
superiority /suːˌpɪərɪˈɒrɪtɪ/
suspension /səˈspen.ʃən/
syntactic /sɪnˈtæktɪk/
tantrum /ˈtæntrəm/
tension /ˈten.ʃən/
terror /ˈterə/
threshold /ˈθreʃ.h əʊld/
throw /θrəʊ/ (threw, thrown)
timing /ˈtaɪ.mɪŋ/
tip /tɪp/
transitional /trænˈzɪʃənəl/
trap /træp/
trip /trɪp/
trust /trʌst/
tug /tʌg/
turmoil /ˈtɜː.mɔɪl/
twitch /twɪtʃ/
undifferentiated /ˌʌndɪfəˈren.ʃɪ.eɪ.tɪd/
unfamiliar /ʌn.fəˈmɪl.i.ər/
upright /ˈʌp.raɪt/
urge /ɜːdʒ/
utter /ˈʌtə/
utterance /ˈʌtərəns/
ventilate /ˈven.tɪ.leɪt/
viewpoint /ˈvjuː.pɔɪnt/
vigour /ˈvɪgə/
wedge /wedʒ/
whine /waɪn/
wrapping /ˈræp.ɪŋ/

Hereditary influences on health promotion of the child
and family; Communication and health assessments
of the child and family; Assessing sleep problems in
children; Review of systems; Initiating a comprehensive
family assessment; Family composition

Text 1
Assessment clues to genetic disorders

Major or minor birth defects (anomalies) and dysmorphic features	cardiac defect, ear or eye abnormalities, micrognathia, forehead prominence, hairline low-set on forehead or nape of neck, wide-set eyes, epicanthal folds, low-set ears
Growth abnormalities	short stature, overgrowth, asymmetric growth, intrauterine growth retardation
Skeletal abnormalities	limb abnormalities, asymmetry, scoliosis, hyperextensible joints, hypotonic or hypertonic muscle tone, pectus excavatum, finger or joint abnormalities
Vision or hearing problems	coloboma, cat's eye, hearing loss, vision loss
Metabolic disorders	unusual odour of breath, urine, or stool
Sexual development abnormalities	ambiguous genitalia, small penis, delayed onset of puberty, primary amenorrhoea, precocious sexual development, large testicles
Skin disorders	unusual pigmentation, café-au-lait spots, dry and scaly skin, skin tumours
Recurrent infection or immune deficiency	ear infections, pneumonia
Developmental and speech delays or loss of milestones	
Cognitive delays	learning disabilities, mild to severe mental retardation
Behavioural disorders	hyperactivity, attention deficit disorder, autistic-like behaviour, aggressive behaviour

Guidelines
Referral regarding genetic counselling
- individuals with a family history of hereditary diseases or birth defects.

- known balanced translocation carriers or parents who have previously had foetus or child with a chromosome abnormality
- couples with a history of multiple miscarriages, stillbirths, or infertility
- individuals at risk for ethnic-related disorders
- pregnant women exposed to teratogenic agents
- pregnant women of advanced maternal age (≥ 35 years)
- disorders in which pregnancy could threaten maternal or foetal life or health.

Exercise 1
Answer the following questions. Prepare short talks and/or dialogues on these topics

1. Describe assessment clues to genetic disorders (birth defects, growth abnormalities, skeletal abnormalities, vision or hearing problems, skin disorders, immune deficiency, metabolic disorders, sexual development abnormalities, speech delays, cognitive delays, behavioural disorders).
2. Describe guidelines for referral regarding genetic counselling.

Exercise 2
Study the following summary and then interpret basic information in English.

1. There is probably a genetic component in all disease processes.
2. Genetic diseases are usually classified as those produced by chromosome aberrations, those caused by a single mutant gene, or those resulting from interaction on genetic and environmental factors (multifactorial).
3. Environmental teratogens and maternal disease may also disrupt foetal development, leading to birth defects.
4. Chromosome aberrations are caused by deviations in either chromosome structure or number.
5. Alterations in chromosome number as a result of unequal distribution of genetic material during gamete formation or early cell division of the zygote.
6. Disorders caused by a single gene are distributed in families according to predictable mendelian principles of inheritance, although there are exceptions based on non-traditional concepts.

Exercise 3
Fill in the missing words. Choose the correct ones.

1. _____ _____ can be _____ __ _____ and can be located on an autosome or an X chromosome.	a dominant or recessive b Mutant genes
2. Variations in gene action include the _____ with which it is manifested (penetrance), the _____ ___ _____ of its expression (expressivity), and the different and seemingly unrelated _____ associated with the basic defect (pleiotropy).	a severity or variability b regularity c effects
3. _____ _____, errors or morphogenic development, may arise __ ___ _____ of development and demonstrate wide variability in _____ _____.	a at any stage b causative factors c Congenital defects
4. Although no cure for _____ _____ is presently available, various _____ _____ are used to _____ __ _____ the basic defect.	a therapeutic measures b modify or correct c genetic disease
5. The objectives of genetic screening are to _____ the presence of disease in individuals, detect _____ _____ of a disease, and monitor the _____ of disease and/or _____ in a population.	a unaffected carriers b incidence c malformations d detect
6. _____ _____ includes screening through ultrasound and maternal serum alpha-fetoprotein (MS AFP) testing, and diagnosis by _____, _____, chorionic villi sampling (CVS), and ___ _____.	a amniocentesis, b ultrasound c DNA testing d Prenatal testing
7. _____ _____ is directed toward providing individuals and families with information needed to ____ _____ about a _____ __ _____ appropriate to them.	a make decisions b Genetic counselling c course of action

8. Nurse's roles in genetic counselling include _____ _____, _____ families, _____ families about their disease and its therapy, and providing _____-__ _____ and support.	a interviewing
	b educating
	c follow-up care
	d identifying cases

Translation 1

1. Birth defects and dysmorphic features are e.g.: cardiac defect, micrognathia, and forehead prominence. 2. Growth abnormalities include: short stature, overgrowth, or asymmetric growth. 3. Skeletal abnormalities present with asymmetry, scoliosis, hyperextensible joints, and hypotonic or hypertonic muscle tone. 4. Vision or hearing problems mean e.g. hearing loss, vision loss. 5. Metabolic disorders cause unusual odour of breath, urine, or stool. 6. In sexual development abnormalities ambiguous genitalia, amenorrhoea, or precocious sexual development can be seen. 7. Following skin disorders may be present: unusual pigmentation, dry and scaly skin. 8. Cognitive delays result in learning disabilities, and mental retardation. 9. Behavioural disorders result in hyperactivity, attention deficit disorder, autistic-like behaviour, aggressive behaviour.

Exercise 4

Match the column with the column B. Try to learn the expressions and/ or sentences by heart.

A

1. Individuals with a family history of hereditary diseases or birth defects ...
2. Genetic diseases are usually classified as ...
3. Chromosome aberrations are caused by ...
4. Alterations in chromosome number are a result of...
5. Congenital defects, errors or morphogenic development ...
6. Genetic counselling is directed toward ...
7. Nurse's roles in genetic counselling include ...

B

a. ... *as well as couples with a history of multiple miscarriages, stillbirths, or infertility need referral regarding genetic counselling.*
b. ... *deviations in either chromosome structure or number.*

c. ...*unequal distribution of genetic material during gamete formation or early cell division of the zygote.*

d. ... *identifying cases, interviewing families, educating families about their disease and its therapy, and providing follow-up care and support.*

e. ... *providing individuals and families with information needed to make decisions about a course of action appropriate to them.*

f. ... *may arise at any stage of development and demonstrate wide variability in causative factors.*

g. ... *those produced by chromosome aberrations, those caused by a single mutant gene, or those resulting from interaction on genetic and environmental factors (multifactorial).*

Text 2
Communication and health assessments of the child and family
Guidelines
Communicating with children

Allow children time to feel comfortable. Avoid sudden or rapid advances, broad smiles, extended eye contact, or other gestures that may be seen as threatening. Talk to the parent if child is initially shy. Communicate through transition objects such as dolls, puppets, or stuffed animals before questioning a young child directly. Give older children the opportunity to talk without the parents present. Assume a position that is at eye level with child. Speak in a quiet, unhurried, and confident voice. Speak clearly, be specific, use simple words, and short sentences. State directions and suggestions positively. Offer a choice only when one exists. Be honest with children. Allow them to express their concerns and fears. Use a variety of communication techniques.

Guidelines
Taking a drug allergy history

Ask the following questions:

- Are you allergic to any medication? If yes, what is (are) the medication(s) you are allergic to?
- What dosage form did you take?
- What type of reaction did you have?
- How soon after the therapy was started did this occur?
- How long ago did the reaction occur?
- Who told you that it was an allergic reaction?
- Have you taken this drug or other drugs of similar class after this reaction occurred? If yes, did you experience similar problems?

Habits to explore during health interview

Behaviour patterns, such as nail-biting, thumb-sucking, pica (habitual ingestion of non-food substances), rituals ("security" blanket or toy), and unusual movements (head-banging, rocking, overt masturbation, walking on toes). Activities of daily living, such as hour of sleep and arising, duration of night-time sleep and naps, type and duration of exercise, regularity of stools and urination, age of toilet training, and occurrences of daytime or night-time bed-wetting. Unusual disposition, as well as response to frustration. Use or abuse of alcohol, drugs, coffee, and cigarettes

Guidelines
Assessing sleep problems in children
General history of chief complaint

Ask parents/child to describe sleep problems; record in their words. Inquire about onset, duration, character, frequency, and consistency of sleep problems:

- circumstances surrounding onset (birth of sibling, start of toilet training, death of significant other, move from crib to bed).
- circumstances that aggravate problem, i.e., over-tiredness, family conflict, or disrupted routine (visitors)
- remedies used to correct problem and results of interventions

24-hour sleep history

Time and regularity of meals
- family members present
- activities afterwards, especially evening meal

Time of night and day sleep periods
- hours of sleep and waking
- hours of being put to bed and taken out of bed
- how bedtime is decided (when child looks tired or at a time decided by parent; do both parents agree on bedtime?)

Pre-bedtime or nap rituals (bath, bottle- or breast-feeding, snack, television, active or quiet playing, story)
- mood before nap or bedtime (wide awake, sleepy, happy, cranky)
- Which parent(s) participates in nap or bedtime rituals?

Nap and bedtime rituals

- Where is child allowed to fall asleep? (own bed or crib, couch, parent's bed, someone's lap, other)
- Is child helped to fall asleep? (rocked, walked, patted, given pacifier or bottle, placed in room with light, television, radio on, other)
- Are patterns consistent each time, or do they vary?
- Does child awake if sleep aids are changed or taken away (placed in own bed, television turned off, other)?
- Does child verbally insist that parents stay in room?

Child's behaviours if refuses to go to sleep or stay in room

- If child complains of fears, how convincing are the fears?

Sleep environment

- Number of bedrooms
- Location of bedrooms, especially in relation to parent(s)' room
- Sensory features (light on, door open or closed, noise level, temperature)

Night wakings

- Time, frequency and duration
- Child's behaviour (call out, cry, come out from room, appear frightened, confused or upset)
- Parent(s)' responses (let child cry, go in immediately, take to own bed, feed, pick up, rock, give pacifier, talk, scold, threaten, other)
- Conditions that re-establish sleep
- Do they always work?
- How long do the interventions take to work?
- Which parent intervenes?
- Do both parents use same or different approach?

Daytime sleepiness

- Occurrence of falling asleep at inappropriate times (circumstances, suddenness and irresistibility of onset, length of sleep, mood on awakening)
- Signs of fatigue (yawning, lying down, as well as overactivity, impulsivity, distractibility, irritability, temper tantrums)

Past sleep history

- Sleep patterns since infancy, especially age when slept during the night, stopped daytime naps, later bedtime

- Response to changes in sleep arrangements (crib to bed, different room or house, other)
- Sleep behaviours (restlessness, snoring, sleepwalking, nightmares, partial wakings (young child may wake confused, crying, and thrashing, but does not respond to parent; falls asleep with intervention if not excessively disturbed)
- Parent(s)' perception of child's sleep habits (good or poor sleeper, light or deep sleeper, needs little sleep)
- Family history of sleep problems (sibling behaviour imitated by child; some sleep disorders, e. g., narcolepsy, and enuresis, tend to recur in families)

Exercise 5
Answer the following questions. Prepare short talks and/or dialogues on these topics

1. How to communicate with children?
2. Speak about guidelines for taking a drug allergy history.
3. What are habits to explore during health interview?
4. What do you know about assessing sleep problems in children (general history, time of night and day sleep periods, nap and bedtime rituals, sleep environment, night wakings, daytime sleepiness, past sleep history)?

Translation 2
1. Communicate through transition objects such as dolls, puppets, or stuffed animals before questioning a young child directly. 2 Speak clearly, be specific, use simple words, and short sentences. 3. Allow them to express their concerns and fears. 4. Habits to explore during health interview are: behaviour patterns, such as nail-biting, thumb-sucking, pica, rituals and unusual movements. 5. Activities of daily living, such as hour of sleep and arising, duration of night-time sleep and naps, type and duration of exercise, regularity of stools and urination, age of toilet training, and occurrences of daytime or night-time bed-wetting. 5. Inquire about onset, duration, character, frequency, and consistency of sleep problems: circumstances surrounding onset, circumstances that aggravate problem, remedies used to correct problem and results of interventions. 6. Ask about pre-bedtime or nap rituals (bath, bottle- or breast-feeding, snack, television, active or quiet playing, story).

Exercise 6
Match the column A with the column B. Try to learn the expressions and/or sentences by heart.

A

1. Is child helped to fall asleep...
2. What are child's behaviours if ...
3. What are sensory features ...
4. Child's behaviour during night wakings ...
5. Parent(s)' responses may be: ...
6. Signs of daytime sleepiness are: ...
7. Past sleep history contains: ...
8. Some sleep disorders, ...

B

a.   *... fatigue (yawning, lying down), as well as overactivity, impulsivity, distractibility, irritability, and temper tantrums).*
b.   *... e. g., narcolepsy, and enuresis, tend to recur in families*
c.   *... sleep patterns since infancy, sleep behaviours (restlessness, snoring, sleepwalking, nightmares, and partial wakings).*
d.   *... (light on, door open or closed, noise level, temperature)?*
e.   *... refuses to go to sleep or stay in room?*
f.   *... let child cry, go in immediately, take to own bed, feed, pick up, rock, give pacifier, talk, scold, threaten, other.*
g.   *... (rocked, walked, patted, given pacifier or bottle, placed in room with light, television, radio on?*
h.   *... (call out, cry, come out from room, appear frightened, confused or upset).*

Text 3
Guidelines
Review of systems

General	overall state of health, fatigue, recent and/or unexplained weight gain or loss (period of time for either), contributing factors (change of diet, illness, altered appetite), exercise tolerance, fevers (time of day), chills, night sweats (unrelated to climatic conditions), frequent infections, general ability to carry out activities of daily living
Integument	pruritus, pigment or other colour changes, acne, eruptions, rashes (location), tendency to bruising, petechiae, excessive dryness, general texture, disorders or deformities of nails, hair growth or loss, hair colour change (for adolescent, use of hair dyes or other potentially toxic substances, such as hair straighteners)

Head	headaches, dizziness, injury (specific details)
Eyes	visual problems (ask about behaviours indicative of blurred vision, such as bumping into objects, clumsiness, sitting very close to the television, holding a book close to the face, writing with head near desk, squinting, rubbing the eyes, bending the head in an awkward position), cross-eye (strabismus), eye infections, oedema of lids, excessive tearing, use of glasses or contact lenses, date of last optic examination
Nose	nosebleeds (epistaxis), constant of frequent running or stuffy nose, nasal obstruction (difficulty in breathing), alteration or loss of sense of smell
Ears	earaches, discharge, evidence of hearing loss (ask about behaviours such as need to repeat requests, loud speech, inattentive behaviour), results of any previous auditory testing
Mouth	mouth-breathing, gum bleeding, toothaches, tooth-brushing, use of fluoride, difficulty with teething (symptoms), last visit to dentist (especially if temporary dentition is complete), response to dentist
Throat	sore throats, difficulty in swallowing, choking (especially when chewing food – may be from poor chewing habits), hoarseness, or other voice irregularities
Neck	pain, limitation of movement, stiffness, difficulty in holding head straight (torticollis), thyroid enlargement, enlarged nodes or other masses
Chest	breast enlargement, discharge, masses, enlarged axillary nodes (for adolescent female, ask about breast self-examination)
Respiratory	chronic cough, frequent colds (number per year), wheezing, shortness of breath at rest or on exertion, difficulty in breathing, sputum production, infections (pneumonia, tuberculosis), date of last chest x-ray examination, and skin reaction from tuberculin testing
Cardiovascular	cyanosis or fatigue on exertion, history of heart murmur or rheumatic fever, anaemia, date of last blood count, blood type, recent transfusion
Gastrointestinal	appetite, food tolerance, elimination habits, nausea, vomiting (not associated with eating, may be indicative of brain tumour or increased intracranial pressure), jaundice or yellowing skin or sclera, belching, flatulence, recent change in bowel habits (blood in stools, change in colour, diarrhoea, and constipation)
Genitourinary	pain on urination, frequency, hesitancy, urgency, haematuria, nocturia, polyuria, unpleasant odour to urine, force of stream, discharge, change in size of scrotum, date of last urinalysis (for adolescent, sexually transmitted disease, type of treatment; for male adolescent, ask about testicular self-examination)

Gynaecologic	menarche, date of last menstrual period, regularity or problems with menstruation, vaginal discharge, pruritus, date and result of last Pap smear (include obstetric history as discussed under birth history when applicable); if sexually active, type of contraception
Musculoskeletal	weakness, clumsiness, lack of coordination, unusual movements, back or joint stiffness, muscle pains or cramps, abnormal gait, deformity, fractures, serious sprains, activity level
Neurological	seizures, tremors, dizziness, loss of memory, general affect, fears, nightmares, speech problems, any unusual habits
Endocrine	intolerance to weather changes, excessive thirst and urination, excessive sweating, salty taste to skin, signs of early puberty

Guidelines
Initiating a comprehensive family assessment

Perform a comprehensive assessment on:

- children receiving comprehensive well-child care
- children experiencing major stressful life events (e. g., chronic illness, disability, parental divorce, or death of a family member)
- children requiring extensive home care
- children with developmental delays
- children with repeated accidental injuries and those with suspected child abuse
- children with behavioural or physical problems that suggest family dysfunction as the aetiology

Family assessment interview
General guidance for family interview

Schedule the interview with the family at a time that is most convenient for all parties, include as many family members as possible; clearly state the purpose of the interview. Begin the interview by asking each person's name and their relationship to each other. Restate the purpose of the interview and the objective. Keep the initial conversation general to put members at ease and to learn the "big picture" of the family. Identify major concerns and reflect these back to the family to be certain that all parties perceive the same message. Terminate the interview with a summary of what was discussed and a plan for additional sessions if needed.

Exercise 7
Answer the following questions. Prepare short talks and/or dialogues on these topics

1. What can you say about body parts and systems (general, integument, head, eyes, nose, ears, mouth, throat, neck, chest, respiratory, gastrointestinal, genitourinary, gynaecologic, musculoskeletal, neurological, endocrine)?
2. What is meant by comprehensive family assessment?
3. Describe general guidance for family interview.

Translation 3

1. Review of systems consists of: general (overall state of health); integument (pruritus, petechiae, dryness, deformities of nails, hair growth or loss, hair colour change); head (headaches, dizziness, injury); eyes (visual problems, blurred vision, squinting, rubbing the eye, oedema of lids, excessive tearing); nose (nosebleeds or stuffy nose, nasal obstruction, loss of sense of smell); ears (earaches, discharge, hearing loss); mouth (mouth-breathing, gum bleeding, toothaches, difficulty with teething); throat (sore throats, difficulty in swallowing, choking, hoarseness). 2. Review of systems also contains: neck (pain, stiffness, thyroid enlargement, enlarged nodes, chest (breast enlargement, discharge, enlarged axillary nodes); respiratory (chronic cough, wheezing, shortness of breath, sputum production); cardiovascular (cyanosis or fatigue, heart murmur or rheumatic fever, anaemia). 3. Review of systems includes: gastrointestinal (blood in stools, diarrhoea, and constipation); genitourinary (pain on urination, frequency, hesitancy, urgency, haematuria, nocturia, polyuria, change in size of scrotum, testicular self-examination); gynaecologic (menarche, last menstrual period, vaginal discharge, last Pap smear, obstetric history, type of contraception, breast self-examination). 4. Further systems are: musculoskeletal (weakness, clumsiness, back or joint stiffness, muscle pains or cramps, gait, fractures, sprains); neurological (seizures, tremors, dizziness, loss of memory, fears, nightmares, speech problems); endocrine (excessive thirst and urination, excessive sweating). 5. Perform a comprehensive assessment on: comprehensive well-child care, stressful life events, home care, developmental delays, suspected child abuse, behavioural or physical problems. 6. General guidance for family interview: clearly state the purpose, identify major concerns, ask each person's name and their relationship to each other. 7. Terminate the interview with a summary and a plan for additional sessions.

Text 4
Structural assessment areas
Family composition
- immediate members of the household (names, ages, and relationships)
- significant extended family members
- previous marriages, separations, death of spouses, or divorces

Home and community environment
- type of dwelling/number of rooms/occupants
- sleeping arrangements
- number of floors, accessibility of stairs, elevators
- adequacy of utilities
- safety features (fire escape, smoke detector, guardrails on windows, use of car restraint)
- environmental hazards (e. g., chipped paint, poor sanitation, pollution, heavy street traffic)
- availability and location of health facilities, schools, play areas
- relationship with neighbours
- recent crises or changes in home
- child's reaction/adjustment to recent stresses

Occupation and education of family members
- types of employment
- work schedules
- work satisfaction
- exposure to environmental/industrial hazards
- sources of income and adequacy
- effect of illness on financial status
- highest degree or grade level attained

Cultural and religious traditions
- religious beliefs and practices
- cultural/ethnic beliefs and practices
- language spoken in home

Assessment questions include:
- Does the family identify with a particular religious/ethnic group? Are both parents from that group?
- How is religious/ethnic background part of family life?

- What special religious/cultural traditions are practised in the home (e. g., food choices and preparation)?
- Where were family members born, and how long have they lived in the country?
- What language does the family speak most frequently?
- Do they speak/understand English?
- What do they believe causes health or illness?
- What religious/ethnic beliefs influence the family's perception of illness and its treatment?
- What methods are used to prevent/treat illness?
- How does the family know when a health problem needs medical attention?
- Who is the person the family contacts when a member is ill?
- Does the family rely on cultural/religious healers or remedies? If so, ask them to describe the type of healer or remedy.
- Who does the family go for support (clergy, medical healer, relatives)?
- Does the family experience discrimination because of their race, beliefs, or practices? Ask them to describe.

Exercise 8
Answer the following question. Prepare a short talk on this topic.

1. What is meant by structural assessment areas (family composition, home and community environment, occupation and education of family members)?

Translation 4

1. Family composition means: members of the household, previous marriages, separations, death of spouses, or divorces. 2. Home and community environment describes: type of dwelling, sleeping arrangements, adequacy of utilities, safety features (fire escape, smoke detector, guardrails on windows, use of car restraint), environmental hazards (e. g., chipped paint, poor sanitation, pollution, heavy street traffic), recent crises or changes in home. 3. Occupation and education of family members characterizes: types of employment, environmental and industrial hazards, and effect of illness on financial status. 4. Cultural and religious traditions include: religious beliefs, cultural and ethnic beliefs, language spoken in home. 5. Questions to be asked include: What special religious or cultural traditions are practised in the home (e. g., food choices and preparation)?; What do they believe causes health or illness and what methods are used

to prevent and treat illness?; Does the family rely on cultural or religious healers or remedies?; Does the family experience discrimination because of their race, beliefs, or practices?

Text 5
Functional assessment areas
Family interactions and roles
 Interactions refer to ways the family members relate to each other. Chief concern is amount of intimacy and closeness among the members, especially spouses. Roles refer to behaviours of people as they assume a different status or position

Observations include:
 • Family members' responses to each other (cordial, hostile, cool, loving, patient, short-tempered)
 • Obvious roles of leadership versa submission
 • Support and attention shown to various members

Assessment questions include:
 • What activities do the family perform together?
 • Whom do family members talk to when something is bothering them?
 • What are members' household chores?
 • Who usually oversees what is happening with the children, such as at school or concerning their health?
 • How easy or difficult it is for the family to change or accept new responsibilities for household tasks?

Power, decision making, and problem solving
 Power refers to individual member's control over others in family; manifested through family decision making and problem solving. Chief concern is clarity of boundaries of power between parents and children. One method of assessment involves offering a hypothetical conflict or problem, such as a child failing school, and asking family how they would handle this situation.

Assessment questions include:
 • Who usually makes the decisions in the family?
 • If one parent makes a decision, can the child appeal to the other parent to change it?

- What input do children have in making decisions or discussing rules?
- Who makes and enforces the rules?
- What happens when a rule is broken?

Exercise 9
Answer the following questions. Prepare short talks and/or dialogues on these topics

1. Characterize family interactions and roles.
2. What do observations include?
3. What questions are included in assessment?
4. What can you say about power, decision making, and problem solving?

Translation 5

1. Family interactions refer to ways the family members relate to each other. 2. Chief concern is amount of intimacy and closeness among the members, especially spouses. 3. Observations include: family members' responses to each other (cordial, hostile, cool, loving, patient, short-tempered). 4. Assessment questions include: What activities do the family perform together? What are members' household chores? Who usually oversees what is happening with the children? 5. Power refers to individual member's control over others in family, manifested through family decision making and problem solving. 6. Assessment questions include: Who usually makes the decisions in the family? Who makes and enforces the rules and what happens when a rule is broken?

Text 6
Communication
Concerned with clarity and directness of communication patterns

Observations include:
- Who speaks to whom?
- If one person speaks for another or interrupts.
- If members appear disinterested when certain individuals speak.
- If there is agreement between verbal and non-verbal messages.
- Further assessment includes periodically asking family members if they understood what was just said and to repeat the message.

Assessment questions include:
- How often do family members wait until others are through talking before "having their say?"
- Do parents or older siblings tend to lecture and preach?
- Do parents tend to talk "down" to the children?

Expression of feelings and individuality

Concerned with personal space and freedom to grow with limits and structure needed for guidance. Observing patterns of communication offers clues to how freely feelings are expressed.

Assessment questions include:
- Is it OK for family members to get angry or sad?
- Who gets angry most of the time? What do they do?
- If someone is upset, how do other family members try to comfort this person?
- Who comforts specific family members?
- When someone wants to do something, such as try out for a new sport or get a job, what is the family's response (offer assistance, discouragement, or no advice)?

Family Apgar

Definition	Function measured by the family Apgar	Relevant open-ended questions
Adaptation is the use of intra-familial and extra-familial resources for problem solving when family equilibrium is stressed during a crisis	How resources are shared, or the degree to which a member is satisfied with the assistance received when family resources are needed.	How have family members aided each other in time of need? In what way have family members received help or assistance from friends and community agencies?
Partnership is the sharing of decision-making and nurturing responsibilities by family members.	How decisions are shared, or the member's satisfaction with mutuality in family communication and problem-solving.	How do family members communicate with each other about such matters as vacations, finances, medical care, large purchases, and personal problems?

Growth is the physical and emotional maturation and self-fulfilment that is achieved by family members through mutual support and guidance.	How nurturing is shared, or the member's satisfaction with the freedom available within the family to change roles and attain physical and emotional growth or maturation.	How have family members changed during the past years? How has this change been accepted by family members? In what ways have family members aided each other in growing or developing independent life-styles? How have family members reacted to your desires for change?
Affection is the caring or loving relationship that exists among family members.	How emotional experiences are shared, or the member's satisfaction with the intimacy and emotional interaction that exists in the family.	How have members of your family responded to emotional expressions such as affection, love, sorrow, or anger?
Resolve is the commitment to devote time to other members of the family for physical and emotional nurturing. It also usually involves a decision to share wealth and space.	How time (and space and money) is shared, or the member's satisfaction with the time commitment that has been made to the family by its members.	How do members of your family share time, space, and money?

Guidelines
Evaluating kinetic family drawings

Note omission of family members; if someone is missing, ask child if everyone in the family has been included in the drawing. Ask child to explain what each family member is doing. Encourage child to tell as much as possible about the drawing. Note signs of physical intimacy or distance, such as people close to each other or touching. Note placement of people in the drawing, such as top or bottom of drawing and proximity to each other. Note facial expressions, such as happy, sad, blank, or bored. Note which members are facing each other or turned away from each other and how they are grouped together.

Exercise 10
Answer the following questions. Prepare short talks and/or dialogues on these topics

1. What do observations of communication include?

2. Describe assessment questions and expression of feelings and individuality.
3. What is meant by family Apgar?
4. What can you say about evaluating kinetic family drawings?
5. Why is noting placement of people in the drawing, such as top or bottom of drawing and proximity to each other important?
6. Why should you note facial expressions, such as happy, sad, blank, or bored?

Translation 6

1. Observations include: who speaks to whom; if there is agreement between verbal and non-verbal messages; if one person speaks for another or interrupts; if parents or older siblings tend to lecture and preach. 2. Observing patterns of communication offers clues to how freely feelings are expressed. 3. When someone wants to do something, what is the family's response (offer assistance, discouragement, or no advice)? 4. Family Apgar characterizes: adaptation (the use of intra-familial and extra-familial resources for problem solving); partnership (the sharing of decision-making and nurturing responsibilities); growth (the physical and emotional maturation); affection (the caring or loving relationship); resolve (the commitment to devote time to other members of the family). 5. Functions measured by the family Apgar are: how resources are shared; how decisions are shared; communication about vacations, finances, medical care, or large purchases; how nurturing is shared; physical and emotional growth or maturation; how emotional experiences are shared; emotional interaction; response to emotional expressions such as affection, love, sorrow, or anger; how time (and space and money) is shared. 6. When evaluating kinetic family drawings: note omission of family members; ask child to explain what each family member is doing; note signs of physical intimacy or distance; note placement of people in the drawing; note facial expressions, such as happy, sad, blank, or bored.

Key 13
Exercise 3
1 b, a; 2 b, a, c; 3 c, a, b; 4 c, a, b; 5 d, a, b, c; 6 d, a, b, c; 7 b, a, c; 8 d, a, b, c

Exercise 4
1a; 2g; 3b; 4g; 5f; 6e; 7d

Exercise 6
1g; 2e; 3d; 4h; 5f; 6a; 7c; 8b

VOCABULARY 13

aberration /ˌæb.əˈreɪ.ʃən/
abuse /əˈbjuːz/
accept /əkˈsept/
accessibility /əkˌses.əˈbɪl.ɪ.ti/
additional /əˈdɪʃ.ən.əl/
adequacy /ˈæd.ə.kwə.si/
advance /ədˈvɑːnt s/
aetiology /ˌiː.tiˈɒl.ə.dʒi/
affection /əˈfek.ʃən/
aggravate /ˈæg.rə.veɪt/
alpha-fetoprotein /ˈælfəˌfiːtəˈprəʊ.tiːn/
alteration /ˌɒl.təˈreɪ.ʃən/
ambiguous /æmˈbɪgjʊəs/
amenorrhoea /ˌeɪ.men.əˈriː.ə/
amniocentesis /ˌæm.ni.əʊ.senˈtiː.sɪs/
appeal /əˈpiːl/
applicable /əˈplɪk.ə.bl̩/
arise /əˈraɪz/ (arose, arisen)
arrangement /əˈreɪndʒ.mənt/
asymmetry /eɪˈsɪm.ə.tri/
attain /əˈteɪn/
attention /əˈten.ʃən/
auditory / ˈɔːdɪtərɪ/
autosome /ˈɔː.təˌsəʊm/
awake /əˈweɪk/
awaken /əˈweɪ.kən/
awkward /ˈɔː.kwəd/
axillary /æˈksɪl.ər.i/
bang /bæŋ/
belch /beltʃ/
bending /bend.ɪŋ/
blank /blæŋk/
blood /blʌd/ count /kaʊnt/
blurred /blɜːd/
bored /bɔːd/
bother /ˈbɒðə/
boundary /ˈbaʊn.dər.i/
bump /ˈbʌmp/
carrier /ˈkær.i.ər/
carry /ˈkær.i/ out /aʊt/
causative /ˈkɔː.zə.tɪv/
chew /tʃuː/
chill /tʃɪl/
chipped /ˈtʃɪpt/
chorionic /ˈkɔːr.ɪ.ən.ɪk/

380

chromosome /ˈkrəʊməˌsəʊm/

clarity /ˈklær.ɪ.ti/

clergy /ˈklɜːdʒɪ/

closeness /kləʊsnɪs/

clue /kluː/

clumsiness /ˈklʌm.zi.nəs/

coloboma /ˌkə.l.əˈbəʊ.mə/

comfort /ˈkʌm.fət/

composition /ˌkɒm.pəˈzɪʃ.ən/

comprehensive /ˌkɒm.prɪˈhen.sɪv/

confident /ˈkɒn.fɪ.dənt/

consistency /kənˈsɪs.tənt .si/

consistent /kənˈsɪs.tənt/ **with** /wɪð/

constipation /ˌkɒnt .stɪˈpeɪ.ʃən/

contraception /ˌkɒntrəˈsepʃən/

contribute /kənˈtrɪb.juːt/

convince /kənˈvɪns/

cool /kuːl/

cordial /ˈkɔːdɪəl/

correct /kəˈrekt/

counselling /ˈkaʊnt .səl.ɪŋ/

couple /ˈkʌp.l/

cramp /kræmp/

cranky /ˈkræŋkɪ/

cross-eyed /krɒs. aɪd/

deficit /ˈdef.ɪ.sɪt/

deformity /dɪˈfɔː.mɪ.ti/

delay /dɪˈleɪ/

detect /dɪˈtekt/

deviation /ˌdiːvɪˈeɪʃən/

disability /ˌdɪs.əˈbɪl.ɪ.ti/

discharge /dɪsˈtʃɑːdʒ/

discouragement /dɪˈskʌr.ɪdʒ.mənt/

discrimination /dɪˌskrɪm.ɪˈneɪ.ʃən/

disinterested /dɪˈsɪn.trə.stɪd/

disrupt /dɪsˈrʌpt/

distractibility /dɪˌstræktəˈbɪl.ə.ti/

disturb /dɪˈstɜːb/

dizziness /ˈdɪz.ɪ.nəs/

dominant /ˈdɒm.ɪ.nənt/

dosage /ˈdəʊ.sɪdʒ/

drawing /ˈdrɔː.ɪŋ/

dryness /draɪnɪs/

dwelling /ˈdwel.ɪŋ/

dye /daɪ/

dysmorphic /disˈmɔːr.fik/

earache /ˈɪə.reɪk/

educate /ˈedjʊˌkeɪt/
elimination /ɪˌlɪm.ɪˈneɪ.ʃən/
enforce /ɪnˈfɔːs/
enlargement /ɪnˈlɑː.dʒ.mənt/
enuresis /ˌen.jʊəˈriː.sɪs/
epicanthal /ˌe.pəˈkan.θəl/
epistaxis /ˌe.pɪˈstæk.sɪs/
equilibrium /ˌiːkwɪˈlɪbrɪəm/
escape /ɪˈskeɪp/
excessive /ekˈses.ɪv/
excessively /ɪkˈsesɪvlɪ/
exertion /ɪgˈzɜːˌʃən/
expressivity /ˌek.ˌspreˈsi.və.ti:/
facility /fəˈsɪl.ɪ.ti/
fail /feɪl/
failing /ˈfeɪ.lɪŋ/
fall /ˈfɔːl/ **asleep** /əˈsliːp/
fatigue /fəˈtiːg/
flatulence /ˈflæt.jʊ.lənts/
fold /fəʊld/
follow-up /ˈfɒl.əʊ.ʌp/
forearm /ˈfɔː.rɑːm/
frequency /ˈfriː.kwən.si/
gait /geɪt/
gamete /ˈgæmiːt/
growth /grəʊθ/
guardrail /ˈgɑːdˌreɪl/
guidance /ˈgaɪ.dəns/
habitual /həˈbɪtjʊəl/
haematuria /ˌhiː.mə.tˈjʊə.ri.ə/
handle /ˈhæn.dəl/
healer /ˈhiːlə/
hearing /ˈhɪə.rɪŋ/ **loss** /lɒs/
hereditary /həˈred.ɪ.tər.i/
hesitancy /ˈhez.ɪ.tən.si/
hoarseness /ˈhɔːsnɪs/
hostile /ˈhɒs.taɪl/
household /ˈhaʊs.həʊld/ **chores** /tʃɔːz/
hyperextensible /ˌhaɪ.pə.rikˈstens.əbəl/
hypertonic /ˌhaɪ.pərˈtɑː.nik/
hypotonic /ˌhaɪ.pəˈtɑː.nik/
inattentive /ˌɪnəˈtentɪv/
incidence /ˈɪnt .sɪ.dənt s/
infertility /ˌɪn.fəˈtɪl.ɪ.ti/
inheritance /ɪnˈherɪtəns/
initially /ɪˈnɪʃ.əl.i/
insist /ɪnˈsɪst/

interaction /ˌɪn.təˈræk.ʃən/
interrupt /ˌɪn.təˈrʌpt/
intervene /ˌɪn.təˈviːn/
intervention /ˌɪn.təˈven.ʃən/
interviewing /ˈɪntəˌvjuːɪŋ/
intimacy /ˈɪntɪməsɪ/
intracranial /ˌɪn.trəˈkrəɪ.ni.əl/
intrauterine /ˌɪn.trəˈjuː.tər.aɪn/
irresistibility /ˌɪrɪˌzɪstəˈbɪlɪtɪ/
jaundice /ˈdʒɔːn.dɪs/
kinetic /kɪˈnetɪk/
lap /læp/
lecture /ˈlek.tʃə/
malformation /ˌmæl.fəˈmeɪ.ʃən/
maturation /ˌmæt.jʊəˈreɪ.ʃən/
memory /ˈmem.ər.i/
menarche /menˈɑː.ki/
Mendelian /menˈdiː.liː.ən/ disorder /dɪˈsɔː.dər/
micrognathia /ˌmaɪ.krəʊˈneɪ.thiː.ə/
miscarriage /ˈmɪsˌkær.ɪdʒ/
modify /ˈmɒd.ɪ.faɪ/
morphogenesis /ˌmɔːr.fəˈdʒe.ni.sɪs/
multifactorial /ˌməl.tiː.fak.ˈtɔːr.iː.əl/
multiple /ˈmʌl.tɪ.pl̩/
murmur /ˈmɜː.mər/
mutant /ˈmjuːtənt/
nape /neɪp/
narcolepsy /ˈnɑː.kə.lep.si/
nocturia /nɒktˈjʊər.ɪ.ə/
node /nəʊd/
nosebleed /ˈnəʊzˌbliːd/
nurture /ˈnɜːtʃə/
objective /əbˈdʒek.tɪv/
obstetrics /ɒbˈstetrɪks/
occupant /ˈɒk.jʊ.pənt/
occurrence /əˈkʌr.ənts/
odour /ˈəʊ.dər/
omission /əʊˈmɪʃ.ən/
overgrowth /ˌəʊ.və.grəʊθ/
oversee /ˌəʊ.vəˈsiː/
over-tiredness /ˌəʊ.vəˈtaɪədnɪs/
pacifier /ˈpæs.ɪ.faɪ.ər/
paint /peɪnt/
Pap smear /ˈpæpˌsmɪərʳ/
participate /pɑːˈtɪs.ɪ.peɪt/
pat /ˈpæt/
pectus excavatum /ˌpek.təs eks.kəˈveɪ.təm/

penetrance /ˈpe.nə.trəns/
perceive /pəˈsiːv/
petechia /pɪˈtiːkɪ.ə/ pl **petechiae**
pica /ˈpaɪ.kə/
pigmentation /ˌpɪɡ.mənˈteɪ.ʃən/
pleiotropy /plaɪ.ˈɑː.trə.piː/
pollution /pəˈluː.ʃən/
polyuria /ˌpɒl.ɪˈjʊə.rɪ.ə/
preach /priːtʃ/
precocious /prɪˈkəʊ.ʃəs/
prominence /ˈprɒm.ɪ.nəns/
provide /prəˈvaɪd/
proximity /prɒkˈsɪm.ɪ.ti/
pruritus /prʊəˈraɪ.təs/
purpose /ˈpɜː.pəs/
recessive /rɪˈses.ɪv/
record /ˈrekɔːd/
referral /rɪˈfɜː.rəl/
refuse /rɪˈfjuːz/
remedy /ˈrem.ə.di/
repeat /rɪˈpiːt/
request /rɪˈkwest/
responsibility /rɪˌspɒn.sɪˈbɪl.ɪ.ti/
restraint /rɪˈstreɪnt/
retardation /ˌriː.tɑːˈdeɪ.ʃən/
rock /rɒk/
rub /rʌb/
running /ˈrʌn.ɪŋ/
sample /ˈsɑːm.pl̩/
sanitation /ˌsæn.ɪˈteɪ.ʃən/
satisfaction /ˌsætɪsˈfækʃən/
scaly /ˈskeɪ.li/
schedule /ˈʃedjuːl/
sclera /ˈsklɪə.rə/
scold /skəʊld/
scoliosis /ˌskɒl.iˈəʊ.sɪs/
scrotum /ˈskrəʊ.təm/ pl **scrotta**
security /sɪˈkjʊə.rɪ.ti/
seemingly /ˈsiː.mɪŋ.li/
seizure /ˈsiː.ʒə/
self-fulfilment /ˌself fʊlˈfɪl.mənt/
serum /ˈsɪə.rəm/ pl **sera**
session /ˈseʃ.ən/
short tempered /ˌʃɔːtˈtem.pəd/
shortness /ˈʃɔːt.nəs/
sleepwalk /ˈsliːpˌwɔːk/
snore /snɔːr/

sorrow /ˈsɒrəʊ/

spot /spɒt/

spouse /spaʊs/

sprain /spreɪn/

sputum /ˈspjuː.təm/ pl sputa

squint /skwɪnt/

state /steɪt/

stature /ˈstætʃ.ər/

stiffness /ˈstɪf.nəs/

stillbirth /ˈstɪlˌbɜː.θ/

stool /stuːl/

strabismus /strəˈbɪz.məs/

straighteners /ˈstreɪ.tᵊn.əz/

stream /striːm/

stuffed /stʌft/

stuffy /ˈstʌfɪ/

submission /səbˈmɪʃ.ən/

suddenness /ˈsʌdənnɪs/

suspected /səˈspek.tɪd/

swallow /ˈswɒl.əʊ/

sweat /swet/

sweating /swet.ɪŋ/

tearing /teər.ɪŋ/

teething /tiː.θɪŋ/

temporary /ˈtem.pər.ər.i/

terminate /ˈtɜː.mɪ.neɪt/

testicle /ˈtes.tɪ.kl̩/

testicular /tesˈtɪk.jə.lər/

texture /ˈteks.tʃər/

thrash /θræʃ/

threaten /ˈθret.ən/

toothache /ˈtuː.θˌeɪk/

tooth-brushing /ˈtuː.θ brʌʃɪŋ/

torticollis /tɔː.tɪˈkɒl.ɪs/

transition /trænˈzɪʃ.ən/

translocation /ˌtrænz.ləʊˈkeɪ.ʃᵊn/

tremor /ˈtrem.ər/

tuberculin /tjuːˈbɔː.kjə.lɪn/

ultrasound /ˈʌl.trə.saʊnd/

unaffected /ˌʌn.əˈfek.tɪd/

unequal /ʌnˈiː.kwəl/

unhurried /ʌnˈhʌrɪd/

unrelated /ˌʌn.rɪˈleɪ.tɪd/

urgency /ˈɜː.dʒən.si/

urinalysis /ˌjʊə.rɪˈnæl.ə.sɪs/

urination /ˌjʊə.rɪˈneɪ.ʃən/

utility /juːˈtɪl.ə.ti/

vaginal /vəˌdʒaɪ.nəl/
variability /ˌveərɪəˈbɪlɪtɪ/
vary /ˈveə.ri/
villus /ˈvɪl.əs/ pl **villi** /ˈvɪl.aɪ/
wheeze /wiːz/
X-ray /ˈeks.reɪ/
yawn /jɔːn/
zygote /ˈzaɪ.ɡəʊt/

Physical and developmental assessment of the child;
Performing paediatric physical examination; Atraumatic
care; Dietary history; Inflammations of the eyelid; Various
patterns of respiration; Effective auscultation; Change in
stooling patterns of newborns; Paediatric symptom checklist

Text 1
Dietary history

- What are the family's usual mealtimes?
- Do family members eat together or at separate times?
- Who does the family grocery shopping and meal preparation?
- How much money is spent to buy food each week?
- How are most foods prepared — baked, broiled, fried, other?
- How often does the family or your child eat out?
- What kinds of restaurants do you go to?
- What kinds of food does your child typically eat at restaurants?
- Does your child eat breakfast regularly?
- Where does your child eat lunch?
- What are your child's favourite foods, beverages, and snacks?
- What are the average amounts eaten per day?
- What foods are artificially sweetened?
- What are your child's snacking habits?
- When are sweet foods usually eaten?
- What are your child's tooth-brushing habits?
- What special cultural practices are followed? What ethnic foods are eaten?
- What foods and beverages does your child dislike?
- How would you describe your child's usual appetite (hearty eater, picky eater)?
- What are your child's feeding habits (breast, bottle, cup, spoon, eats by self, needs assistance, any special devices)?
- Does your child take vitamins or other supplements? Do they contain iron or fluoride?
- Are there any known or suspected food allergies? Is your child on a special diet?

- Has your child lost or gained weight recently?
- Are there any feeding problems (excessive fussiness, spitting up, colic, difficulty sucking or swallowing?
- Are there any dental problems or appliances, such as braces, that affect eating?
- What types of exercise does your child do regularly?
- Is there a family history of cancer, diabetes, heart disease, high blood pressure, or obesity?

Additional questions for infants

What was the infant's birth weight? When did it double? Triple?
Was the infant premature?
Are you breast-feeding or have you breast-fed your infant? For how long?
If you use a formula, what is the brand?
- How long has the infant been taking it?
- Are you giving the infant cow's milk (whole, low-fat, skimmed)?
- When did you start?
- How much does the infant drink a day?
- Do you give your infant extra fluids (water, juice)?
- If the infant takes a bottle to bed at nap or night-time, what is in the bottle?
- At what age did you start cereal, vegetables, meat or other protein sources, fruit/juice, finger food, table food?
- Do you make your own baby food or use commercial foods, such as infant cereal?
- Does the infant take a vitamin/mineral supplement? If so, what type?
- Has the infant shown an allergic reaction to any food(s)? If so, list the foods and describe the reaction.
- Does the infant spit up frequently, have unusually loose stools, or have hard, dry stools? If so, how often?
- How often do you feed your infant?
- How would you describe your infant's appetite?

Exercise 1
Answer the following questions. Prepare short talks and/or dialogues on these topics

1. How to take dietary history?
2. What are additional questions for infants?

Exercise 2
Study the following summary and then interpret basic information in English.

1. Communication, the most important skill nurses must possess in the care of children, has verbal, nonverbal, and abstract components.
2. To effectively establish a setting for communication, nurses must make an appropriate introduction, clarify their role and the purpose of the interview, and ensure privacy and confidentiality.
3. When communicating with parents, nurses need to encourage parental involvement, listen carefully, use silence, and be empathic.
4. Communication with children must reflect their development stage.
5. Verbal communication techniques include the third-person technique, use of "I" messages, facilitative responding, storytelling, bibliotherapy, the use of "what if" questions, and other word games.
6. Nonverbal communication with children may take the form of writing, drawing, magic, and play.

Exercise 3
Fill in the missing words. Choose the correct ones.

1. The objectives of performing _____ _____ are to identify pertinent information, determine the _____ _____, analyse ____ _____ _____, secure the past history, and _____ a family and sexual history.	a chief complaint b the present illness, c record d health history
2. _____ _____ is the collection of data about family composition and relationships among members; it focuses on home and community environment, _____ ___ _____, and cultural and religious _____.	a occupation and education b Family assessment c traditions
3. The family function interview examines, _____ ___ _____, power, _____ _____, _____ _____, communication, and expression of feelings and individuality.	a decision making b interaction and roles c problem solving
4. Nutritional assessment is performed by determination of _____ _____, clinical _____, and _____ analysis.	a examination b biochemical c dietary intake

Translation 1

1. You should ask these questions to take dietary history: How are most foods prepared – baked, broiled, fried, other?; Does your child eat breakfast regularly?; Where does your child eat lunch?; What are your child's favourite foods, beverages, and snacks?; What foods and beverages does your child dislike?; What are your child's feeding habits (breast, bottle, cup, spoon, eats by self, needs assistance, any special devices)?; Are there any known or suspected food allergies?; Are there any feeding problems (excessive fussiness, spitting up, colic, difficulty sucking or swallowing? 2. Additional questions for infants are: Are you breast-feeding or have you breast-fed your infant? For how long? Are you giving the infant cow's milk (whole, low-fat, skimmed)?; Do you give your infant extra fluids (water, juice)?; 3. At what age did you start cereal, vegetables, meat or other protein sources, fruit/juice, finger food, table food?; Does the infant spit up frequently, have unusually loose stools, or have hard, dry stools?; How often do you feed your infant? 4. To effectively establish a setting for communication, nurses must make an appropriate introduction, clarify their role and the purpose of the interview, and ensure privacy and confidentiality. 5. Communication with children must reflect their development stage. 6. Nonverbal communication with children may take the form of writing, drawing, magic, and play. 7. The objectives of performing a health history are to identify pertinent information, determine the chief complaint, analyse the present illness, secure the past history, and record a family and sexual history. 8. The family function interview examines interaction and roles, power, decision making, problem solving, communication, and expression of feelings and individuality.

Text 2
Guidelines
Performing paediatric physical examination
Perform examination in appropriate, non-threatening area.
- Have room well lit, and decorated with neutral colours.
- Have room temperature comfortably warm.
- Place all strange and potentially frightening equipment out of sight.
- Have some toys, dolls, stuffed animals and games available for child.
- If possible, have rooms decorated and equipped for different-age children.
- Provide privacy, especially for school-age children and adolescents.

Provide time for play and becoming acquainted. **Observe behaviours** that signal child's readiness to cooperate:

- talking to nurse,
- making eye contact,
- accepting offered equipment,
- allowing physical touching,
- choosing to sit on examining table rather than parent's lap

If signs of readiness are not observed, use the following techniques:

- Talk to parent while essentially "ignoring" child; gradually focus on child or favourite object, such as a doll.
- Make complimentary remarks about child, such as appearance, dress, or a favourite object.
- Tell a funny story or play a simple magic trick.
- Have a nonthreatening "friend" available, such as a hand puppet to "talk" to child for the nurse.

If child refuses to cooperate, use the following techniques:

- Assess reason for uncooperative behaviour; consider that a child who is unduly afraid may have had a previous traumatic experience.
- Try to involve child and parent in process.
- Avoid prolonged explanations about examining procedure.
- Use a firm, direct approach regarding expected behaviour.
- Perform examination as quickly as possible.
- Have attendant gently restrain child.
- Minimize any disruptions or stimulation – limit number of people in room, use isolated room, use quiet, calm, confident voice.

Begin examination in a nonthreatening manner for young children or children who are fearful:

- Use those activities that can be presented as games, such as test for cranial nerves or parts of developmental screening tests.
- Use approaches such as "Simon says" to encourage child to make a face, squeeze a hand, stand on one foot, and so on.
- Use "paper-doll" technique: Lay child supine on an examining table or floor that is covered with a large sheet of paper. Trace around child's body outline. Use body outline to demonstrate what will be examined, such as a drawing a chart and listening with the stethoscope before performing the activity on child.

If several children in the family will be examined, begin with the most cooperative child to provide modelling of desired behaviour. Involve a child in examination process:

- Provide choices, such as sitting on table or in parent's lap.
- Allow child to handle or hold equipment.
- Encourage child to use equipment on a doll, family member, or examiner.
- Explain each step of the procedure in simple language.

Examine child in a comfortable and secure position:
- sitting in parent's lap
- sitting upright if in respiratory distress

Proceed to examine the body in an organized sequence (usually head to toe) with the following exceptions:

- Alter sequence to accommodate needs of different-age children
- Examine painful areas last
- In emergency situation, examine vital functions (airway, breathing and circulation, and injured area first.
- Reassure child throughout examination, especially about bodily concerns that arise during puberty
- Discuss findings with family at end of examination.
- Praise child for cooperation during examination; give reward such as a small toy or sticker.

Guidelines
Measuring triceps, skinfold thickness

- With child's right arm flexed 90 degrees at elbow, mark midpoint between acromion and olecranon on posterior aspect of arm.
- With arm hanging freely, grasp a fold of skin between thumb and forefinger 1 cm above midpoint.
- Gently pull fold away from underlying muscle and continue to hold until measurement is completed.
- Place calliper jaws over skinfold at midpoint mark; if a plastic calliper is used, apply pressure with thumb to align lines of calliper; follow directions for using other callipers.
- Estimate reading to nearest 1.0 mm, 2 to 3 seconds after applying pressure.
- Take measurements until duplicates agree within 1 mm.

Exercise 4
Answer the following questions. Prepare short talks and/or dialogues on these topics

1. How to perform paediatric physical examination?
2. Speak about suitable techniques to use.
3. What to do if child refuses to cooperate?
4. How to proceed in emergency situation?
5. Describe measuring triceps, and skinfold thickness.

Translation 2

1. Perform examination in appropriate, non-threatening area. 2. Have some toys, dolls, stuffed animals and games available for child. 3. If possible, have rooms decorated and equipped for different-age children. 4. Observe behaviours that signal child's readiness to cooperate: talking to nurse, making eye contact, allowing physical touching. 5. Make complimentary remarks about child, such as appearance, dress, or a favourite object. 6. Perform examination as quickly as possible. 7. Minimize any disruptions or stimulation – limit number of people in room, use isolated room, use quiet, calm, confident voice. 8. If several children in the family will be examined, begin with the most cooperative child to provide modelling of desired behaviour. 9. Explain each step of the procedure in simple language. 10. Proceed to examine the body in an organized sequence (usually head to toe). 11. In emergency situation, examine vital functions (airway, breathing and circulation), and injured area first. 12. Praise child for cooperation during examination; give reward such as a small toy or sticker.

Text 3
Atraumatic care
Reducing young children's fears
    Young children, especially preschoolers, fear intrusive procedures because of their poorly defined body boundaries. Therefore, avoid invasive procedures, such as measuring rectal temperature, whenever possible.

Guidelines
Observing behaviour

1. What is the child's overall personality — calm, anxious, tense, content, outgoing, shy, talkative, aggressive, introverted, stable, or moody?
2. Is the child active, sedentary, fidgety, or restless?

3. Does the child have a long attention span, or is the child easily distracted?

4. Does the child sit quietly on the examining table or parent's lap, or does the child climb, run, open doors, and otherwise explore the environment?

5. How does the child react to commands — with fear or willingness to obey?

6. How advanced is the child's ability to follow requests? Can the child follow two or three commands in succession without the need for repetition? Is the child attentive to requests, or must they be repeated several times?

7. Is the child cooperative, belligerent, or argumentative?

8. What is the child's response to delayed gratification or frustration? Is the child able to withstand momentary discomfort and wait for the requests to be met?

9. In what tone of voice does the child make requests or talk to the parents?

10. Does the child seek approval and gain satisfaction from it?

11. Does the child use eye-to-eye contact during conversation?

12. Does the child agree with the parent's answers or find reasons to disagree, interrupt, or argue? What is the child's reaction to the nurse — respectful, friendly, reserved, apprehensive, or uninterested?

13. Is the child interested in the surroundings? Does the child look around the room, ask questions about unfamiliar objects, seem to enjoy exploring them, or attempt to break or destroy them?

14. Can the child follow directions for using the instruments, or imitate their use? Is the child quick or slow to grasp explanations?

Inflammations of the eyelid

Hordeolum or stye	Internal stye	Chalazion	Marginal blepharitis	Dacryocystit
inflammation of sebaceous glands near lashes, usually on lower lid; painful, red swollen areas	acute inflammation of meibomian glands of upper lid; if upper lid is everted, stye appears as a yellow line across the tarsus (edge of the eyelid)	granulomas or cysts of internal sebaceous glands; localized, nontender; firm, discrete swellings covered with freely movable skin	inflammation of edge of lid; red, scaly, crusted lid edges; may include pustules around base of lashes and pus from meibomian glands	is inflammation and blockage of lacrimal sac or duct; swelling, redness, and pain, below and to nasal side of inner canthus with purulent discharge

Various patterns of respiration
- **Tachypnoea** — increased rate
- **Bradypnea** — decreased rate
- **Apnoea** — cessation of breathing
- **Hyperpnoea** — increased depth
- **Hypoventilation** — decreased depth (shallow) and irregular rhythm
- **Hyperventilation** — increased rate and depth
- **Kussmaul breathing** — hyperventilation, gasping and laboured respiration, usually seen in diabetic coma or other states of respiratory acidosis.
- **Cheyne-Stokes respirations** — gradually increasing rate and depth with periods of apnoea
- **Biot breathing** — periods of hyperpnoea alternating with apnoea (similar to Cheyne-Stokes except that depth remains constant)
- **Seesaw (paradoxic) respirations** — chest falls on inspiration and rises on inspiration
- **Agonal** — last gasping for breaths before death

Guidelines
Effective auscultation
- Make sure child is relaxed and not crying, talking, or laughing. Record if child is crying.
- Check that room is comfortable and quiet.
- Warm stethoscope before placing it against skin.
- Apply firm pressure on chest piece but not enough to prevent vibrations and transmission of sound.
- Avoid placing stethoscope over hair or clothing, moving it against skin, breathing on tubing, or sliding fingers over chest piece, which may cause sounds that falsely resemble pathologic findings.
- Use a symmetric and orderly approach to compare sounds.

Classification of normal breath sounds

Vesicular breath sounds	Bronchovesicular breath sounds	Bronchial breath sounds
• Heard over entire surface of lungs, with exception of upper interscapular area and area beneath manubrium.	• Heard over manubrium and in upper interscapular regions where trachea and bronchi bifurcate.	• Heard only over trachea and suprasternal notch. • Inspiratory phase is short, and expiratory phase is long.

• Inspiration is louder, longer, and higher pitched than expiration. • Sound is soft swishing noise.	• Inspiration is louder and higher in pitch than in vesicular breathing.	

Exercise 5
Answer the following questions. Prepare short talks and/or dialogues on these topics

1. Speak about guidelines for observing behaviour.
2. Describe inflammations of the eyelid.
3. What do you know about various patterns of respiration?
4. Describe effective auscultation.
5. What can you say about classification of normal breath sounds?

Translation 3

1. Young children, especially preschoolers, fear intrusive procedures, therefore avoid invasive procedures if possible. 2. Observing behaviour includes following questions: What is the child's overall personality - calm, anxious, tense, content, outgoing, shy, talkative, aggressive, introverted, stable, or moody?; Does the child sit quietly on the examining table or parent's lap, or does the child climb, run, open doors, and otherwise explore the environment?; Can the child follow two or three commands in succession without the need for repetition?; Is the child able to withstand momentary discomfort and wait for the requests to be met?; What is the child's reaction to the nurse – respectful, friendly, reserved, apprehensive, or uninterested?; Does the child look around the room, ask questions about unfamiliar objects, seem to enjoy exploring them, or attempt to break or destroy them?; Can the child follow directions for using the instruments, or imitate their use?; Is the child quick or slow to grasp explanations? 3. Various patterns of respiration are: tachypnoea, bradypnea, apnoea, hyperpnoea, hypoventilation, hyperventilation, Kussmaul breathing, Cheyne-Stokes respirations, Biot breathing, seesaw (paradoxic) respirations, agonal respirations. 4. These are guidelines for effective auscultation: make sure child is relaxed and not crying, talking, or laughing; warm stethoscope before placing it against skin; avoid placing stethoscope over hair or clothing, moving it against skin, breathing on tubing, or sliding fingers over chest piece, which may cause sounds that falsely resemble pathologic findings. 5. Classification of normal breath sounds distinguishes: vesicular breath sounds, bronchovesicular breath sounds, and bronchial breath sounds.

Text 4
Paediatric symptom checklist
- Complains of aches or pains
- Spends more time alone
- Tires easily, little energy
- Fidgety, unable to sit still
- Has trouble with a teacher
- Less interested in school
- Acts as if driven by a motor
- Daydreams too much
- Distracted easily
- Is afraid of new situations
- Feels sad, unhappy
- Is irritable, angry
- Feels hopeless
- Has trouble concentrating
- Less interest in friends
- Fights with other children
- Absent from school
- School grades dropping
- Is down on himself or herself
- Visits physician, but physician finds nothing wrong
- Has trouble with sleeping
- Worries a lot
- Wants to be with you more than before
- Feels he or she is bad
- Takes unnecessary risks
- Gets hurt frequently
- Seems to be having less fun
- Acts younger than children his or her age
- Does not listen to rules
- Does not show feelings
- Does not understand other people's feelings
- Teases others
- Blames others for his or her troubles
- Takes things that do not belong to him or her
- Refuses to share

Tests for sensory discrimination	Tests for cerebellar function
• Touch the skin with a pin or piece of cotton and ask child to describe the different sensations. • Place a cold or warm object on the skin (the rubber and metal heads of the reflex hammer work well) and have child differentiate between them.	• **Finger to nose test** – with child's arm extended, ask child to touch the nose with the index finger with the eyes open and then closed. • **Heel to shin test** – while standing, have child run the heel of one foot down the shin or anterior aspect of the tibia of the other leg, both with the eyes opened and then closed.
• Touch different parts of the body simultaneously and see if child can localize both points.	• **Romberg test** – with the eyes closed, have child stand with the heels together; falling or leaning to one side is abnormal and is called Romberg sign.

Exercise 6
Answer the following questions. Prepare short talks and/or dialogues on these topics

1. What does paediatric symptom checklist include?
2. What can you say about tests for sensory discrimination and tests for cerebellar function?

Exercise 7
Study the following summary and then interpret basic information in English.

1. The most common approach to examining children follows a head-to-toe sequence.
2. Growth measurements during the physical examination focus on length, height, weight, skinfold thickness, and arm and head circumference. Assessment of growth is measured against standard growth charts to determine a child's status in comparison with other children of the same age.
3. Measurements of temperature, pulse, respiration, and blood pressure require accurate assessment techniques to provide useful data.
4. The general appearance of a child is a cumulative, subjective impression of physical appearance, state of nutrition, behaviour, personality, interactions with parents and nurse, posture, development, and speech.
5. Assessment of the skin, which primarily involves inspection and palpation, focuses on colour, texture, temperature, moisture, and turgor. The nurse needs to be aware of both physiologic and ethnic factors that may affect these areas.
6. In assessment to the lymph nodes, the nurse examines, by palpation, the part of the body in which the glands are located.
7. The head is inspected for shape, symmetry, mobility, and head control.
8. Assessment of the neck includes palpation of the trachea and thyroid gland.

Exercise 8
Fill in the missing words. Choose the correct ones.

1. Examination of the eyes includes placement and _____, _____ of external and internal structures, and _____ _____.	a vision testing b inspection c alignment
2. Ears are examined for _____ ___ _____, inspection of external and internal structures, and _____ _____.	a placement and alignment b auditory testing
3. The lungs are examined by methods of inspection, _____, _____, and _____.	a palpation b auscultation c percussion
4. Auscultation is the most important _____ for examining ___ _____.	a the heart b procedure
5. Heart _____ are classified as _____, _____, and _____ and should be evaluated for location, time, intensity, and _____.	a innocent, b functional, c organic d loudness e murmurs
6. _____ assessment follows an _____ _____ of inspection, auscultation, percussion, and palpation, since _____ may _____ normal abdominal sounds.	a orderly sequence b palpation c distort d Abdominal
7. Examination of the _____ may be _____-_____ in the child, and the nurse must _____ transferring personal anxiety.	a avoid b anxiety-provoking c genitalia
8. _____ assessment addresses behaviour, cognitive-perceptual development, _____ _____, _____ ___ _____ functioning, reflexes, cranial nerves, and soft signs.	a motor functioning b sensory and cerebellar c Neurological

Translation 4

1. The child complains of aches or pains, tires easily, has little energy, is fidgety, unable to sit still, is distracted easily, is irritable and angry. 2. The child also daydreams too much, has trouble concentrating, has trouble with sleeping, visits physician, but physician finds nothing wrong. 3. The child does not listen to rules, takes unnecessary risks and gets hurt frequently. 4. In tests for sensory discrimination you should: touch the skin with a pin or piece of cotton, place a cold or warm object on the skin, touch different parts of the body. 5. Tests for cerebellar function include: finger to nose test, heel to shin test and Romberg test. 6. The most common approach to examining children follows a head-to-toe sequence. 7. Growth measurements during the physical examination focus on length, height, weight, skinfold thickness, and arm and head circumference. 8. Measurements of temperature, pulse, respiration, and blood pressure require accurate assessment techniques to provide useful data. 9. The general appearance of a child is an impression of physical appearance, state of nutrition, behaviour, personality, posture, development, and speech. 10. Assessment of the skin focuses on colour, texture, temperature, moisture, and turgor.

Exercise 9

Match the column A with the column B. Try to learn the expressions and/or sentences by heart.

A

1. In assessment to the lymph nodes, the nurse ...
2. The head is inspected for ...
3. Assessment of the neck includes ...
4. Examination of the eyes and ears includes ...
5. The lungs are examined by methods ...
6. Heart murmurs should be evaluated for ...
7. Abdominal assessment follows ...
8. Neurological assessment addresses ...

B

a. ... *an orderly sequence of inspection, auscultation, percussion, and palpation.*
b. ... *of inspection, palpation, percussion, and auscultation.*
c. ... *placement and alignment, inspection of external and internal structures, and vision and auditory testing.*
d. ... *location, time, intensity, and loudness.*
e. ... *shape, symmetry, mobility, and head control.*

f. ... *behaviour, motor functioning, sensory and cerebellar functioning, reflexes, cranial nerves.*
g. ... *examines the part of the body in which the glands are located.*
h. ... *palpation of the trachea and thyroid gland.*

Text 5
Change in stooling patterns of newborns

Meconium	Transitional stools	Milk stool
Infant's first stool; composed of amniotic fluid and its constituents, intestinal secretions, shed mucosal cells, and possibly blood (ingested maternal blood or minor bleeding of alimentary tract vessels).	Usually appear by third day after initiation of feeding; greenish brown to yellowish brown, thin, and less sticky than meconium; may contain some milk curds.	Usually appears by fourth day. **In breast-fed infants'** stools are yellow to golden, are pasty in consistency, and have an odour similar to that of sour milk.
Passage of meconium should occur within the first 24 to 48 hours, although it may be delayed up to 7 days in very-low-birth-weight infants.		**In formula-fed infants'** stools are pale yellow to light brown, are firmer in consistency, and have a more offensive odour.

Clusters of neonatal behaviours in Brazelton neonatal behavioural assessment scale

Habituation	ability to respond to and then inhibit responding to discrete stimulus (light, rattle, bell, pin-prick) while asleep
Orientation	quality of alert states and ability to attend to visual and auditory stimuli while alert
Motor performance	quality of movement and tone
Range of state	measure of general arousal level or arousability of infant
Regulation of state	how infant responds when aroused
Autonomic stability	signs of stress (tremors, startles, skin colour) related to homeostatic (self-regulating) adjustment of the nervous system
Reflexes	assessment of several neonatal reflexes

Guidelines
Assessing attachment behaviour
- When the infant is brought to the parents, do they reach out for the child and call the child by name?
- Do the parents speak about the child in terms of identification — whom the infant looks like; what appears special about their child over other infants?

- When parents are holding the infant, what kind of body contact is there — do parents feel at ease in changing the infant's position; are fingertips or whole hands used; are there parts of the body they avoid touching or parts of the body they investigate and scrutinize?
- When the infant is awake, what kinds of stimulation do the parents provide — do they talk to the infant, to each other, or to no one; how do they look at the infant — direct visual contact, avoidance of eye contact, or looking at other people or objects?
- How comfortable do the parents appear in terms of caring for the infant? Do they express any concern regarding their ability to disgust for certain activities, such as changing diapers?
- What type of affection do they demonstrate to the newborn, such as smiling, stroking, kissing, or rocking?
- If the infant is fussy, what kinds of comforting techniques do the parents use, such as rocking, swaddling, talking, or stroking?

Tests used in assessing gestational age

Posture	With infant quiet and in a supine position, observe degree of flexion in arms and legs. Muscle tone and degree of flexion increase with maturity. Full flexion of the arms and legs = 4
Square window	With thumb supporting back of arm below wrist, apply gentle pressure with index and third fingers on dorsum of hand without rotating infant's wrist. Measure angle between base of thumb and forearm. Full flexion (hand lies flat on ventral surface of forearm) = 4
Arm recoil	With infant supine, fully flex both forearms on upper arms, hold for 5 seconds; pull down on hands to fully extend and rapidly release arms. Observe rapidity and intensity of recoil to a state of flexion. A brisk return to full flexion = 4
Popliteal angle	With infant supine and pelvis flat on a firm surface, flex lower leg on thigh and then flex thigh on abdomen. While holding knee with thumb and index finger, extend lower leg with index finger of other hand. Measure degree of angle behind knee (popliteal angle). An angle of less than 90 degrees = 5
Scarf sign	With infant supine, support head in midline with one hand; use other hand to pull infant's arm across the shoulder so that infant's hand touches shoulder. Determine location of elbow in relation to midline. Elbow does not reach midline = 4
Heel to ear	With infant supine and pelvis flat on a firm surface, pull foot as far as possible up toward ear on same side. Measure distance of foot from ear on same side. Measure distance of foot from ear and degree of knee flexion (same as popliteal angle). Knees flexed with a popliteal angle of less than 10 degrees = 4

Exercise 10
Answer the following questions. Prepare short talks and/or dialogues on these topics

1. Describe change in stooling patterns of newborns.
2. What do you know about clusters of neonatal behaviours in Brazelton neonatal behavioural assessment scale?
3. What can you say about assessing attachment behaviour?
4. Which tests are used in assessing gestational age?

Translation 5

1. Meconium, infant's first stool is composed of amniotic fluid, intestinal secretions, shed mucosal cells, and possibly blood. 2. Transitional stools usually appear by third day after initiation of feeding; greenish brown to yellowish brown, thin, and less sticky than meconium. 3. In breast-fed infants' stools are yellow to golden, are pasty in consistency, and have an odour similar to that of sour milk. 4. In formula-fed infants' stools are pale yellow to light brown, are firmer in consistency, and have a more offensive odour. 5. Habituation is ability to respond to and then inhibit responding to discrete stimulus (light, rattle, bell, pin-prick) while asleep. 6. Orientation is ability to attend to visual and auditory stimuli while alert. 7. Motor performance is quality of movement and tone. 8. Autonomic stability includes signs of stress (tremors, startles, skin colour) related to homeostatic (self-regulating) adjustment of the nervous system. 9. In assessing attachment behaviour you should observe: When parents are holding the infant, what kind of body contact is there?; When the infant is awake, what kinds of stimulation do the parents provide?; Do the parents express any concern regarding their ability to disgust for certain activities, such as changing diapers?; What type of affection do they demonstrate to the newborn, such as smiling, stroking, kissing, or rocking?; What kinds of comforting techniques do the parents use, such as rocking, swaddling, talking, or stroking? 10. Tests used in assessing gestational age include: posture, square window, arm recoil, popliteal angle, scarf sign, heel to ear.

Key 14
Exercise 3
1 d, a, b, c; 2 b, a, c; 3 b, a, c; 4 c, a, b

Exercise 8

1 b, c, a; 2 a, b; 3 a, c, b; 4 b, a; 5 e, a, b, c, d; 6 d, a, b, c; 7 c, b, a; 8 c, a, b

Exercise 9

1g; 2e; 3h; 4c; 5b; 6d; 7a; 8f

VOCABULARY 14

acquainted /əˈk.weɪn.tɪd/
acromion /əˈkrəʊ.mi.ən/ pl **acromia** /əˈkrəʊ.mi.ə/
adjustment /əˈdʒʌst.mənt/
advanced /ədˈvɑːnst/
agonal /ˈəg.əʊ.nəl/
alert /əˈlɜːt/
align /əˈlaɪn/
alignment /əˈlaɪn.mənt/
alimentary /ˌæl.menˈtə.rɪ/
amniotic /ˌæm.niˈɒt.ɪk/
angle /ˈæŋgəl/
anterior /ænˈtɪə.ri.ər/
apnoea /ˈæp.ni.ə/
appliance /əˈplaɪ.əns/
apprehensive /ˌæp.rɪˈhen.sɪv/
approval /əˈpruː.vəl/
argue /ˈɑːg.juː/
argumentative /ˌɑːgjʊˈmen.tə.tɪv/
arousability /əˈraʊz.əˈbɪl.ɪ.tɪ/
arousal /əˈraʊzəl/
aroused /əˈraʊzd/
artificially /ˌɑː.tɪˌfɪʃ.iˈæl.ɪ/
at /æt/ **ease** /iːz/
atraumatic /ˈeɪ.trə.ˈmat.ik/
attend /əˈtend/
attendant /əˈten.dənt/
attention /əˈten.tʃən/ **span** /spæn/
attentive /əˈten.tɪv/
auscultation /ˌɔː.skəlˈteɪ.ʃən/
average /ˈæv.ər.ɪdʒ/
avoidance /əˈvɔɪ.dəns/
away /əˈweɪ/
belligerent /bəˈlɪdʒ.ər.ənt/
beverage /ˈbev.ər.ɪdʒ/
bifurcate /ˈbaɪ.fə.keɪt/
blame /bleɪm/
blepharitis /ˌblef.ə.ˈraɪ.təs/
brace /breɪs/
brand /brænd/
Brazelton /breɪˈzel.tɒn/ **scale** /ˈskeɪl/
broil /brɔɪl/
bronchial /ˈbrɒŋ.ki.əl/
bronchovesicular /ˈbrɒŋ.kə.vəˈsɪk.jə.lər/
calliper /ˈkæl.ɪpə/
canthus /ˈkan.θəs/ pl **canthi** /ˈkan.ˌθaɪ/

cerebellar /ˌser.ə.ˈbe.lər/
cessation /sesˈeɪ.ʃən/
chalazion /kə.ˈleɪ.zi:.ən/ pl **chalazia** /zi:ə/
checklist /ˈtʃek.lɪst/
chest piece /tʃest.pi:s/ hrudník
Cheyne-Stokes /cheɪn.i:.ˌstəʊks/ **respirations** /ˌrespə.ˈreɪʃənz/
chief /tʃif/
circumference /sə.ˈkʌm.fər.əns/
colic /ˈkɒl.ɪk/
commercial /kə.ˈmɜ:.ʃəl/
compare /kəm.ˈpeər/
comparison /kəm.ˈpær.ɪ.sən/
complaint /kəm.ˈpleɪnt/
complimentary /ˌkɒmplɪ.ˈmen.tə.rɪ/
cotton /ˈkɒt.ən/
cranial /ˈkreɪ.ni.əl/
crusted /ˈkrʌs.tɪd/
cumulative /ˈkju:.mjʊ.lə.tɪv/
curd /kɜ:d/
dacryocystitis /ˈdæk.ˌkrɪəʊ.sɪs.taɪ.tis/
daydream /ˈdeɪ.dri:m/
dental /ˈden.təl/
destroy /dɪ.ˈstrɔɪ/
determine /dɪ.ˈtɜ:.mɪn/
differentiate /ˌdɪfə.ˈrenʃieɪt/
disagree /ˌdɪs.ə.ˈgri:/
discrete /dɪs.ˈkri:t/
disgust /dɪs.ˈgʌst/
dislike /dɪs.ˈlaɪk/
disruption /dɪs.ˈrʌp.ʃən/
distract /dɪ.ˈs.trækt/
dorsum /ˈdɔ:.səm/ pl **dorsa**
double /ˈdʌb.l̩/
drop /drɒp/
elbow /ˈelbəʊ/
estimate /ˈes.tɪ.meɪt/
extended /ɪk.ˈsten.dɪd/
falsely /ˈfɒl.sli/
fearful /ˈfɪə.fəl/
fidgety /ˈfɪdʒ.ɪ.ti/
fight /faɪt/
flexion /flek.ʃən/
fluid /ˈflu:.ɪd/
fluoride /ˈflʊə.raɪd/
forearm /ˈfɔ:.rɑ:m/
formula /ˈfɔ:.mjʊ.lə/
fried /fraɪd/

fussiness /ˈfə.siː.nəs/

fussy /ˈfʌsɪ/

gasp /gɑːsp/

grade /greɪd/

granuloma /græn.jəˈləʊ.mə/

grasp /grɑːsp/

gratification /ˌɡræt.ɪ.fɪˈkeɪ.ʃən/

habit /ˈhæb.ɪt/

habituation /həˌbɪtʃ.uˈeɪ.ʃ°n/

hammer /ˈhæm.ər/

hearty /ˈhɑː.ti/

heel /hiːl/

hopeless /ˈhəʊp.ləs/

hordeolum /hɔːr.ˈdiː.ə.ləm/ pl hordeola /-lə/

hyperpnoea /ˌhaɪ.pəˈpni.ə/

hypoventilation /ˌhaɪ.pəʊˌven.tɪˈleɪ.ʃən/

imitate /ˈɪm.ɪ.teɪt/

impression /ɪmˈpreʃ.ən/

inhibit /ɪnˈhɪb.ɪt/

innocent /ˈɪnəsənt/

inspection /ɪnˈspek.ʃən/

instrument /ˈɪn.strə.mənt/

interscapular /ˌɪn.tərˈskæp.jə.ləʳ/

introvert /ˈɪn.trə.vɜːt/

intubate /ɪnˈtjuː.beɪt/

invasive /ɪnˈveɪ.sɪv/

involvement /ɪnˈvɒlv.mənt/

iron /aɪən/

irritable /ˈɪr.ɪ.tə.bļ/

jaw /dʒɔː/

Kussmaul /ˈkus.ˌmaul/ breathing /ˈbriː.ðɪŋ/

laboured /ˈleɪ.bəd/

lacrimal /ˈlæk.rɪm.əl/ sac /sæk/

lash /læʃ/

lean /liːn/

localize /ˈləʊ.kəl.aɪz/

loose /luːs/

loudness /laʊd.nəs/

low pitched /ˌləʊˈpɪtʃt/

lymph /lɪmf/ node /nəʊd/

manubrium /məˈnuː.bri.əm/

marginal /ˈmɑː.dʒɪnəl/

maturity /məˈtjʊə.rɪ.ti/

measurement /ˈmeʒ.ə.mənt/

meconium /mɪˈkəʊ.nɪ.əm/

meibomian /maɪˈbəʊ.miː.ən/ gland /glænd/

metal /ˈmet.əl/

midpoint /ˈmɪd.pɔɪnt/

moisture /ˈmɔɪs.tʃər/

momentary /ˈməʊ.mən.tər.i/

moody /ˈmuː.di/

movable /ˈmuːvəbəl/

movement /ˈmuːv.mənt/

mucosal /mjuːˈkəʊ.səl/

nonthreatening /ˌnɒn.ˈθret.ᵊn.ɪŋ/

notch /nɒtʃ/

obey /əʊˈbeɪ/

orderly /ˈɔː.dəl.i/

outgoing /ˈaʊtˌɡəʊɪŋ/

outline /ˈaʊt.laɪn/

palpation /pælˈpeɪ.ʃən/

paradoxic /ˌpærəˈdɒksɪk/

pattern /ˈpæt.ən/

perceptual /pəˈseptjʊəl/

percussion /pəˈkʌʃ.ən/

personality /ˌpɜː.sənˈæl.ə.ti/

pertinent /ˈpɜːtɪnənt/

picky /ˈpɪkɪ/

pin /pɪn/

possess /pəˈzes/

posterior /pɒsˈtɪə.ri.ər/

posture /ˈpɒs.tʃər/

power /ˈpaʊə/

premature /ˈprem.ə.tʃər/

pull /pʊl/

purulent /ˈpjʊə.rʊ.lənt/

pus /pʌs/

pustule /ˈpʌstjuːl/

quietly /ˈkwaɪətlɪ/

reading /ˈriː.dɪŋ/

recoil /rɪˈkɔɪl/

reflect /rɪˈflekt/

remark /rɪˈmɑːk/

repetition /ˌrepɪˈtɪ.ʃən/

resemble /rɪˈzem.bl̩/

respectful /rɪˈspektfəl/

restless /ˈrest.ləs/

restrain /rɪˈstreɪn/

reward /rɪˈwɔːd/

Romberg /romˈbərg/ **sign** /saɪn/

rubber /ˈrʌbə/

scarf /skɑːf/

scrutinize /ˈskruːtɪˌnaɪz/

sebaceous /sɪˈbeɪʃəs/

secure /sɪˈkjʊə/
sedentary /ˈsed.ən.tər.i/
seesaw /ˈsiːˌsɔː/
self-regulating /ˌself.ˈreg.jə.leɪt.ɪŋ/
sensation /senˈseɪ.ʃən/
sensory /ˈsen.sər.i/
sequence /ˈsiː.kwəns/
shallow /ˈʃæləʊ/
shed /ʃed/
shin /ʃɪn/
simultaneously /ˌsɪm.əlˈteɪ.ni.əs.li/
skim /skɪm/
skin fold /ˈskɪn.ˌfəʊld/
slide /slaɪd/
slide /slaɪd/ (slid, slid)
spit up /spɪt ʌp/
stable /ˈsteɪ.bl̩/
startle /ˈstɑː.tl̩/
sticky /ˈstɪk.i/
stroke /strəʊk/
stye /staɪ/
subjective /səbˈdʒek.tɪv/
succession /səkˈseʃ.ən/
suck /sʌk/
supine /ˈsuː.paɪn/
supplement /ˈsʌp.lɪ.mənt/
suprasternal /ˌsuː.prəˈstɜː.nəl/
surface /ˈsɜː.fɪs/
swaddle /ˈswɒdəl/
swish /swɪʃ/
tarsus /ˈtɑː.səs/ pl tarsi /ˈtɑːr.ˌsaɪ/
tease /tiːz/
thickness /ˈθɪk.nəs/
thigh /θaɪ/
thyroid /ˈθaɪə.ˌrɔɪd/
tibia /ˈtɪb.i.ə/ pl tibiae
tire /taɪər/
tone /təʊn/
transitional /trænˈzɪʃənəl/
transmission /trænzˈmɪʃ.ən/
triple /ˈtrɪp.l̩/
tubing /ˈtjuː.bɪŋ/
turgor /ˈtɜːgə/
uncooperative /ˌʌn.kəʊˈɒp.ər.ə.tɪv/
underlying /ˌʌn.dəˈlaɪ.ɪŋ/
unduly /ʌnˈdjuːlɪ/
ventral /ˈvent.rəl/

vesicular /vəˈsɪk.jə,lər/
vibration /vɑɪˈbreɪˌʃən/
whole /həʊl/
willingness /ˈwɪl.ɪŋ.nəs/
withstand /wɪðˈstænd/
worry /ˈwʌr.i/

Health promotion of the newborn and family; Physical examination of the newborn; Health problems of the newborn; The high-risk newborn and family; Signs of stress or fatigue in neonates; Conditions caused by defects in physical development

Text 1
Guidelines
Physical examination of the newborn
- Provide a normothermic and non-stimulating examination area. Undress only body area examined to prevent heat loss.
- Proceed in an orderly sequence (usually head to toe) with the following exceptions. Perform all procedures that require quiet first, such as auscultating the lungs, heart, and abdomen. Perform disturbing procedures, such as testing reflexes, last. Measure head, chest, and length at same time to compare results.
- Proceed quickly to avoid stressing infant. Check that equipment and supplies are working properly and are accessible.
- Comfort infant during and after examination; involve parent in the following: talk softly; hold infant's hands against chest; swaddle and hold; give pacifier or gloved finger to suck.

Guidelines
Ophthalmia neonatorum prophylaxis
Clean the eyelids with sterile cotton and sterile water if needed.

- Separate lids and apply 2 drops or a 1 to 2 cm ribbon of ointment in each conjunctival sac.
- Massage lids to ensure spread of the medication.
- Wipe excess medication from eye with sterile cotton 1 minute after application.
- Do not rinse eyes with sterile normal saline.

Advantages of human milk vs cow's milk:

- Contains adequate (not excessive) protein; has greater quantities of certain amino acids, including cystine and taurine
- Contains more lactalbumin (produces easily digested curds) than casein (produces large, hard curds)
- Contains more lactose, which in the gut stimulates growth of microorganisms, which synthesize some B vitamins and produce organic acids that may retard growth of harmful bacteria
- Contains more monounsaturated fatty acids, which enhance absorption of fat and calcium
- Contains adequate (not excessive) minerals with exception of fluoride (low in both)
- Amounts of iron and zinc are low but more readily absorbed
- Contains less calcium and phosphorus but a more favourable ratio of the minerals, which prevents excessive calcium excretion
- Contains adequate amount of vitamin A, B complex, and E; vitamin C content depends on maternal intake; vitamin D is low, but more readily absorbed (vitamins C, D, and E are low in cow's milk, but K is higher)
- Contains growth modulators that modify growth or maturation
- Offers several immunologic benefits; contains various immunoglobulins (Ig); macrophages, granulocytes, T- and B-cell lymphocytes, and other factors that inhibit bacterial growth
- Has laxative effect
- Is economical, readily available, and sanitary
- Has psychological benefits of close bond between infant and mother during feeding

Exercise 1
Answer the following questions. Prepare short talks and/or dialogues on these topics

1. Describe physical examination of the newborn.
2. What do you know about ophthalmia neonatorum prophylaxis?
3. Speak about advantages of human milk vs cow's milk.

Exercise 2
Study the following summary and then interpret basic information in English.

1. Transition from foetal or placental circulation to independent respiration is the most important physiologic change required of the newborn.

| 2. Chemical and thermal factors help initiate the neonate's first respiration. |
| 3. Circulatory changes in the neonate result from shifts in pressure of the heart and major vessels and from functional closures of the foetal shunts. |
| 4. The newborn's large surface area, thin layer of subcutaneous fat, and unique mechanism for producing heat predispose the newborn to excessive heat loss. |
| 5. The infant's high rate of metabolism is closely correlated with the rate of fluid exchange, which is seven times greater in the infant than in the adult. |
| 6. The skin and mucous membranes the reticuloendothelial system, and antibodies are the first, second, and third lines to defence against infection. |
| 7. Apgar scoring, the initial assessment of the newborn, focuses on heart rate, respiratory effort, muscle tone, reflex irritability, and colour. |

Exercise 3
Fill in the missing words. Choose the correct ones.

1. Physical assessment of the newborn includes assessment of clinical gestational age, general _____, general _____, _____-___-____ assessment, and _____-_____ attachment, or bonding.	a parent-infant b appearance c measurements d head-to-toe
2. _____ _____ focuses on localized reflexes and _____, muscle tone, head control, and movement and is best accomplished during the general _____ _____.	a Neurologic assessment b physical examination c posture
3. Behavioural assessment of newborns with the Brazelton Neonatal behavioural _____ _____ examines responses to seven categories: _____, orientation, _____ _____, range of state, regulation of state, autonomic regulation and _____.	a habituation b motor performance c reflexes d Assessment Scale
4. An instrument for assessing the _____ _____ between parent and infant is the Nursing Child Assessment _____ _____.	a reciprocal interchange b Feeding Scale
5. Physical care to the newborn includes maintaining _____ _____, maintaining _____ body temperature, _____ from infection and injury, and providing _____ _____.	a stable b patent airway c optimum nutrition d protecting

6. Although the attachment, or _____, process primarily affects _____ ___ _____, _____ also play an important role.	a infants and parents
	b siblings
	c bonding
7. With short _____ _____, teaching needs to begin before birth and continue after _____ with telephone and/or home _____ ___.	a discharge
	b maternity admissions
	c follow up
8. An _____ _____ of discharge teaching is ensuring the newborn's safe _____ home.	a transportation
	b essential aspect

Translation 1

1. Provide a normothermic and non-stimulating examination area. 2. Proceed in an orderly sequence (usually head to toe), perform auscultating the lungs, heart, and abdomen first. 3. Measure head, chest, and length at same time to compare results. 4. Check that equipment and supplies are working properly and are accessible. 5. Comfort infant during and after examination. 6. In ophthalmia neonatorum prophylaxis clean the eyelids with sterile cotton and sterile water if needed and apply ointment in each conjunctival sac. 7. Advantages of human milk vs cow's milk: human milk contains adequate protein; has greater quantities of certain amino acids; contains more lactalbumin; more lactose; more monounsaturated fatty acids; contains adequate minerals; adequate amount of vitamin A, B complex, and E; contains growth modulators; offers several immunologic benefits; is economical, readily available, and sanitary; has psychological benefits. 8. Transition from foetal or placental circulation to independent respiration is the most important physiologic change required of the newborn.

Exercise 4
Match the column A with the column B. Try to learn the expressions and/or sentences by heart.

A

1. Circulatory changes in the neonate result from …
2. Apgar scoring, the initial assessment of the newborn, focuses on …
3. Physical assessment of the newborn includes …
4. Neurologic assessment focuses on …
5. Behavioural assessment of newborns examines responses to seven categories …

6. Physical care to the newborn includes ...

B

a. ... *localized reflexes and posture, muscle tone, head control, and movement.*

b. ... *assessment of clinical gestational age, general measurements, general appearance, head-to-toe assessment.*

c. ... *maintaining a patent airway, maintaining a stable body temperature, protecting from infection and injury, and providing optimum nutrition.*

d. ... *heart rate, respiratory effort, muscle tone, reflex irritability, and colour.*

e. ... *shifts in pressure of the heart and major vessels and from functional closures of the foetal shunts*

f. ... *habituation, orientation, motor performance, range of state, regulation of state, autonomic regulation and reflexes.*

Text 2
Health problems of the newborn
Types of physical injuries at birth

Soft tissue injury	Head injury	Neurologic injury
erythema, abrasion, petechiae, ecchymoses, subcutaneous fat necrosis,	skull moulding, caput succedaneum, subgaleal haemorrhage,	subdural or epidural haematoma, facial paralysis, brachial palsy,
subconjunctival (scleral) haemorrhage, retinal haemorrhage, haemorrhage into abdominal organ(s)	cephalohematoma, fracture (depressed, or linear), intracranial haemorrhage	phrenic nerve palsy (diaphragmatic paralysis), spinal cord injury

Common types of soft tissue injury

Erythema and abrasion	usually the result of the application of forceps; discolouration is the same configuration as the instrument
Petechiae	non-raised pinpoint haemorrhages caused by a sudden increase and then release of pressure during passage through the birth canal; may be seen on the chest, face, and head
Ecchymoses	small haemorrhagic areas (larger than petechiae) that may occur after traumatic, rapid (or "precipitate"), or breech delivery

Subcutaneous fat necrosis	clearly outlined masses located in the subcutaneous tissues that are firm to the overlying skin but movable over the underlying tissue; most likely caused by traumatic manipulation during delivery
Subconjunctival (scleral) haemorrhages	the result of rupture of capillaries in the sclera from pressure on the foetal head during delivery; most common location is the limbus of the iris
Retinal haemorrhages	flame-shaped, irregular, or round areas of bleeding in the retina from excessive pressure on the foetal head during delivery; extensive areas may indicate subdural haematoma or brain trauma

Family focus
Phototherapy and parent-infant interaction

The traditional use of phototherapy has evoked concerns regarding a number of psycho-behavioural issues, including parent-infant separation, potential social isolation, decreased sensorineural stimulation, altered biologic rhythms, altered feeding patterns, and activity changes. Parental anxiety is greatly increased, particularly at the sight of the newborn blindfolded and until special lights. The interruption of breast-feeding for phototherapy is a potential deterrent to successful maternal-infant attachment and interaction. Because research has demonstrated that bilirubin catabolism occurs primarily within the first few hours of the initiation of phototherapy, there is increased support for the removal of the infant from treatment for feeding and holding. Intermittent phototherapy may be just as effective as continuous therapy when used correctly. The benefits of stopping phototherapy for parental feeding and holding outweigh concerns related to the clearance of bilirubin.

Exercise 5
Answer the following questions. Prepare short talks and/or dialogues on these topics

1. Characterize types of physical injuries at birth.
2. Speak about common types of soft tissue injury.
3. What can you say about phototherapy and parent-infant interaction?

Exercise 6
Study the following summary and then interpret basic information in English.

1. Problems of the newborn may be attributed to birth injuries, infections, immature physiologic systems, and inborn errors of metabolism.
2. The forces of labour and delivery my cause soft tissue injury, head trauma, fractures, and paralysis.
3. The most common forms of paralysis in the newborn are facial nerve, brachial plexus, and phrenic nerve palsies.
4. Common skin problems of the newborn include erythema toxicum, candidiasis, bullous impetigo, and "birthmarks," especially port-wine stains and haemangiomas.
5. Because of immature physiologic status, infants may be predisposed to hyperbilirubinemia, hypoglycaemia, hyperglycaemia, and hypocalcaemia.
6. Hyperbilirubinemia is classified according to the two types of bilirubin: unconjugated and conjugated. In the newborn it may result from excess production of bilirubin and/or decreased capacity of the liver to conjugate bilirubin.

Exercise 7
Fill in the missing words. Choose the correct ones.

1. The _____ _____ of unconjugated hyperbilirubinemia has been _____. However, much controversy surrounds __ ___ ____ it should be used.	a phototherapy b if and when c primary treatment
2. _____ _____ of the newborn is characterized by abnormally _____ _____ of red blood cells as a result of blood _____ between mother and foetus.	a rapid destruction b incompatibility c Haemolytic disease
3. _____ can often __ _____ with the initiation of early _____.	a be prevented b Hypoglycaemia c feedings
4. _____ disease of the newborn is characterized by _____ from the umbilicus or circumcision site, _____ __ _____ stools, haematuria, _____ on skin and scalp, and epistaxis.	a oozing b bloody or black c ecchymoses d Haemorrhagic
5. The most significant inborn _____ __ _____ are congenital _____, phenylketonuria, and galactosemia.	a hypothyroidism b errors of metabolism

6. _____ _____ is required to treat _____ hypothyroidism.	a Thyroid replacement b congenital
7. _____ _____ is the treatment of choice for _____ and _____. However, even with strict control, outcomes for these children are less favourable than previously thought.	a phenylketonuria b galactosemia c Dietary control

Translation 2

1. Types of physical injuries at birth are: soft tissue injury (erythema, abrasion, petechiae, ecchymoses, subconjunctival or retinal haemorrhage, haemorrhage into abdominal organs); head injury (subgaleal haemorrhage, cephalohematoma, fracture, intracranial haemorrhage); neurologic injury (subdural or epidural haematoma, facial paralysis, brachial palsy, and spinal cord injury). 2. Common types of soft tissue injury are: discolouration, pinpoint haemorrhages, small haemorrhagic areas, outlined masses located in the subcutaneous tissues, rupture of capillaries in the sclera, flame-shaped, irregular, or round areas of bleeding in the retina. 3. The traditional use of phototherapy has evoked concerns regarding parent-infant separation, altered feeding patterns, and activity changes. 4. There is increased support for the removal of the infant from treatment for feeding and holding. 5. Intermittent phototherapy may be just as effective as continuous therapy. 6. Problems of the newborn may be attributed to birth injuries, infections, immature physiologic systems, and inborn errors of metabolism.

Exercise 8
Match the column A with the column B. Try to learn the expressions and/or sentences by heart.

A

1. The forces of labour and delivery may cause …
2. Common skin problems of the newborn include …
3. In the newborn hyperbilirubinemia may result from …
4. Haemolytic disease of the newborn is characterized by …
5. Haemorrhagic disease of the newborn is characterized by …
6. Thyroid replacement is required to treat …
7. Dietary control is the treatment of choice …

B

a.   *... excess production of bilirubin and/or decreased capacity of the liver to conjugate bilirubin.*

b.   *... soft tissue injury, head trauma, fractures, and paralysis.*

c.   *... congenital hypothyroidism.*

d.   *... oozing from the umbilicus or circumcision site, bloody or black stools, and haematuria.*

e.   *... abnormally rapid destruction of red blood cells as a result of blood incompatibility between mother and foetus*

f.   *... for phenylketonuria and galactosemia.*

g.   *... erythema toxicum, candidiasis, bullous impetigo, and "birthmarks".*

Text 3
The high-risk newborn and family
Guidelines
Physical assessment
General assessment

Using electronic scale, weigh daily, or more often if ordered. Measure length and head circumference periodically. Describe general body shape and size, posture at rest, ease of breathing, presence and location of oedema. Describe any apparent deformities. Describe any signs of distress: poor colour, mouth open, head bobbing, grimace, furrowed brow.

Respiratory assessment

Describe shape of chest (barrel, concave), symmetry, presence of incisions, chest tubes, or other deviations. Describe use of accessory muscles: nasal flaring or substernal, intercostal, or subclavicular retractions. Determine respiratory rate and regularity. Auscultate and describe breath sounds; stridor, crackles, wheezing, wet diminished sounds, areas of absence of sound, grunting, diminished air entry, equality of breath sounds. Determine whether suctioning is needed. Describe cry if not intubated. Describe ambient oxygen and method of delivery; if intubated, describe size of tube, type of ventilator and settings, and method of securing tube. Determine oxygen saturation by pulse oximetry and partial pressure of oxygen and carbon dioxide by transcutaneous oxygen ($tcPO_2$), and transcutaneous carbon dioxide ($tcPCO_2$).

Cardiovascular assessment

Determine heart rate and rhythm. Describe heart sounds, including any murmurs. Determine the point of maximum intensity (PMI), the point where the heartbeat sounds and palpates loudest (a change in the point of maximum intensity may indicate a mediastinal shift). Describe infant's colour (may be of cardiac, respiratory, or hematopoietic origin): cyanosis, pallor, plethora, jaundice, mottling). Assess colour of nail beds, mucous membranes, lips. Determine blood pressure. Indicate extremity used and cuff size; check each extremity at least once. Describe peripheral pulses, capillary refill (<2 to 3 seconds), peripheral perfusion (mottling). Describe monitors, their parameters, and whether alarms are in "on" position.

Gastrointestinal assessment

Determine presence of abdominal distention: increase in circumference, shiny skin, evidence of abdominal wall erythema, visible peristalsis, visible loops of bowel, status of umbilicus. Determine any signs of regurgitation, and time related to feeding; character and amount of residual if gavage fed; if nasogastric tube in place, describe type of suction, drainage (colour, consistency, pH, guaiac). Describe amount, colour, consistency and odour or any emesis. Palpate liver margin. Describe amount, colour, and consistency of stools; check for occult blood and/or reducing substances if ordered or indicated by appearance of stool. Describe bowel sounds: presence or absence (must be present if feeding).

Genitourinary assessment

Describe any abnormalities of genitalia. Describe amount (as determined by weight), colour, pH, lab stick findings, and specific gravity of urine (to screen for adequacy of hydration). Check weight (the most accurate measure for assessment of hydration).

Neurologic-musculoskeletal assessment

Describe infant's movements: random, purposeful, jittery, twitching, spontaneous, elicited; level of activity with stimulation; evaluate based on gestational age. Describe infant's position or attitude: flexed, extended. Describe reflexes observed: Moro, sucking, Babinski, plantar reflex, and other expected reflexes. Determine level of response and consolability. Determine changes in head circumference (if indicated); size and tension of fontanelles, suture lines. Determine pupillary responses in infant > 32 weeks of gestation.

Temperature

Determine skin and axillary temperature. Determine relationship to environmental temperature.

Skin assessment

Describe any discolouration, reddened area, signs of irritation, blisters, abrasions, or denuded areas, especially where monitoring equipment, infusions, or other apparatus come in contact with skin; also check and note any skin preparation used (e. g., povidone-iodine tape). Determine texture and turgor of skin: dry, smooth, flaky, peeling, etc. Describe any rash, skin lesion, or birthmarks. Determine whether intravenous infusion catheter or needle is in place and observe for signs of infiltration. Describe parenteral infusion lines: location, type (arterial, venous, peripheral, umbilical, peripheral central venous); type of infusion (medication, saline, dextrose, electrolyte, lipids, total parenteral nutrition); type of infusion pump and rate of flow; type of needle (butterfly, catheter); appearance of insertion site.

Components of a care plan to overcome feeding resistance

Stimulate normal feeding interactions. Hold and cuddle infant in "en face" feeding position. Engage in eye contact with infant. Engage in verbal interaction with infant. Provide tactile stimulation. Begin with torso and progress to head and neck. Apply firm, consistent pressure. Use palm or hand or textured object (e. g., washcloth). Gradually move toward mouth, cheeks, and lips. Stroke oral area from cheeks to lips. Pace according to child's tolerance. Overcome oral hypersensitivity (sensitivity to intraoral stimulation). Provide oral stimulation as above. When external oral stimulation is tolerated, attempt massage of gums and tongue (use finger or soft rubber item). Massage gums from centre and move toward molar region, and move gradually from anterior to posterior. Withdraw stimulus and close child's mouth if child gags. Encourage oral exploration. Assist child in mouthing hands, fingers, toes, or soft rubber toys. Play oral games (e. g., blowing a kiss, kissing an object — toy, animal). Provide oral feedings. Introduce small volumes as early as possible. Offer feedings consistently (water, formula). Avoid force feeding. Provide feeding stimulation during tube feedings. Hold child in feeding position. Provide oral stimulation during bolus feedings. Give oral feedings before tube feedings. Give bolus feedings in response to hunger when possible rather than on predetermined schedule. Provide non-nutritive sucking to encourage use of oral musculature.

Exercise 9
Answer the following questions. Prepare short talks and/or dialogues on these topics

1. What do you know about general assessment and physical assessment?

2. What can you say about respiratory assessment and cardiovascular assessment?
3. Describe gastrointestinal assessment and genitourinary assessment.
4. Characterize neurologic-musculoskeletal assessment and skin assessment.
5. What are components of a care plan to overcome feeding resistance?

Translation 3

1. In general assessment: weigh daily, measure length and head circumference periodically, describe general body shape and size, posture at rest, ease of breathing, presence and location of oedema, and apparent deformities. 2. Describe any signs of distress: poor colour, mouth open, head bobbing, grimace, furrowed brow. 3. Describe shape of chest, symmetry, use of accessory muscles (nasal flaring or substernal, intercostal, or subclavicular retractions). 4. Auscultate and describe breath sounds; stridor, crackles, wheezing, wet diminished sounds, areas of absence of sound, grunting, and determine whether suctioning is needed. 5. Determine oxygen saturation by pulse oximetry and partial pressure of oxygen and carbon dioxide. 6. Determine heart rate and rhythm, heart sounds, including any murmurs. 7. Describe infant's colour (may be of cardiac, respiratory, or hematopoietic origin), cyanosis, pallor, plethora, jaundice, mottling. 8. Determine presence of abdominal distention: increase in circumference, shiny skin, evidence of abdominal wall erythema, visible peristalsis, visible loops of bowel, status of umbilicus. 9. Describe amount, colour, consistency and odour or any emesis, describe amount, colour, and consistency of stools and check for occult blood. 10. Describe any abnormalities of genitalia.

Exercise 10
Match the column A with the column B. Try to learn the expressions and/or sentences by heart.

A
1. Describe infant's movements:
2. Describe infant's position
3. Determine changes in
4. Describe any discolouration,
5. Determine texture and turgor of skin:
6. Determine whether intravenous infusion
7. Describe parenteral infusion lines (arterial, venous, peripheral, umbilical, peripheral central venous);
8. Stimulate normal feeding interactions,

9. When external oral stimulation is tolerated,
10. Assist child in mouthing
11. Offer feedings consistently (water, formula)
12. Provide non-nutritive sucking

B

a. ... *head circumference, size and tension of fontanelles, and suture lines.*
b. ... *dry, smooth, flaky, peeling, etc.*
c. ... *catheter or needle is in place and observe for signs of infiltration-*
d. ... *engage in eye contact and verbal interaction with infant and provide tactile stimulation.*
e. ... *attempt massage of gums and tongue.*
f. ... *or attitude: flexed, extended.*
g. ... *to encourage use of oral musculature.*
h. ... *but avoid force feeding.*
i. ... *hands, fingers, toes, or soft rubber toys.*
j. ... *type of infusion (medication, saline, dextrose, electrolyte, lipids, total parenteral nutrition).*
k. ... *reddened area, signs of irritation, blisters, abrasions, or denuded areas.*
l. ... *random, purposeful, jittery, twitching, spontaneous, elicited and level of activity with stimulation.*

Text 4
Signs of stress or fatigue in neonates

Autonomic stress	Changes in state	Behavioural changes
• acrocyanosis • deep, rapid respirations • regular rapid heart rate	• dull or sleep state • crying or fussy • glassy-eyed or strained alertness	• unfocused and uncoordinated eyes • limp arms and legs • flaccid shoulders dropped back • hiccoughs • sneezes • yawning • straining having a bowel movement

Behavioural manifestations of developmental organization
Motor stability behaviours

Smooth, well-modulated posture and well-modulated tone; synchronous smooth movements with efficient motoric strategies: hand clasping, foot clasping, finger folding, hand-to-mouth manoeuvres, grasping, suck searching and sucking, handholding, tucking

State stability and attention regulation behaviours

Clear, robust sleep states; rhythmic, robust crying; good self-quieting or consolability; robust, focused, shiny-eyed alertness with intent or animated facial expressions, including: frowning, cheek softening, mouth pursing to "ooh face", cooing, attentional smiling

Factors that affect growth and development of preterm infants

- past history
- gestational age at birth
- head circumference, weight, and length at birth
- length of growth delay
- days necessary to regain birth weight
- measurements at term rate
- head circumference, weight, length at discharge from hospital
- medical diagnosis, its severity, treatment, and response
- length of hospitalization

Possible causes of neonatal apnoea

- anaemia, polycythaemia
- airway obstruction with mucus of poor positioning
- dehydration, cooling or overheating
- hypercapnia or hypocapnia,
- hypoglycaemia
- hypocalcaemia
- hyponatremia
- sepsis, meningitis
- seizures
- increased vagal tone (in response to suctioning nasopharynx, gavage tube insertion, reflux of gastric contents, endotracheal intubation)
- periodic breathing
- CNS depression from pharmacologic agents
- intraventricular haemorrhage
- patent ductus arteriosus, congestive heart failure
- depression following maternal obstetric sedation
- infants with respiratory distress, pneumonia
- inborn errors of metabolism such as hyperammonaemia
- congenital defects of the upper airways

Manifestations observed in neonatal sepsis

General signs	• infant generally "not doing well" • poor temperature control – hypothermia, hyperthermia (rare)
Circulatory system	• pallor, cyanosis, or mottling, cold, clammy skin, hypotension, oedema, abnormal heartbeat – bradycardia, tachycardia
Respiratory system	• irregular respirations, apnoea, or tachypnoea, cyanosis, grunting, dyspnoea, retractions
Central nervous system	• diminished activity – lethargy, hyporeflexia, coma; increased activity – irritability, tremors, seizures; full fontanel; increased or decreased tone; abnormal eye movements
Gastrointestinal system	• poor feeding, vomiting, diarrhoea or decreased stooling, abdominal distention, hepatomegaly, hemoccult-positive stools
Hematopoietic system	• jaundice, pallor, petechiae, ecchymosis, splenomegaly

Causes of neonatal seizures

Metabolic	hypoglycaemia, hyperglycaemia, hypocalcaemia, hypomagnesemia, pyridoxine deficiency, aminoacidurias, hyperammonemia
Toxic and electrolyte	hypernatremia, hyponatremia, narcotic withdrawal, uraemia, bilirubin encephalopathy
Prenatal infections	toxoplasmosis, syphilis, cytomegalovirus, herpes simplex, hepatitis
Postnatal infections	bacterial meningitis, viral meningoencephalitis, sepsis, brain abscess
Trauma at birth	hypoxic brain injury, intracranial haemorrhage, subarachnoid, epidural haemorrhage, intraventricular haemorrhage of prematurity
Malformations	central nervous system agenesis, hydrocephalopathy, par encephalopathy, tuberous sclerosis
Miscellaneous	degenerative disease, benign familial neonatal seizures

Exercise 11
Answer the following questions. Prepare short talks and/or dialogues on these topics

1. Describe signs of stress or fatigue in neonates.
2. Characterize behavioural manifestations of developmental organization.

3. What factors affect growth and development of preterm infants?
4. What are possible causes of neonatal apnoea?
5. What manifestations are observed in neonatal sepsis?
6. What are causes of neonatal seizures?

Exercise 12
Study the following summary and then interpret basic information in English.

1. High-risk neonates may be defined as newborns, regardless of gestational age or birth weight, who have a greater than average chance of morbidity or mortality because of conditions or circumstances superimposed on the normal course of events associated with birth and adjustment to extrauterine existence.
2. Identification of high-risk newborns may occur during any one of the following stages: preconceptual, prenatal, natal, or postnatal.
3. High-risk infants may be classified according to size, gestational age, and morbidity factors.
4. Newborn intensive care units are categorized according to the population served and degree of treatment.
5. General management of the newborn entails immediate care; protection from infection; monitoring physiologic data, including heart rate, respiratory activity, temperature, and blood pressure; laboratory data; and systematic assessment of the high-risk infant.
6. Assessment of the newborn includes a general assessment, respiratory assessment, cardiovascular assessment, gastrointestinal assessment, genitourinary assessment, neurologic-musculoskeletal assessment, skin assessment, and temperature.
7. Because their metabolic processes are immature, high-risk newborns are placed in a heated environment to help control thermoneutrality.
8. Because of the immature, fragile skin of premature infants, the nurse should use caution when applying topical preparations and, when possible, avoid bandages or dressings.

Exercise 13
Fill in the missing words. Choose the correct ones.

1. Meeting the high-risk infant's _____ _____ requires specific knowledge of the infant's _____ _____, and _____ _____ methods of feeding.	a particular needs b physiologic characteristics c nutritional needs

2. Delayed development in ____-____ neonates is a concern; _____ interventions are individualized to _____ the effects.	a developmental b ameliorate c high-risk
3. Parental involvement in the care of high-risk infants is important, and nurses should help to _____ parent-infant _____ by guiding them to support groups and home _____ _____.	a relationships b health teaching c facilitate
4. Prematurity _____ ___ the largest number of _____ to an NICU.	a admissions b accounts for
5. Several severe _____ _____ place the infant at high risk: _____ of prematurity, RDS syndrome, extraneous air syndromes, _____ _____ and BPD. Therapeutic management of RDS includes _____ _____ and _____ _____.	a assisted ventilation b apnoea c meconium aspiration d respiratory conditions e oxygen therapy
6. Newborns are highly _____ to infection, particularly _____.	a septicaemia b susceptible
7. _____ complications in the high-risk infant may include patent ductus arteriosus and persistent pulmonary _____.	a Cardiovascular b hypertension
8. Neurologic disturbances in the high-risk newborn may include perinatal hypoxic-ischaemic _____ _____, periventricular-intraventricular haemorrhage, _____ _____, and neonatal _____.	a intracranial haemorrhage b seizures c brain injury
9. Maternal conditions that _____ _ _____ to the newborn include _____ and _____ _____.	a diabetes b pose a threat c substance abuse

Translation 4

1. Signs of stress or fatigue in neonates are: autonomic stress (deep, rapid respirations, regular rapid heart rate); changes in state (dull or sleep state, crying or fussy); behavioural changes (unfocused eyes, limp arms

and legs, hiccoughs, sneezes, yawning, straining and bowel movement). 2. Behavioural manifestations of developmental organization include: motor stability behaviours, state stability and attention regulation behaviours. 3. Factors that affect growth and development of preterm infants are: past history, gestational age at birth, head circumference, weight, and length at birth, medical diagnosis, its severity, treatment, and response. 4. Possible causes of neonatal apnoea include: airway obstruction, anaemia, polycythaemia, dehydration, cooling or overheating, hypercapnia or hypocapnia, hypoglycaemia, hypocalcaemia, hyponatremia, sepsis, meningitis, seizures, increased vagal tone, CNS depression, intraventricular haemorrhage, congestive heart failure, respiratory distress, pneumonia, inborn errors of metabolism, and congenital defects of the upper airways. 5. These are manifestations observed in neonatal sepsis: general signs (infant generally "not doing well"); circulatory system (pallor, cyanosis, or mottling, cold, clammy skin, hypotension, oedema, bradycardia, tachycardia); respiratory system (apnoea, or tachypnoea, cyanosis, grunting, dyspnoea, retractions), central nervous system (lethargy, hyporeflexia, coma, irritability, tremors, seizures, full fontanel, increased or decreased tone, abnormal eye movements); gastrointestinal system (poor feeding, vomiting, diarrhoea or decreased stooling, hepatomegaly, hemoccult-positive stools); and hematopoietic system (jaundice, pallor, petechiae, ecchymosis, splenomegaly). 6. Causes of neonatal seizures may be metabolic (uraemia, bilirubin encephalopathy, hypoglycaemia, hyperglycaemia, hypocalcaemia, hypomagnesemia, pyridoxine deficiency, amino-acidurias, and hyperammonaemia). 7. Prenatal infections include toxoplasmosis, syphilis, cytomegalovirus, herpes simplex, hepatitis and postnatal infections include bacterial meningitis, viral meningoencephalitis, sepsis, and brain abscess.

Exercise 14
Study the following summary and then interpret basic information in English.

1. Trauma at birth means: hypoxic brain injury, intracranial haemorrhage, subarachnoid, epidural haemorrhage, and intraventricular haemorrhage of prematurity.
2. There can also be: malformations (central nervous system agenesis, hydro-encephalopathy, par encephalopathy, tuberous sclerosis) and miscellaneous conditions (degenerative disease, neonatal seizures).
3. Identification of high-risk newborns may occur during any one of the following stages: preconceptual, prenatal, natal, or postnatal.
4. General management of the newborn entails immediate care, protection from infection, monitoring physiologic data, including heart rate, respiratory activity, temperature, and blood pressure.

5. Assessment of the newborn includes: a general assessment, respiratory assessment, cardiovascular assessment, gastrointestinal assessment, genitourinary assessment, neurologic-musculoskeletal assessment, skin assessment, and temperature.
6. Because of the immature, fragile skin of premature infants, the nurse should use caution when applying topical preparations.
7. Meeting the high-risk infant's nutritional needs requires specific knowledge of physiologic characteristics.
8. Several severe respiratory conditions place the infant at high risk: apnoea of prematurity, RDS, meconium aspiration syndrome, extraneous air syndromes, and BPD.
9. Therapeutic management of RDS includes oxygen therapy and assisted ventilation.
10. Cardiovascular complications in the high-risk infant may include patent ductus arteriosus and persistent pulmonary hypertension.
11. Neurologic disturbances include hypoxic-ischaemic brain injury, periventricular-intraventricular haemorrhage, intracranial haemorrhage, and neonatal seizures.
12. Maternal conditions include diabetes and substance abuse.

Text 5
Conditions caused by defects in physical development
Guidelines
Identifying latex allergy

Does the child have any symptoms, such as sneezing, coughing, rashes, or wheezing, when handling rubber products (Balloons, tennis balls, adhesive bandage strips) or when in contact with rubber hospital products such as gloves or catheters?

- Has your child ever had an allergic reaction during surgery?
- Does the child have a history of rashes, asthma, or allergic reactions to medication or foods, especially milk, kiwi, bananas, or chestnuts?
- How would you identify or recognize an allergic reaction in your child?
- What would you do if an allergic reaction occurred?
- Has anyone ever discussed latex or rubber allergy or sensitivity with you?
- Has the child had any allergy testing?
- When did the child last come in contact with any type of rubber product? Were you present?

Selected items possible containing latex

Medical items	Nonmedical items
Adhesive bandage strips; airways masks; anaesthesia circuits; blood pressure cuffs and tubing; bulb syringe; catheters; chux (washable rubber); crutches (axillary, hand pads); dressings; elastic bandages; electrode pads; endotracheal tubes; finger cots; gloves (sterile and examining, surgical and medical); intravenous tubing, injection ports, bags, burets; Jobst spandex products; medication vials; nasogastric (NG) tubes; penrose drains; PRN adapter (heparin lock); stethoscope	Art supplies (paint, markers, glue); Balloons; balls; cleaning/kitchen glove; condoms; dental dams and equipment, diaphragms; elastic exercisers; elastic on legs, waist or clothing, rubber pants, possibly disposable diapers; feeding nipples; foam rubber lining on splints, braces; infant tooth-brush-massager; pacifier; racquet handles; rubber bands; water toys, swim, scuba equipment.
tubing; suction tubing; syringes; tape (cloth adhesive paper); theraband strips and tubes; tourniquet; urodynamics rectal pressure catheters; wheelchair cushions, tires	

Major features of foetal alcohol syndrome

Facial features	Neurologic	Behaviour	Growth
• short palpebral fissures • hypoplastic philtrum (ventrical ridge in upper lip) • thinned upper lip • short, upturned nose, hypoplastic maxilla • micrognathia or prognathia in adolescence • retrognathia in infancy	• mental retardation • motor retardation • microcephaly • poor coordination • hypotonia • hearing disorders	• irritability (infancy), • hyperactivity (child)	• prenatal growth retardation, • persistent postnatal growth lag, especially in boys

Exercise 15
Answer the following questions. Prepare short talks and/or dialogues on these topics

1. How to identify latex allergy?
2. Characterize items containing latex.
3. Describe major features of foetal alcohol syndrome (facial features, neurologic, behaviour, growth).

Exercise 16
Study the following summary and then interpret basic information in English.

1. Congenital malformations or anomalies, or birth defects, are present at birth and are the result of genetic or nongenetic influences.
2. Typical reactions of parents to an infant with a physical defect include grief over "loss" of a perfect child, shock, and withdrawal.
3. The nurse's primary roles in care of an infant with a physical defect are caregiver, provider of family support, and supplier of information.
4. Surgery initiates a number of physiologic responses, including cardiovascular, respiratory, endocrine, renal, gastrointestinal, immune, neurologic, and fluid and electrolyte.
5. Nurses must be sensitive to pain in the neonate, be alert for signs of pain, and intervene appropriately.
6. One of the largest groups of congenital anomalies includes those associated with the embryonic neural tube, the most common of which are spina bifida occulta and myelomeningocele
7. Folic and supplementation in women before and during pregnancy prevents many causes of neural tube defects, anencephaly, and spina bifida.
8. Care of the infant and child with myelomeningocele requires both immediate and long-term professional supervision. Associated problems include infection, neurologic damage, impaired renal function, musculoskeletal impairment, and latex allergy.

Exercise 17
Fill in the missing words. Choose the correct ones.

1. _____ is a symptom of an underlying brain pathology, demonstrated by impaired absorption of _____ _____ (CSF) or _____ to the flow of CSF within the ventricles.	a cerebrospinal fluid b obstruction c Hydrocephalus
2. Therapy for hydrocephalus involves _____ of the hydrocephalus, treatment of the underlying _____ _____ if possible, prevention and/or treatment of complications, and management of problems related to _____ _____.	a brain pathology b relief c psychomotor development
3. Treatment of developmental _____ of the hip involves maintaining the _____ __ ___ _____ correctly positioned in the acetabulum by means of _____ _____, usually the Pavlik harness.	a head of the femur b external device c dysplasia

4. Treatment of _____ involves manual overcorrection of the _____, maintenance of the correction until normal _____ _____ is gained, and to detect possible _____-__ _____ recurrence of the deformity.	a muscle balance b deformity c follow-up observation d clubfoot
5. _____ ____ deformities are repaired at the earliest opportunity; _____ _____ repair is usually delayed to take _____ of growth changes.	a cleft palate b advantage c Cleft lip
6. Management of cleft palate involves a multidisciplinary approach to care involving professionals from _____, _____, _____, social work, _____, speech therapy, and audiology.	a surgery b medicine c nursing d dentistry
7. Major _____ _____ with infants born with either cleft involve feeding. _____-_____ is possible and is _____ if this is the mother's choice.	a Breast-feeding b encouraged c nursing challenges
8. Tracheooesophageal _____ consists of an abnormal connection between the _____ and the _____, placing the untreated infant at risk for life-threatening aspiration.	a trachea b fistula c oesophagus
9. Anorectal defects are often associated with other _____ _____, such as those involving the _____ _____ and _____.	a kidneys b gastrointestinal tract c congenital anomalies
10. Defects involving herniation through the _____ _____ range from a simple _____ _____ to complex _____.	a umbilical hernia b abdominal wall c gastroschisis

11. _____ _____ defects are repaired early to _____ normal function and _____ adjustment.	a promote
	b psychological
	c Genitourinary tract
12. With cases of _____ _____, an appropriate _____ is established as early as possible.	a gender
	b ambiguous genitalia

Translation 5

1. Does the child have any symptoms, such as sneezing, coughing, rashes, or wheezing, when handling rubber products (Balloons, tennis balls, adhesive bandage strips) or when in contact with rubber hospital products such as gloves or catheters? 2. Does the child have a history of rashes, asthma, or allergic reactions to medication or foods, especially milk, kiwi, bananas, or chestnuts? 3. Selected items containing latex are: medical items (adhesive bandage strips, dressings, elastic bandages, airways masks, blood pressure cuffs and tubing, bulb syringe, catheters, electrode pads, endotracheal tubes, gloves, injection ports, bags, medication vials, stethoscope tubing, suction tubing, syringes, tourniquets, urodynamics, rectal pressure catheters, wheelchair cushions, and tires. 3. Nonmedical items include: paint, markers, glue, Balloons, balls, cleaning/kitchen glove, condoms, dental dams, diaphragms, elastic on legs, waist or clothing, rubber pants, disposable diapers, pacifier, water toys, and swim equipment. 4. Major features of foetal alcohol syndrome are: facial features (thinned upper lip, upturned nose, hypoplastic maxilla, micrognathia or prognathia, retrognathia); neurologic (mental and motor retardation, microcephaly, hypotonia, hearing disorders); behaviour (irritability, hyperactivity); growth (prenatal growth retardation, persistent postnatal growth lag, especially in boys). 5. Congenital malformations or anomalies are the result of genetic or nongenetic influences. 6. The nurse's primary roles are: caregiver, provider of family support, and supplier of information.

Exercise 18
Match the column A with the column B. Try to learn the expressions and/or sentences by heart.
A
1. Surgery initiates a number of physiologic responses, including:
2. One of the largest groups of congenital anomalies
3. Folic and supplementation prevents
4. Hydrocephalus is a symptom of an underlying brain pathology,

5. Therapy for hydrocephalus involves relief of the hydrocephalus, treatment of the underlying brain pathology,
6. Treatment of developmental dysplasia of the hip
7. Treatment of clubfoot involves
8. Cleft lip deformities are repaired at the earliest opportunity,
9. Tracheooesophageal fistula consists of an abnormal connection
10. Anorectal defects are often associated with other congenital anomalies,
11. Defects involving herniation through the abdominal wall

B

a. ... *includes those associated with the embryonic neural tube.*
b. ... *anencephaly, and spina bifida.*
c. ... *prevention and/or treatment of complications, and management of problems related to psychomotor development.*
d. ... *cardiovascular, respiratory, endocrine, renal, gastrointestinal, immune, neurologic, and fluid and electrolyte.*
e. ... *cleft palate repair is usually delayed.*
f. ... *involves maintaining the head of the femur correctly positioned.*
g. ... *range from a simple umbilical hernia to complex gastroschisis.*
h. ... *between the oesophagus and the trachea.*
i. ... *such as those involving the gastrointestinal tract and kidneys.*
j. ... *manual overcorrection of the deformity.*
k. ... *demonstrated by impaired absorption of cerebrospinal fluid (or obstruction to the flow of CSF within the ventricles).*

Key 15
Exercise 3
1 c, b, d, a; 2 a, c, b; 3 d, a, b, c; 4 a, b; 5 b, a, d, c; 6 c, a, b; 7 b, a, c; 8 b, a

Exercise 4
1c; 2f; 3d; 4e; 5b; 6a

Exercise 7
1 c, a, b; 2 c, a, b; 3 b, a, c; 4 d, a, b, c; 5 b, a; 6 a, b; 7 c, a,

Exercise 8
1b; 2g; 3a; 4e; 5d; 6c; 7f;

Exercise 10

1l; 2f; 3a; 4k; 5b; 6c; 7j; 8d; 9e; 10i; 11h; 12g

Exercise 13
1 c, b, a; 2 c, a, b; 3 c, a, b; 4 b, a; 5 d, b, c, a, e; 6 b, a; 7 a, b; 8 c, a, b; 9 b, a, c

Exercise 17
1 c, a, b; 2 b, a, c; 3 c, a, b; 4 d, b, a, c; 5 c, a, b; 6 a, b, d, c; 7 c, a, b; 8 b, c, a; 9 c, b, a; 10 b, a, c; 11 c, a, b; 12 b, a

Exercise 18
1d; 2a; 3b; 4k; 5c; 6f; 7j; 8e; 9h; 10i; 11g

VOCABULARY 15

abrasion /əˈbreɪ.ʒən/
accessible /əkˈses.ə.bl̩/
accessory /əkˈses.ər.i/
acetabulum /ˌæ.sɪˈtæb.jə.ləm/ pl acetabula
acrocyanosis /ˌækrəʊˌsaɪəˈnəʊ.sɪs/
adapter /əˈdæp.tər/
adhesion /ədˈhiː.ʒən/
admission /ədˈmɪʃ.ən/
advantage /ədˈvɑːn.tɪdʒ/
airway /ˈeə.weɪ/
alarm /əˈlɑːm/
altered /ˈɒl.tərd/
ambient /ˈæm.bi.ənt/
ambiguous /æmˈbɪgjʊəs/
aminoaciduria /əˌmiːnəʊˈæ.sɪd.ju.ə.riə/
anaemia /əˈniː.mi.ə/
anaesthesia /ˌænɪsˈθiːzɪə/
anencephaly /æn.en.ˈse.fə.liː/
animate /ˈæn.ɪ.mət/
anomaly /əˈnɒm.ə.li/
anorectal /æn.əʊ.ˈrek.təl/
apparent /əˈpær.ənt/
apply /əˈplaɪ/
aspiration /ˌæspɪˈreɪʃən/
attribute /ˈæt.rɪ.bjuːt/
audiology /ˈɔːdɪˈɑː.lədʒiː/
axillary /æˈksɪl.ər.i/
Babinski's /bəˈbin.skiː z/ reflex /ˈriː.fleks/
band /bænd/
bandage /ˈbæn.dɪdʒ/
barrel /ˈbær.əl/
bilirubin /ˌbɪl.ɪˈruː.bɪn/
birthmark /ˈbɜːθˌmɑːk/
blindfold /ˈblaɪnd.fəʊld/
blister /ˈblɪs.tər/
bob /bɒb/
bolus /bəʊ.ləs/
bond /bɒnd/
borderline /ˈbɔːr.dər.laɪ n/ personality /ˌpɜː.sənˈæl.ə.ti/ disorder BPD /dɪsˈɔːdə/
bowel /ˈbaʊ.əl/ movement /ˈmuːv.mənt/
brachial /ˈbreɪ.ki.əl/
bradycardia /ˌbræd.ɪˈkɑːdi.ə/
brow /braʊ/
bulb /bʌlb/ syringe /sɪˈrɪndʒ/
bullous /ˈbʊ.ləs/

burette /bjʊˈret/
butterfly /ˈbʌt.ə.flaɪ/
candidiasis /ˌkan.dəˈdaɪ.ə.səs/ pl. **candidiases** /ˌkan.dəˈdaɪ.ə.ˌsiːz/
capillary /kəˈpɪl.ər.i/ **refill** /ˈriː.fɪl/
caput /ˈkeɪp.ˌuːt/
carbon /ˈkɑː.bən/ **dioxide** /daɪˈɒk.saɪd/
casein /ˈkeɪ.ˌsiːn/
catabolism /kəˈta.bə.ˌli.zəm/
cephalhaematoma /ˌsefəlˌhiːməˈtəʊmə/
challenge /ˈtʃæl.ɪndʒ/
chux /tʃʌks/
circuit /ˈsɜːkɪt/
circumcision /ˌsɜːkəmˈsɪ.ʒən/
clammy /ˈklæm.i/
clasp /klɑːsp/
clearance /klɪər.əns/
cleft /kleft/ **lip** /lɪp/
cleft /kleft/ **palate** /ˈpæl.ət/
closure /ˈkləʊ.ʒə/
cloth /klɒθ/
clubfoot /klʌb.fʊt/
coma /ˈkəʊ.mə/
comfort /ˈkʌm.fət/
concave /ˈkɒnkeɪv/
condom /ˈkɒn.dɒm/
configuration /kənˌfɪg.əˈreɪʃən/
congenital /kənˈdʒen.ɪ.təl/
conjugate /kənˈdʒʌ.gət/
conjunctival /ˌkɒn.dʒʌŋkˈtaɪ.vəl/ **sac** /sæk/
consistency /kənˈsɪs.tənt .si/
consolability /kənˈsəʊl.əˈbɪlɪtɪ/
continuous /kənˈtɪn.ju.əs/
controversy /ˈkɒntrəˌvɜːsɪ/
coo /kuː/
cooling /ˈkuː.lɪŋ/
correlate /ˈkɒrɪˌleɪt/
course /kɔːs/
crackle /ˈkræk.l̩/
crutch /krʌtʃ/
cuddle /ˈkʌd.l̩/
cuff /kʌf/
cushion /ˈkʊʃ.ən/
cyanosis /ˌsaɪəˈnəʊ.sɪs/
cystine /sɪs.tɪn/
cytomegalovirus /ˌsaɪ.təʊ.ˌmeg.ə.lə.ˈvaɪ.rəs/
dam /dæm/
decrease /dɪˈkriːs/

defence /dɪ'fent s/ ̈

deformity /dɪ'fɔː.mɪ.ti/

delivery /dɪ'lɪv.ər.i/

dentistry /'dentɪstrɪ/

denude /dɪ'njuːd/

depressed /dɪ'prest/

destruction /dɪ'strʌk.ʃən/

deterrant /dɪ'ter.ənt/

deviation /ˌdiː.vɪ'eɪʃən/

dextrose /'dek.strəʊs/

diaper /'daɪəpə/

diaphragm /'daɪ.ə.fræm/

diaphragmatic /ˌdaɪə.fræg'mæt.ɪk/

discharge /dɪs'tʃɑːdʒ/

discolouration /dɪsˌkʌlə'reɪʃən/

disposable /dɪ'spəʊ.zə.bəl/

distention /dɪ'sten.ʃən/

disturb /dɪ'stɜːb/

drain /dreɪn/

drainage /'dreɪ.nɪdʒ/

dressing /'dres.ɪŋ/

drop /drɒp/

ductus arteriosus /'dək.təs.ɑːr.ˌtir.iː.'əʊ.səs/

dull /dʌl/

dysplasia /dɪs'pleɪ.zi.ə/

dyspnoea /dɪs.pniː.ə/

ecchymosis /ˌeki'məʊ.sɪs/ pl **ecchymoses** /ˌe.ki.'məʊ.ˌsiːz/

elicit /ɪ'lɪs.ɪt/

emesis /e'mɪ.sɪs/

encephalopathy /enˌsef.ə'lɒp.ə.θi/

endotracheal /en.dɒ.trə'kiː.əl/

engage /ɪn'geɪdʒ/

enhance /ɪn'hɑːns/

epidural /ˌep.ɪ'djʊə.rəl/

epistaxis /ˌe.pɪ.'stæk.sɪs/

equality /ɪ'kwɒl.ɪ.ti/

erythema /ˌer.ɪ'θiː.mə/

essential /ɪ'sen.ʃəl/

exception /ɪk'sep.ʃən/

excessive /ek'ses.ɪv/

excretion /ɪk'skriː.ʃən/

exerciser /'ek.sər.ˌsaɪ.zər/

exploration /ˌek.splə'reɪ.ʃən/

extraneous /ɪk'streɪnɪəs/

extraordinary /ɪk'strɔː.dənrɪ/

favourable /'feɪ.vər.ə.bl̩/

feeding /ˌfiː.dɪŋ/

438

femur /ˈfiː.mər/ pl **femora**

finger /ˈfɪŋ.gə/ **cot** /ˈkɑːt/

fissure /ˈfɪʃ.ər/

fistula /ˈfɪs.tʃə.lə/ pl **fistulae**

flaccid /ˈflæksɪd/

flaky /ˈfleɪkɪ/

flame-shaped /fleɪm ʃeɪpt/

flexed /flekst/

foam /fəʊm/

folding /fəʊldɪŋ/

follow-up /ˈfɒl.əʊ.ʌp/

fontanelle /ˌfɒn.təˈnel/

force /fɔːs/

forceps /ˈfɔː.seps/

fragile /ˈfrædʒ.aɪl/

frown /fraʊn/

furrowed /ˈfʌrəʊd/

galactosemia /gə.ˌlak.tə.ˈsiː.miː.ə/

gastroschisis /ˌgæs.trəʊˌs.kə.səs/

gavage /gə.ˈvɑːʒ/

glue /gluː/

granulocyte /ˌgræn.jə.lə.saɪt/

gravity /ˈgræv.ɪ.ti/

grimace /ˈgrɪ.məs/

grunt /grʌnt/

guaiacol /ˈgwaɪ.ˌakel/

gum /gʌm/

haemangioma /ˌhiː.ˌman.dʒiː.ˈəʊ.mə/

haematoma /ˌhiː.məˈtəʊ.mə/ **pl haematomata**

haematuria /ˌhiː.mə.tˈjʊə.ri.ə/

haemolytic /ˌhiː.məˈlɪ.tɪk/

handhold /ˈhænd.ˌhəʊld/

heartbeat /ˈhɑːt.biːt/

hematopoietic /hi.ˌma.tə.pɔːiˈe.tik/

hemoccult test /ˈhiː.mə.ˌkəlt test/

heparin /he.pə.rɪn/

hepatomegaly /ˌhɛp.ə.toʊˈmɛg.ə.li/

herniation /ˌhɜː.niˈeɪˌʃən/

herpes /ˈhɜː.piːz/ **simplex** /ˈsɪm.pleks/

hiccough /ˈhɪk.ʌp/

hydrocephalus /ˌhaɪ.drəˈsef.ə.ləs/

hyperammonaemia /ˌhaɪ.pə.ˌram.ə.ˈniː.miː.ə/

hyperbilirubinemia /ˌhaɪ.pə.ˌbil.iː.ˌrʊ.bin.ˈiː.miː.ə/

hypercapnia /ˌhaɪ.pə.kæp.niə/

hyperglycaemia /ˌhaɪ.pər.glaɪ.ˈsiː.miː.ə/

hypocalcaemia /ˌhaɪ.pəʊ.kælˈsiː.mi.ə/

hypocapnia /ˌhaɪ.pəʊˈkæp.nɪ.ə/

hypoglycaemia /ˌhaɪ.pəʊ.glaɪˈsiː.mi.ə/
hyponatremia /ˌhaɪ.pəʊˈnetriːmɪ.ə/
hypoplastic /ˌhaɪ.pəʊ.ˈpla.stɪk/
hyporeflexia /ˌhaɪ.pəʊˈ.riː.ˈflek.siː.ə/
hypotension /ˌhaɪ.pəʊˈten.ʃən/
hypothyroidism /ˌhaɪ.pəʊˈθaɪ.rɔɪd.ɪsm/
hypotonia /ˌhaɪpəʊˈtəʊ.niə/
hypoxic-ischaemic /haɪˈpɒk.sɪk ɪsˈkiː.mɪk/ **IgA** /ˌaɪ.dʒiː.ˈeɪ/
immunoglobulin /ɪˌmjuː.n.əʊˈglɒb.jə.lɪn/
immunoglobulin E /ɪˌmjuː.n.əʊˈglɒb.jə.lɪn/
immunologic /ɪm.jə.nəˈlɒdʒ.ɪ.k/
impaired /ɪmˈpeəd/
impetigo /ˌɪm.pəˈtaɪ.gəʊ/
incompatibility /ˌɪn.kəmˌpætəˈbɪlɪtɪ/
infiltration /ˌɪn.fɪlˈtreɪ.ʃən/
insertion /ɪnˈsɜː.ʃən/
intent /ɪnˈtent/
interchange /ˌɪn.təˈtʃeɪndʒ/
intercostal /ˌɪn.təˈkɒs.təl/
intermittent /ˌɪn.təˈmɪt.ənt/
intracranial /ˌɪn.trəˈkreɪ.ni.əl/
intraventricular /ɪn.trə.venˈtrɪk.jə.lər/
intubate /ɪnˈtjʊːbeɪt/
iris /ˈaɪrɪs/
irregular /ɪˈreg.jə.lər/
irritability /ˌɪr.ɪ.təˈbɪl.ɪ.ti/
jittery /ˈdʒɪ.tə.rɪ/
Jobst spandex /ˈspæn.deks/
labstick /ləˈbstɪk/
lactalbumin /ˌlak.ˌtal.ˈbjʊ.mən/
lactose /ˈlæk.təʊs/
lag /læg/
laxative /ˈlæk.sə.tɪv/
lesion /ˈliː.ʒən/
lethargy /ˈle.θ.ə.dʒi/
life-threatening /ˈlaɪfˌθret.ən.ɪŋ/
limbus /ˈlim.bəs/
limp /lɪmp/
linear /ˈlɪn.i.ər/
lining /ˈlaɪn.ɪŋ/
lock /lɒk/
loop /luːp/
lymphocyte /ˈlim.fə.saɪt/
macrophage /ˈmæk.rəˈfeɪdʒ/
manipulation /məˌnɪp.jʊˈleɪ.ʃən/
manoeuvre /məˈnuːvə/
margin /ˈmɑː.dʒɪn/

marker /mɑːk.ər/
mask /mɑːsk/
mass /mæs/
massager /ˈmæsɑːʒə/
maternity /məˈtɜː.nə.ti/ pad /pæd/
maternity /məˈtɜː.nə.ti/ ward /wɔːd/
maxilla /mæˈksɪ.lə/
mediastinal /ˌmiː.di.əsˈtaɪ.nəl/
meningitis /ˌmen.ɪnˈdʒaɪ.tɪs/
meningoencephalitis /məˌnɪŋ.gəʊ.ən.ˌse.fə.ˈlaɪ.təs/
micrognathia / ˌmaɪ.krəʊ.ˈneɪ.thiː.ə/
miscellaneous /ˌmɪs.əlˈeɪ.ni.əs/
modify /ˈmɒd.ɪ.faɪ/
modulator /ˈmɑː.jə.ˌleɪ.tər/
molar /ˈməʊlə/
monounsaturated /ˌmɒn.əʊ.ʌnˈsætʃ.ᵊr.eɪ.tɪd/
Moro /ˈmɔːr.ˌəʊ/ reflex /ˈriː.fleks/
mottling /ˈmɒt.l̩ɪŋ/
moulding /ˈməʊl.dɪŋ/
mucous membrane /ˌmjuː.kəsˈmem.breɪn/
multidisciplinary /ˌmʌl.ti.dɪs.əˈplɪn.ᵊr.i/
murmur /ˈmɜː.mər/
musculature /ˈmʌs.kjʊ.lə.tʃər/
myelomeningocele /ˌmaɪ.ə.ləʊ.menˈɪŋ.gə.si:l/
nasal /ˈneɪ.zəl/ flaring / fleər.ɪŋ/
nasogastric /ˈneɪ.zəˈgæs.trɪk/
necrosis /ˈnek.rəʊ.sɪs/
neonatorum /ˌniː.ə.nə.ˈtəʊr.əm/
neural /ˈnjʊə.rəl/ tube /tjuːb/
nipple /ˈnɪp.l̩/
non raised /ˌnɒn reɪzd/
normothermia /ˌnɔːr.məʊ.ˈthər.miə/
nursing /ˈnɜː.sɪŋ/
occult /əˈkʌlt/
oedema /ɪˈdiː.mə/
oesophagus /ɪˈsɒf.ə.gəs/
ointment /ˈɔɪnt.mənt/
oozing /uːz.ɪŋ/
ophthalmia /ɑːf.ˈthal.miː.ə/
outweigh /ˌaʊtˈweɪ/
overcome /ˌəʊ.vəˈkʌm/
overcorrection /ˌəʊ.və.kəˈrek.ʃᵊn/
overheating /ˌəʊvəˈhiːtɪŋ/
overlying /ˌəʊ.vəlˈaɪ.ɪŋ/
pace /peɪs/
pacifier /ˈpæs.ɪ.faɪ.ər/
pallor /ˈpæl.ər/

palpebral /ˈpæl.pɪ.brəl/
palsy /ˈpɔːl.zi/
pants /pænts/
paralysis /pəˈræl.ə.sɪs/
parencephalopathy /ˈpɑːr.ˌen.kef.əˈlɒp.ə.θi/
parenteral /pəˈren.tə.rəl/
partial /ˈpɑː.ʃəl/
particularly /pəˈtɪk.jʊ.lə.li/
passage /ˈpæs.ɪdʒ/
Pavlik /pɒvˈlɪk/ **harness** /ˈhɑː.nəs/
peel /piːl/
Penrose /ˈpen.ˌrəʊz/ **drain** /dreɪn/
perfusion /pəˈfjuː.ʒən/
peripheral /pəˈrɪf.ər.əl/
peristalsis /ˌper.ɪˈstæl.sɪs/
periventricular /ˌper.ɪ.venˈtrɪk.jə.ləʳ/
petechia /pɪˈtiː.kɪ.ə/ pl petechiae
phenylketonuria /ˌfe.nəl.ˌkiː.tᵊn.ˈjʊə.rɪə/
philtrum /ˈfil.trəm/ pl **philtra** /-trə/
phototherapy /ˈfəʊ.təʊ.θer.ə.pi/
phrenic /ˈfren.ɪk/
pin-point, pinpoint /ˈpɪn.pɔɪnt/
place /pleɪs/
plantar /plænt.ə/ **reflex** /ˈriː.fleks/
plethora /ˈpleθ.ᵊr.ə/
polycythaemia /ˌpɑː.liː.ˌsaɪ.ˈthiː.miː.ə/
port /pɔːt/
pose /pəʊz/
povidone /ˈpəʊ.və.ˌdəʊn/ **iodine** /ˈaɪ.ə.ˌdaɪn/
precipitate /prɪˈsɪp.ɪ.teɪt/
preconceptual /ˌpriː.kənˈsep.tʃu.əl/
predetermined /ˌpriː.dɪˈtɜː.mɪnd/
predispose /ˌpriː.dɪˈspəʊz/
prematurity /priː məˈtjʊə.rɪ.ti/
preparation /ˌprepəˈreɪʃən/
pressure /ˈpreʃ.ə/
proceed /prəˈsiːd/
prognathia /ˈprɒg.nə.θɪ.ə/
prophylaxis /ˌprɒf.ɪˈlæk.sɪs/
pulse /pʌls/ **oximetry** /ˈɒk.sɪ.m.ɪ.tri/
pupillary /pjuː.pɪl.ər.i/
purposeful /ˈpɜː.pəsfəl/
purse /pɜːs/
pyridoxine /ˌpir.ə.ˈdɑːk.ˌsiːn/
random /ˈrændəm/
rash /ræʃ/
ratio /ˈreɪ.ʃi.əʊ/

reciprocal /rɪˈsɪprəkəl/
rectal /ˈrek.təl/
recurrence /rɪˈkʌr.əns/
redden /ˈred.ən/
regurgitation /rɪˌɡɜː.dʒɪˈteɪ.ʃən/
residual /rɪˈzɪd.ju.əl/
resistance /rɪˈzɪs.tənt s/
respiratory /ˈre.spə.rə.ˌtɔːr.iː/ **distress** /dɪˈstres/ **syndrome** /sɪn.ˌdrəʊm/
retardation /ˌriː.tɑːˈdeɪ.ʃən/
reticuloendothelial /rɪˌtɪk.jəˈleˌen.dəʊˈθiː.li.əl/
retinal /ˈret.ɪ.nəl/
retraction /rɪˈtræk.ʃən/
retrognathia /ˈreˌtrəʊˈnath.iː.ə/
ribbon /ˈrɪbən/
ridge /rɪdʒ/
rinse /rɪns/
robust /rəʊˈbʌst/
round /raʊnd/
rupture /ˈrʌp.tʃər/
saline /ˈseɪ.laɪn/
saturation /ˌsæt.jʊˈreɪ.ʃən/
scale /skeɪl/
schedule /ˈʃedjuːl/
scleral /ˈsklɪə.rəl/
sclerosis /skləˈrəʊ.sɪs/ pl **scleroses**
secure /sɪˈkjʊə/
seizure /ˈsiː.ʒə/
self-quieting /ˌself ˈkwaɪ.ət.ɪŋ/
sensorineural /senˈsə.ri.ˌnuːrˈəl/
separate /ˈsep.ər.ət/
sepsis /ˈsep.sɪs/
septicaemia /ˌsep.tɪˈsiː.mi.ə/
severity /sɪˈver.ɪ.ti/
shift /ʃɪft/
shiny /ˈʃaɪ.ni/
shunt /ʃʌnt/
smooth /smuːð/
sneeze /sniːz/
specific /spəˈsɪf.ɪk/
spina bifida /ˌspaɪ.nəˈbɪf.ɪ.də/
spinal /ˈspaɪ.nəl/ **cord** /kɔːd/
splenomegaly /ˌspliː.nəʊˈmeɡ.ə.lɪ/
splint /splɪnt/
spread /spred/
stain /steɪn/
state /steɪt/
stimulation /ˌstɪm.jʊˈleɪ.ʃən/

stool /stuːl/
straining /streɪn.ɪŋ/
stridor /straɪd.ər/
strip /strɪp/
subarachnoid /ˌsʌb.əˈræk.nɔɪd/
subclavicular /sʌbˈkləˈvɪk.jə.ləʳ/
subconjunctival /ˌsʌbˌkɒn.dʒæŋk.ˈtɪ.vəl/
subcutaneous /ˌsʌb.kjʊˈteɪ.ni.əs/
subdural /sʌbˈdjʊ.ə.rəl/
subgaleal /ˌsʌb.geɪ.lɪ.əl/
substernal /sʌbˈstɜː.nəl/
succedaneum /sʌkse.deɪni:.um/
suction /ˈsʌk.ʃən/
superimposed /ˌsuːpərɪmˈpəʊzd/
surgery /ˈsɜː.dʒər.i/
susceptible /səˈsep.tɪ.bl̩/
suture /ˈsuː.tʃər/
synthesize /ˈsɪnθɪˌsaɪz/
syringe /sɪˈrɪndʒ/
tachycardia /ˌtæk.ɪˈkɑː.di.ə/
tachypnoea /ˌtæk.ɪˈpnɪə/
tactile /ˈtæk.taɪl/
tape /teɪp/
taurine /ˈtɔː.riːn/
tension /ˈten.ʃən/
theraband /ˌθer.əˈbænd/
thin /θɪn/
topical /ˈtɒp.ɪ.kəl/
tourniquet /ˈtʊə.nɪ.keɪ/
toxoplasmosis /ˌtɒk.səʊ.plæzˈməʊ.sɪs/
trachea /trəˈkiː.ə/
tracheooesophageal /træk.iˈɒ ɪˌsɒf.əˈdʒi.əl/
transcutaneous /trænzˌkjuːˈteɪ.ni.əs/
transition /trænˈzɪʃ.ən/
tremor /ˈtrem.ər/
tube /tjuːb/
tuberous /ˈtʃuː.bə.rəs/ **sclerosis** /skləˈrəʊ.sɪs/
tuck /tʌk/
twitching /twɪtʃ.ɪŋ/
umbilical /ʌmˈbɪl.ɪ.kəl **hernia** /ˈhɜː.ni.ə/
umbilicus /ʌmˈbɪl.ɪ.kəs/
unconjugated /ˈkɒn.dʒə.geɪt.ɪd/
unfocused /ʌnˈfəʊkəst/
unique /juːˈniːk/
upturned /ʌpˈtɜːnd/
urodynamics /ˌjʊə.rəʊ.daɪˈnæm.ɪks/
ventilator /ˈven.tɪ.leɪ.tər/

ventrical /ˈventrɪkəl/
ventricle /ˈven.trɪ.kl̩/
vial /vaɪl/
washcloth /ˈwɒʃˌklɒθ/
wheelchair /ˈwiːl.tʃeər/
wheeze /wiːz/
withdraw /wɪðˈdrɔː/
yawn /jɔːn/

Family home care; The child with fever; Balance and imbalance of body fluid; Conditions that produce fluid and electrolyte imbalance; Emergency treatment of shock; The child with renal dysfunction

Text 1

The child with fever.

Call immediately if:

- Child is < 2 months of age.
- Fever is > 40.5°C.
- Child is crying inconsolably.
- Child is difficult to awaken.
- Child is confused or delirious.
- Child has had a seizure.
- Child has a stiff neck.
- Child has purple spots on the skin.
- Breathing is difficult, and child does not feel better after nose is cleared.
- Child is acting very sick.
- Child has underlying risk factor for serious infection (e. g., sickle cell disease)

Call during office hours if:

- Child is 2 to 4 months old (unless fever is due to a diphtheria-pertussis-tetanus (DPT) vaccination)
- Fever is 40° to 40.5°C, especially if child is < 2 years old.
- Burning pain occurs with urination.
- Fever has been present for > 72 hours
- Fever has been present for > 24 hours without an obvious cause or location of infection.
- Fever disappeared for > 24 hours and then returned.
- Child has a history of febrile seizures.
- Parents have other questions.

Atraumatic care
Skin/vessel, punctures and multiple blood samples
To reduce the pain and distress associated with heel, fingers, venous, or arterial punctures.

- Apply EMLA topically over the site if time permits (at least 60 minutes) or use buffered lidocaine (injected intradermally near vein with 30-gauge needle) to numb the skin.
- Use nonpharmacological methods of pain and anxiety control (e. g., ask child to take a deep breath when the needle is inserted and again when the needle is withdrawn; ask child to count slowly and then faster and louder if pain is felt.
- Emphasize that blood entering syringe or tube does not hurt.
- Reassure young children that you did not "take their blood" away and that they have a lot more inside.
- Place small bandage over puncture site to make removal easy and less painful and to reassure young children that their blood will not leak out.

For multiple blood samples:
- Use an intermittent infusion device ("heparin lock") to collect additional samples from existing intravenous line; consider peripherally inserted central catheters (PICCs) early, not as a last resort.
- Coordinate care to allow several tests to be performed on one blood sample using micro-methods of testing.
- Anticipate tests (i.e. type and cross-match for blood transfusion) and ask laboratory to save blood for additional testing.

Contrary to popular belief, a study of children ages 3 to 6 years found that asking them not to look at the "finger stick", to avoid the site of blood or applying a decorated bandage did not lessen their rating of pain intensity.

Guidelines
Nasogastric, orogastric, or gastrostomy medication administration in children

1. Use elixir or suspension (rather than tablets) preparations of medication whenever possible.
2. Dilute viscous medication or syrup, if possible, with a small amount of water.

3. If administering tablets, crush tablet to a very fine powder and dissolve drug in a small amount of warm water.
4. Never crush enteric-coated or sustained-release tablets or capsules.
5. Avoid oily medications because they tend to cling to side of tube.
6. Do not mix medication with enteral formula unless fluid is restricted. If adding a drug:
7. Check with pharmacist for compatibility.
8. Shake formula well and observe for any physical reaction (e. g. separation, precipitation).
9. Label formula container with name of medication, dosage, date, and time infusion started.
10. Have medication at room temperature.
11. Measure medication in calibrated cup or syringe.
12. Check for correct placement of nasogastric or orogastric tube.
13. Attach syringe (with adaptable tip but without plunger) to tube.
14. Pour medication into syringe.
15. Unclamp tube and allow medication to flow by gravity.
16. Adjust height of container to achieve desired flow rate (e. g., increased height for faster flow).
17. As soon as syringe is empty, pour in water to flush tubing.
18. Amount of water depends on length and gauge of tubing.
19. Determine amount before administering any medication by using a syringe to completely fill an unused nasogastric or orogastric tube with water. The amount of flush solution is usually 1½ times this volume.
20. With certain drug preparations (e. g., suspensions), more fluid may be needed.
21. If administering more than one drug at the same time, flush the tube between each medication with clear water.
22. Clamp tube after flushing, unless tube is left open.

Exercise 1
Answer the following questions. Prepare short talks and/or dialogues on these topics

1. When should you call the doctor for a child with fever?
2. What is meant by atraumatic care?
3. Speak about nasogastric, orogastric, or gastrostomy medication administration in children.

Exercise 2
Study the following summary and then interpret basic information in English.

1. Informed consent is valid when the person is capable of giving consent (is over the age of majority and is competent), the person is supplied with information needed to make an intelligent decision, and the person acts voluntarily when exercising freedom of choice.
2. Informed consent is needed for major surgery, minor surgery, and diagnostic tests and medical treatments with an element of risk.
3. Most parents and children want to be together during stressful procedures and should be offered this opportunity, with guidance on how the parent can comfort the child.
4. In the performance of a procedure the nurse should expect success, involve the child when possible in the procedure, provide distraction, and allow for expression of feelings.
5. In giving postprocedural support, the nurse should encourage children to express their feelings and praise them for completion of the procedure.
6. Six stressful times before and after surgery that produce anxiety in children are the day of admission, blood tests, the afternoon of the day before surgery, injection of preoperative medication, transportation to the operating room, and return from the post-anaesthesia care unit.
7. Assessment of compliance entails measuring factors that affect compliance (through clinical judgement, self-reporting, and direct observation), monitoring therapeutic response, taking pill counts, and performing chemical assay.

Exercise 3
Fill in the missing words. Choose the correct ones.

1. _____ strategies may be classified as _____, educational, and _____.	a behavioural b organizational c Compliance
2. Knowledge of the sick child's _____ _____ and _____ foods can help in _____ adequate nutrition.	a favourite b maintaining c eating habits
3. Control of fever may be accomplished by _____ means, administration of cool compresses; hyperthermia is controlled by environmental means (minimum clothing, increased ___ _____, hypothermia mattress, and/or ____ _____).	a air circulation b cool compressions c pharmacological

4. _____ _____ may be based on one of three basic systems: category-specific isolation precautions, disease-specific isolation precautions, or universal precautions. Only the system of _____ _____, especially body substance isolation _____ _____, when the infected person is undiagnosed.	a provides protection b universal precautions c Infection control
5. _____ _____ in the hospital setting is _____ _____ and can be achieved through environmental measures, infection control measures, limit-setting, and ____ _____.	a Ensuring safety b safe transportation c major concern
6. _____ are used cautiously and typically require _____ _____.	a medical order b Restraints
7. Factors that affect ____ _____ determination are _____ ___ _____, difficulty in evaluating drug response, and ____ _____ area.	a body surface b drug dosage c growth and maturation
8. Family teaching regarding _____ _____ include telling parents why the child is receiving the drug, its _____ _____, and the _____, _____, and length of time the drug is to be administered.	a possible effects b medication administration c amount, d frequency
9. The major forms of _____ feeding for children are _____ feeding and _____ feeding.	Gavage Gastrostomy gastric
10. In the care of children with _____, nurses play an important role in family support and _____ in care of the stoma site.	a ostomies b instruction

Translation 1

1. In the child with fever call the doctor immediately if: breathing is difficult, child is crying inconsolably, is difficult to awaken, is confused or delirious, has had a seizure, has a stiff neck, has purple spots on the skin, or has underlying risk factor. 2. Call during office hours if: child is 2 to 4 months old, burning pain occurs with urination, fever disappeared for > 24 hours and then returned, or child has a history of febrile seizures. 3. To

reduce the pain and distress associated with heel, fingers, venous, or arterial punctures: apply EMLA topically, use nonpharmacological methods of pain and anxiety control, emphasize that blood entering syringe or tube does not hurt, place small bandage over puncture site. 4. For multiple blood samples use an intermittent infusion device, coordinate care to allow several tests to be performed on one blood sample and ask the laboratory to save blood for additional testing. 5. These are guidelines for nasogastric, orogastric, or gastrostomy medication administration in children: use elixir or suspension preparations, dilute viscous medication or syrup with a small amount of water, crush tablet to a very fine powder and dissolve drug in a small amount of warm water. 6. Never crush enteric-coated or sustained-release tablets or capsules, avoid oily medications, do not mix medication with enteral formula, check with pharmacist for compatibility. 7. Shake formula well, label formula container with name of medication, dosage, date, and time infusion started. 8. Have medication at room temperature, measure medication in calibrated cup or syringe. 9. Check for correct placement of nasogastric or orogastric tube, attach syringe to tube, pour medication into syringe, unclamp tube and allow medication to flow by gravity. 10. Adjust height of container to achieve desired flow rate, as soon as syringe is empty, pour in water to flush tubing. 10. With certain drug preparations (e. g., suspensions), more fluid may be needed. 11. If administering more than one drug at the same time, flush the tube between each medication with clear water.

Text 2
Balance and imbalance of body fluids
Origins of inadequate gas exchange
- Factors that depress the respiratory centre, such as head injury, depressant or narcotizing drugs, and infections of the central nervous system
- Factors that affect the lung proper, such as obstructive pulmonary disease, pneumonia, cystic fibrosis, acute pulmonary oedema, atelectasis, and occlusion of respiratory passages
- Factors that interfere with the bellows action of the chest wall, including trauma to the chest wall, skeletal diseases or deformities, and diseases of the thoracic muscles or their innervation (e. g., muscular dystrophy or muscular atrophy)

Conditions that produce hyperventilation
- Primary central nervous system stimulation resulting from emotions, including hysteria, fear, apprehension, pain, anxiety;

central nervous system infection (encephalitis); and certain drug reactions, such as early salicylate intoxication (a primary respiratory stimulant); mechanical ventilation
- Reflex central nervous system stimulation from peripheral chemoreceptors as a result of hypoxia, which provides the stimulus for hyperventilation at high altitudes; fever or high environmental temperatures; congestive heart failure; and anaemia.
- Reflex central nervous system stimulation from intrathoracic stretch receptors, which is believed to be the cause of hyperventilation in localized pulmonary disease
- Pulmonary disorders: inhalation of irritants, asthma, pneumonia, and pulmonary oedema

Metabolic acidosis
Strong acid is gained by:
- gain of exogenous acid (e. g. ammonium chloride) by ingestion or infusion (e. g. salicylates, methanol, ethylene glycol)
- incomplete oxidation of fatty acids, which occurs in conditions such as diabetic ketoacidosis, starvation (including patients receiving nothing by mouth for therapeutic purposes)
- incomplete oxidation of carbohydrate that produces large amounts of lactic acid as a result of primary lactic acidosis (rare) or secondary to tissue hypoxia from excessive exercise, serious trauma, and severe infection.
- inability of the renal system to excrete the normal, ongoing volume of inorganic acid metabolites, which results from the azotemic acidosis of advanced renal failure, renal tubular acidosis, and potassium-sparring diuretics.

Base bicarbonate is lost by:
losses from the gastrointestinal tract — secretions distal to the pyloric sphincter contain large amounts of bicarbonate, which may be lost during conditions that produce diarrhoea or vomiting, fistula drainage, and suction losses as a result of inappropriate bicarbonate excretion in the kidneys because of renal tubular acidosis.

Metabolic alkalosis
Loss of acid can result from the following:
- in children the most common cause of hydrogen ion depletion is loss of hydrochloric acid (HCl) incident, to hypertrophic pyloric stenosis. The infant produces large amounts of HCl which is

vomited with repeated feedings. HCl is also lost in enteral tube drainage.
- less often, hydrogen ions are lost through the kidneys in diuretic therapy, potassium depletion, or administration of adrenocortical hormones.

A gain in base is usually iatrogenic and relatively uncommon in children but can result from the following:
- gain of exogenous bicarbonate from ingestion or infusion
- oxidation of salts or organic acid from infusion or ingestion of lactate, citrate, or acetate.

Exercise 4
Answer the following questions. Prepare short talks and/or dialogues on these topics

1. What do you know about origins of inadequate gas exchange?
2. Which conditions produce hyperventilation?
3. Characterize metabolic acidosis.
4. Characterize metabolic alkalosis.

Exercise 5
Study the following summary and then interpret basic information in English.

1. Water distribution and maintenance are determined by solutes, physical forces, internal control mechanisms, and boundary organs through which external exchanges occur.
2. Infants are subject to fluid depletion because of their relatively greater surface area, their high rate of metabolism, and their immature kidney function.
3. Management of fluid volume disturbances focuses on the following areas: volume of body fluids, osmolality, hydrogen ion status, electrolyte deficits, and disturbances in mineral skeleton and body equilibrium.
4. Fluid disturbances experienced by children are dehydration, water intoxication, and oedema.
5. Dehydration may be classified as isotonic, hypotonic, and hypertonic.
6. Parenteral fluid therapy is initiated to meet ongoing daily physiologic losses, restore previous deficits, and replace ongoing abnormal losses.
7. Fluid gains or losses from the interstitial spaces depend on the following factors: venous hydrostatic pressure, colloidal osmotic pressure, semipermeable capillary wall, tissue tension, and lymphatic flow.

Exercise 6
Fill in the missing words. Choose the correct ones.

1. Oedema formation is caused by increased _____ _____, capillary _____, diminished _____ _____, lymphatic _____, or decreased tissue tension.	a plasma proteins b permeability c venous pressure d obstruction
2. Disturbances in _____-_____ _____ are _____ acidosis, respiratory alkalosis, _____ acidosis, and metabolic alkalosis.	a respiratory b metabolic c acid-base balance
3. Respiratory _____ may result from factors that depress the respiratory centre, factors that affect the _____, and factors that _____ with the bellows action of the _____ _____.	a chest wall b interfere c acidosis d lung
4. Respiratory _____ results primarily from _____ nervous system _____.	a stimulation b central c alkalosis
5. Metabolic acidosis is a lowered _____ __ caused by any process that _____ base bicarbonate concentration or increases metabolic acid _____.	a reduces b formation c plasma pH
6. Metabolic alkalosis is an _____ plasma pH that occurs when there is a reduction of _____ ___ concentration or an excess of _____ _____.	a hydrogen ion b elevated c base bicarbonate
7. Nursing assessment of _____ ___ _____ disturbances entails observation of _____ _____, vital signs, daily weights, _____ ___ _____ measurement, and review of relevant laboratory results.	a intake and output b fluid and electrolyte c general appearance

8. Long-term _____ _____ is accomplished by intermittent intravenous devices; central _____ _____, including short-term (_____, _____, and _____), short-term to moderate-term (peripherally _____ central catheter), and long-term (tunnelled) catheters and ports; or implanted ports.	a subclavian, femoral, and jugular b inserted c venous access d venous catheters
9. Intravenous _____ provides total _____ _____ when _____ via the gastrointestinal tract is impossible, inadequate, or hazardous.	a feeding b nutritional needs c alimentation
10. Before _____ home total _____ _____, the following factors are assessed: parent's ability to _____ the procedure, existence of family support systems, _____ of nearby pharmacies, and insurance coverage.	a parenteral nutrition b initiating c availability d perform

Translation 2

1. Origins of inadequate gas exchange are: factors that depress the respiratory centre, factors that affect the lung proper, and factors that interfere with the bellows action of the chest wall. 2. Conditions that produce hyperventilation are: primary central nervous system stimulation, reflex central nervous system stimulation from peripheral chemoreceptors, reflex central nervous system stimulation from intrathoracic stretch receptors, and pulmonary disorders. 3. Strong acid in metabolic acidosis is gained by: gain of exogenous acid by ingestion or infusion, incomplete oxidation of fatty acids, incomplete oxidation of carbohydrate, and inability of the renal system to excrete the normal, ongoing volume of inorganic acid metabolites. 4. Base bicarbonate is lost by: losses from the gastrointestinal tract, and losses as a result of inappropriate bicarbonate excretion in the kidneys. 5. Loss of acid in metabolic alkalosis can result from the following: loss of hydrochloric acid (HCl) incident, or hydrogen ions are lost through the kidneys in diuretic therapy.

Text 3
Conditions that produce fluid and electrolyte imbalance
Consequences of diarrhoea

Dehydration
- voluminous losses of fluid in frequent, watery stools
- losses when there is also vomiting
- reduced fluid intake resulting from nausea or anorexia
- increased insensible losses from fever, hyperpnea, and sometimes high environmental temperature
- continued (although diminished) obligatory renal losses

Electrolyte imbalance
- losses of sodium, chloride, and potassium, and in some cases bicarbonate
- inadequate replacement of electrolytes when hypotonic or hypertonic solutions are used

Metabolic acidosis
- increased absorption of short-chain fatty acids produced in the colon from bacterial fermentation or unabsorbed dietary carbohydrates
- accumulation of lactic acid from tissue hypoxia secondary to hypovolaemia
- loss of bicarbonate in stools
- ketosis from fat metabolism when glycogen stores are depleted in untreated diarrhoeal dehydration or inadequate carbohydrate intake; may result in malnutrition

Causes of acute diarrhoea
Infection and parasitic infestation
- Bacteria, viruses, parasites

Associated with:
- upper respiratory tract infections
- urinary tract infections
- otitis media

Dietary causes:
- overfeeding
- introduction of new foods

- reinstituting milk too soon after diarrhoeal episode
- osmotic diarrhoea from excess sugar in formula
- excessive ingestion of sorbitol or fructose

Medications:
- antibiotics, laxatives

Toxic causes
Ingestion of:
- heavy metals (arsenic, lead, mercury)
- organic phosphates

Functional causes
- irritable bowel syndrome

Other causes
- necrotizing enterocolitis
- Hirschsprung enterocolitis

Factors that predispose to diarrhoea
Age. As a general rule, the younger the child, the greater the susceptibility and the more severe the diarrhoea. Diarrhoea occurs more frequently in infancy, is a lesser threat in early childhood, and usually constitutes only a minor problem in older children.

Impaired health. Malnourished or debilitated children are more susceptible and tend to have more severe diarrhoea.

Environment. Diarrhoea occurs with greater frequency where there is crowding, substandard sanitation, poor facilities for preparation and refrigeration of food, and generally inadequate health care education. The frequency of diarrhoea in infancy is closely related to the ingestion of contaminated milk; there is a lower incidence of diarrhoea in breast-fed infants.

Causes of chronic diarrhoea
Malabsorptive causes
- celiac disease
- pancreatic insufficiency (cystic fibrosis, chronic pancreatitis, Schwachman syndrome)
- short bowel syndrome

- lactose intolerance
- congenital enzyme deficiency (sucrase-iso-maltase deficiency)

Allergic causes
- allergic gastroenteropathy
- eosinophilic gastroenteritis

Immunodeficiency
- acquired hypoglobulinemia
- Wiskott Aldrich syndrome
- agammaglobulinemia
- severe combined immunodeficiency disease
- thymic hypoplasia
- selective IgA deficiency
- acquired immunodeficiency syndrome (AIDS)

Inflammatory bowel disease
- ulcerative colitis
- Crohn disease

Endocrine causes
- hyperthyroidism
- congenital adrenal hyperplasia
- Addison disease

Motility disorders
- Hirschsprung disease
- intestinal pseudo-obstruction

Parasitic infestations
- *Ascaris*
- *Giardia*

Other causes
- radiation enteritis
- protein-losing enteropathy (Ménétrier disease, intestinal lymphangiectasia)
- secretory tumours (gastrinoma, carcinoma)

Exercise 7
Answer the following questions. Prepare short talks and/or dialogues on these topics

1. Which conditions produce fluid and electrolyte imbalance?
2. Describe consequences of diarrhoea.
3. What are causes of acute diarrhoea?
4. Which factors predispose to diarrhoea?
5. What are causes of chronic diarrhoea?
6. Describe inflammatory bowel disease.

Translation 3

1. Consequences of diarrhoea are: dehydration, electrolyte imbalance, and metabolic acidosis. 2. Causes of acute diarrhoea are: infection and parasitic infestation, dietary causes, medications, toxic causes, or functional causes. 3. Factors that predispose to diarrhoea are: age, impaired health, and environment. 4. Causes of chronic diarrhoea are: malabsorptive causes, allergic causes, immunodeficiency, inflammatory bowel disease, endocrine causes, motility disorders, or parasitic infestations.

Text 4
Emergency treatment
Shock
Ventilation
- Establish airway – be prepared for intubation. Administer oxygen, usually 100% by mask.

Fluid administration
- Restore blood or fluid volume as ordered.

Cardiovascular support
- Administer vasopressors, especially epinephrine subcutaneously, may repeat if needed

General support
- Keep child flat with legs raised above level of heart. Keep child warm and calm.

In addition:
Septic shock — administer broad-spectrum antibiotics intravenously.

Anaphylaxis — remove allergen if possible; may place tourniquet above the site of injection.

Common allergens associated with anaphylaxis
Drugs/medical products
Antibiotics, analgesics, local anaesthetics, chemotherapeutic agents, antiepileptic drugs, diagnostic contrast media, latex

Foods
Milk and milk products, nuts and seeds, legumes (peanuts, soybeans, beans, lentils), eggs, seafood (fish, shellfish), wheat, citrus fruits, strawberries, chocolate

Venoms
Hymenoptera (bee, yellow jacket, hornet, wasp, fire ant), snake, jellyfish, spider

Biologic agents
Allergen extracts, antisera (snake, tetanus, diphtheria), enzymes, hormones, immune globulin (gamma-globulin, blood, plasma)

Possible manifestations of anaphylactic reaction
Cardiovascular
Tachycardia, dysrhythmia, hypotension, relative hypovolemia

Respiratory
Rhinitis — sneezing, nasal itching, rhinorrhoea, laryngeal oedema — stridor, bronchospasm —cough, wheezing

Gastrointestinal
Nausea and vomiting, abdominal pain, diarrhoea

Cutaneous (skin)
Diffuse flushing, feeling of warmth
Urticaria (itching of skin and raised rash — hives)
Angioedema — periorbital, perioral

Central nervous system/other
Sense of impending doom, sometimes loss of consciousness, headache, seizures

Emergency treatment

Burns

Minor burns

- Stop the burning process: apply cold water to the burn or hold the burned area under cold running water.
- Do not disturb any blisters that form.
- Do not apply anything to the wound.
- Cover with a clean cloth if risk of damage or contamination.
- Remove burned clothing and jewellery.

Major burns

Stop the burning process: flame burns — smother the fire; place victim in the horizontal position; roll victim in a blanket or similar object; avoid covering the head.

- Assess for an adequate airway and breathing.
- If not breathing, begin mouth-to-mouth resuscitation.
- Remove burned clothing and jewellery.
- Cover wound with a clean cloth.
- Transport to medical aid.
- Begin IV and oxygen therapy.

Outline of major burn management

- Ascertain the adequacy of the airway and provide oxygen, intubation, and ventilatory support as indicated.
- Insert a large-bore intravenous line, preferably through unburned skin, to deliver fluids at a sufficiently rapid rate to effect resuscitation.
- Remove clothing and jewellery and examine for secondary trauma.
- Obtain an admission weight.
- Insert a nasogastric tube to empty stomach content and maintain gastric decompression.
- Insert an indwelling Foley catheter to obtain specimens and monitor hourly output.
- Evaluate the burn wound and determine the extent and depth of injury.
- Calculate fluid requirements and establish the appropriate regimen.
- Provide intravenous medication for control of pain and anxiety only after adequate oxygenation is ensured and fluid resuscitation is initiated.
- Obtain baseline laboratory studies.

- Perform escharotomy and/or fasciotomy of the chest and extremities for constricting circumferential eschar or elevated compartment pressures, and impaired circulation.
- Apply topical antimicrobials and dressings to the burn wounds.
- Obtain a history regarding the injury and other pertinent data.
- Administer appropriate tetanus prophylaxis.

Methods of burn wound management
Exposure — wounds are left open to air; crust forms on partial-thickness wounds and eschar forms on full-thickness burns.

Open — topical antimicrobial agent is applied directly to the wound surface, and the wound is left uncovered.

Modified — antimicrobial is applied directly or impregnated into thin gauze and applied to the wound; gauze or net secures the area.

Occlusive — antimicrobial is impregnated in gauze or applied directly to the wound; multiple layers of bulky gauze are placed over the primary layer and secured with gauze or net.

Exercise 8
Answer the following questions. Prepare short talks and/or dialogues on these topics

1. Describe emergency treatment of shock.
2. Which are common allergens associated with anaphylaxis?
3. Speak about possible manifestations of anaphylactic reaction.
4. Describe emergency treatment of burns.
5. Outline major burns management.
6. Characterize methods of burn wound management.

Exercise 9
Study the following summary and then interpret basic information in English.

1. Gastrointestinal disorders of childhood that frequently cause fluid depletion and electrolyte disturbance are diarrhoea and vomiting.
2. The four general types of mechanisms of diarrhoea are secretory, cytotoxic, osmotic, and dysenteric diarrhoea.
3. The treatment for acute diarrhoea consists primarily of oral rehydration and provision of an adequate diet.

4. Burns are caused by thermal, electrical, chemical, or radioactive agents.
5. The severity of burn injury is assessed on the basis of the percentage of body surface area burned, depth, location, age, etiologic agent, concomitant injuries, and general health.
6. Emergency measures for severe burns include stopping the burning process; assessing for airway, breathing, and circulation; covering the burn; transporting the child to the hospital; and providing reassurance to the child and family.
7. Management of minor burns consists of facilitating wound healing, relieving discomfort, and preventing complications.
8. Management of major burn injuries involves facilitating wound healing, relieving discomfort, replacing destroyed skin, preventing and/or treating complications, and providing rehabilitation
9. Active participation by the child and family is important in the care of the child with thermal trauma

Translation 4

1. Emergency treatment of shock includes: ventilation, fluid administration, cardiovascular support, and general support. 2. Common allergens associated with anaphylaxis are: drugs/medical products, foods, venoms, biologic agents. 3. Possible manifestations of anaphylactic reaction can be: cardiovascular, respiratory, gastrointestinal, cutaneous, or central nervous system. 4. Emergency treatment of minor burns needs: to stop the burning process, not to disturb any blisters, cover with a clean cloth, and remove burned clothing and jewellery. 5. Emergency treatment of major burns needs: to assess for an adequate airway and breathing, if not breathing, begin mouth-to-mouth resuscitation, and begin IV and oxygen therapy. 6. Outline of major burn management: provide oxygen, intubation, and ventilatory support as indicated, insert a large-bore intravenous line, obtain an admission weight. 7. Insert a nasogastric tube, insert an indwelling, Foley catheter, determine the extent and depth of injury. 8. Calculate fluid requirements, provide intravenous medication, obtain baseline laboratory studies. 9. Perform escharotomy and/or fasciotomy, apply topical antimicrobials and dressings, obtain a history, and administer appropriate tetanus prophylaxis. 10. These are methods of burn wound management: wounds are left open to air, topical antimicrobial agent is applied directly to the wound surface, antimicrobial is applied directly or impregnated into thin gauze and applied to the wound.

Text 5
The child with renal dysfunction
Signs and symptoms of urinary tract disorders or disease at different ages
Neonatal period (birth to 1 month)

Poor feeding, vomiting, failure to gain weight, rapid respiration (acidosis), respiratory distress, spontaneous pneumothorax or pneumomediastinum, frequent urination, screaming on urination, poor urinary stream, jaundice, seizures, dehydration, other anomalies or stigmata, enlarged kidneys or bladder

Infancy (1 to 24 months)

Poor feeding, vomiting, failure to gain weight, excessive thirst, frequent urination, straining or screaming on urination, foul-smelling urine, pallor, fever, persistent diaper rash, seizures (with or without fever), dehydration, enlarged kidneys or bladder

Childhood (2 to 14 years)

Poor appetite, vomiting, growth failure, excessive thirst, enuresis, incontinence, frequent urination, painful urination, swelling of face, seizures, pallor, fatigue, blood in urine, abdominal or back pain, oedema, hypertension, tetany

Classification of urinary tract infections or inflammations

- **Bacteriuria** — presence of bacteria in the urine
- **Asymptomatic bacteriuria** — significant bacteriuria with no evidence of clinical infection
- **Symptomatic bacteriuria** — bacteriuria accompanied by physical signs of urinary infection (dysuria, suprapubic discomfort, haematuria, fever)
- **Recurrent UTI** — repeated episode of bacteriuria or symptomatic UTI
- **Persistent UTI** — persistence of bacteriuria despite antibiotic treatment
- **Febrile UTI** — bacteriuria accompanied by fever and other physical signs of urinary infection: presence of a fever typically implies a pyelonephritis
- **Cystitis** — inflammation of the bladder
- **Urethritis** inflammation of the urethra
- **Pyelonephritis** — inflammation of the upper urinary tract and kidneys

- **Urosepsis** — febrile urinary tract infection coexisting with systemic signs of bacterial illness; blood culture reveals presence of urinary pathogen
- **Processes of fluid and electrolyte movement Osmosis** — passive movement of water from a solution of lower concentration to a solution of higher concentration of particles.
- **Diffusion** — random movement of particles from an area of greater concentration to an area of lower concentration
- **Ultrafiltration** — movement of fluid, under pressure, through filtering material with minute pores

Exercise 10
Answer the following questions. Prepare short talks and/or dialogues on these topics

1. Describe signs and symptoms of urinary tract disorders or disease at different ages (neonatal period, infancy, childhood).
2. What can you say about classification of urinary tract infections or inflammations?
3. Characterize processes of fluid and electrolyte movement.

Exercise 11
Study the following summary and then interpret basic information in English.

1. The main function of the kidney is to maintain the composition and volume of body fluids in equilibrium.
2. Common inflammatory disorders of the genitourinary tract include urinary tract infection, nephrotic syndrome, and acute glomerulonephritis.
3. Management of UTIs is directed at eliminating infection, detecting and correcting functional or anatomic abnormalities, preventing recurrences, and preserving renal function.
4. Vesicoureteral reflux is the retrograde blow of bladder urine into the ureters
5. Common features of acute glomerulonephritis are oliguria, oedema, hypertension, circulatory congestion, haematuria, and proteinuria.
6. Therapeutic management of acute glomerulonephritis is maintenance of fluid balance, treatment of hypertension, and antibiotic therapy.
7. Nephrotic syndrome is characterized by increased glomerular permeability to protein.

Exercise 12

Fill in the missing words. Choose the correct ones.

1. Management of _____ _____ is aimed at reducing excretion of protein, reducing or preventing _____ _____ by tissues, and _____ _____ and other complications; dietary control; corticosteroid therapy; immunosuppressant therapy; use of _____; and use of _____.	a fluid retention b preventing infection c nephrotic syndrome d diuretics e antimicrobials
2. Primary functions of the distal _____ _____ are of urine _____, _____ secretion, and selective and differential _____ of sodium, chloride, and water.	a reabsorption b acidification c potassium d renal tubules
3. The most common _____ _____ _____ are renal tubular acidosis and nephrogenic _____ _____.	a diabetes insipidus b renal tubular disorders
4. Management of _____-_____ syndrome is aimed at control of haematologic _____ and complications of _____ _____.	a manifestations b renal failure c haemolytic-uremic
5. In _____ renal failure, management is directed at determining treatment of the _____ _____, management of complications of renal failure, and _____ _____.	a supportive therapy b underlying cause c acute
6. Abnormalities in _____ renal failure are _____ _____ retention, water and sodium _____, hyperkalaemia, acidosis, _____ ___ _____ disturbance, anaemia, hypertension, and growth disturbances.	a waste product b retention c chronic d calcium and phosphorus
7. When the child will need _____ _____, the nurse educates the family about the disease, its implications, the _____ _____, possible _____ _____ of the disease and the treatment and technical aspects of the procedure.	a therapeutic plan b home dialysis c psychological effects

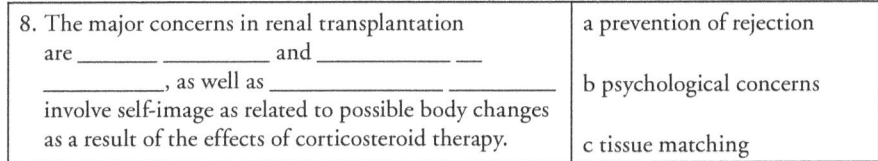

8. The major concerns in renal transplantation are _____ _____ and _____ __ _____, as well as _____ _____ involve self-image as related to possible body changes as a result of the effects of corticosteroid therapy.	a prevention of rejection b psychological concerns c tissue matching

Translation 5

1. Signs and symptoms of urinary tract disorders or disease are: poor feeding, vomiting, failure to gain weight, rapid respiration (acidosis), respiratory distress, spontaneous pneumothorax or pneumomediastinum, frequent urination, screaming on urination, poor urinary stream, jaundice, seizures, dehydration, other anomalies or stigmata, and enlarged kidneys or bladder. 2. In infancy signs and symptoms are also: excessive thirst, frequent urination, straining or screaming on urination, foul-smelling urine, pallor, fever, persistent diaper rash, seizures (with or without fever), dehydration, enlarged kidneys or bladder. 3. In childhood signs and symptoms are e.g.: enuresis, incontinence, frequent urination, painful urination, swelling of face, seizures, pallor, fatigue, blood in urine, abdominal or back pain, oedema, hypertension, tetany. 4. Urinary tract infections or inflammations also include: asymptomatic bacteriuria, symptomatic bacteriuria, recurrent UTI, persistent UTI, febrile UTI, cystitis, urethritis, and pyelonephritis. 5. Processes of fluid and electrolyte movement are: osmosis, diffusion, ultrafiltration.

Key 16
Exercise 3
1 c, b, a; 2 c, a, b; 3 c, a, b; 4 c, b, a; 5 a, c, b; 6 b; a; 7 a, b; 8 b, c, a; 9 b, a, c, d; 10 a, b

Exercise 6
1 c, b, a, d; 2 c, a, b; 3 c, d, b, a; 4 c, b, a; 5 c, a, b; 6 b, a, c; 7 b, c, a; 8 c, d, a, b; 9 c, b, a; 10 b, a, d, c

Exercise 12
1 c, a, b, d, e; 2 d, b, c, a; 3 b, a; 4 c, a, b; 5 c, b, a; 6 c, a, b, d; 7 b, a, c; 8 c, a, b

VOCABULARY 16

accumulation /əˌkjuːmjʊˈleɪʃən/
acetate /ˈæsɪˌteɪt/
acidification /əˌsɪd.ɪ.fɪˈkeɪʃᵊn/
acidosis /ˌæs.ɪˈdəʊ.sɪs/
acquired /əˌkwaɪ.əd/
Addison /ædˈɪ.sən/ **disease** /dɪˈziːz/
adequacy /ˈæd.ə.kwə.si/
administer /ədˈmɪn.ɪ.stər/
adrenal /əˈdriː.nəl/
adrenocortical /ædˌriː.nəˈkɒː.ti.kəl/
agammaglobulinemia /eɪ.gamˈæ.glɒb.jə.lɪˈniː.mi.ə/
alimentation /ˌælɪ.menˈteɪʃən/
alkalosis /ˌælkəˈləʊ.sɪs/
altitude /ˈæl.tɪ.tjuːd/
ammonium chloride /əˈməʊ.ni.əm ˈklɔːraɪd/
angioedema /ænˌdʒɪˈdiːm.ə/
ant /ænt/ mravenec
anticipate /ænˈtɪs.ɪ.peɪt/
antimicrobial /ˌæn.ti.ˈmaɪ.krəʊ.baɪ.əl/
antipyretic /ˈæn.tɪpaɪəˈret.ɪk/
antiserum /æn.tiˌsɪə.rəm/ pl **antisera**
apprehension /ˌæp.rɪˈhen.ʃən/
arsenic /ˈɑː.sən.ɪk/
Ascaris /ˈæs.kə.rɪs/
ascertain /ˌæs.əˈteɪn/
assay /a.ˈseɪ/
assess /əˈses/
asymptomatic /əˌsɪmp.təˈmæt.ɪk/
atelectasis /ˌætəˈlek.tə.sɪs/
atraumatic /ˈeɪ.trə.ˈmat.ik/
atrophy /ˈæt.rə.fi/
availability /əˌveɪ.ləˈbɪl.ɪ.ti/
awaken /əˈweɪ.kən/
azotemic /ˌaɪ.zəʊ.tiː.mik/
bacteriuria /bækˈtɪə.riːˈjʊə.ri.ə/
bandage /ˈbæn.dɪdʒ/
bellows /ˈbeləʊz/
blanket /ˈblæŋ.kɪt/
blister /ˈblɪs.tər/
boundary /ˈbaʊn.dər.i/
buffer /ˈbʌf.ər/
bulky /ˈbʌl.ki/
calibrate /ˈkælɪˌbreɪt/
capsule /ˈkæp.sjuːl/
cautiously /ˈkɔːˌʃəs.li/

celiac /ˈsiː.liː.ˌak/
chemoreceptor /ˌkiː.məʊ.rɪˈsep.tər/
circumferential /səˈkʌm.fər.ən.ʃəl/
citrate /ˈsaɪ.treɪt/
closely /ˈkləʊ.sli/
coated /ˈkəʊ.tɪd/
colloidal /ˈkɒ.lɒ.ɪd.əl/
colon /ˈkəʊ.lɒn/
compartment /kəmˈpɑː.t.mənt/
compatibility /kəmˌpætəˈbɪlɪtɪ/
compliance /kəmˈplaɪ.ənt s/
composition /ˌkɒm.pəˈzɪʃ.ən/
compress /kəmˈpres/
concern /kənˈsɜːn/
concomitant /kənˈkɒ.mɪ.tənt/
congenital /kənˈdʒen.ɪ.təl/
consent /kənˈsent/
constitute /ˈkɒn.stɪ.tjuːt/
constrict /kənˈstrɪkt/
contamination /kənˌtæm.ɪˈneɪ.ʃən/
correct /kəˈrekt/
cover /ˈkʌv.ə/
coverage /ˈkʌv.ər.ɪdʒ/
cross-match /krɒs mætʃ/
crush /krʌʃ/
crust /krʌst/
cutaneous /kjuːˈteɪ.ni.əs/
cystic fibrosis /ˌsɪs.tɪk.faɪˈbrəʊ.sɪs/
cystitis /sɪˈstaɪ.tɪs/
cytotoxic /ˌsaɪ.təʊˈtɒk.sɪk/
debilitate /dɪˈbɪl.ɪ.teɪt/
decompression /ˌdi.kəmˈpre.ʃən/
deficit /ˈdef.ɪ.sɪt/
delirious /dɪˈlɪr.ɪəs/
depleted /dɪˈpliː.tɪd/
depletion /dɪˈpliː.ʃən/
depressant /dɪˈpres.ənt/
depth /depθ/
diaper /ˈdaɪəpə/ **rash** /ræʃ/
differential /ˌdɪf.əˈren.t ʃəl/
diffuse /dɪˈfjuːz/
dilute /daɪˈluːt/
diphtheria /dɪfˈθəɪr.i.ə/
disappear /ˌdɪs.əˈpɪər/
dissolve /dɪˈzɒlv/
distal /ˈdɪs.təl/
disturb /dɪˈstɜːb/

disturbance /dɪˈstɜː.bəns/

doom /duːm/

dysentery /ˈdɪs.ənˌter.i/

dystrophy /ˈdɪs.trə.fi/

eliminate /ɪˈlɪm.ɪ.neɪt/

elixir /ɪˈlɪk.sɪər/

encephalitis /ˌen.kef.əˈlaɪ.tɪs/

ensure /ɪnˈʃɔːr/

entail /ɪnˈteɪl/

enteral /ˈen.tə.rəl/

enteric /enˈtər.ɪk/

enteritis /ˌen.təˈraɪ.təs/

enterocolitis /ˌen.tə.rəʊ.kə.ˈlaɪ.təs/

enuresis /ˌen.jʊəˈriː.sɪs/

eosinophilic /ˌiː.əˈsɪn.ə.fɪl.ɪk/

equilibrium /ˌiːkwɪˈlɪbrɪəm/

eschar /ˈɛskɑː/

escharotomy /ˌes.kɑːˈrɒt.ə.mɪ/

ethylene /ˈeθ.ɪ.liːn/ **glycol** /ˈglaɪ.kɒl/

etiologic /ˌiː.ti.ə.ˈlɑː.dʒik/ **agent** /ˈeɪ.dʒᵊnt/

evaluate /ɪˈvæl.ju.eɪt/

exchange /ɪksˈtʃeɪndʒ/

excrete /ɪkˈskriːt/

exogenous /ekˈsɑdʒ.ə.nəs/

fasciotomy /ˈfæʃ.i.ɒ.tə.mi/

febrile /ˈfiː.braɪl/

femoral /ˈfem.ər.əl/

fermentation /ˌfɜr.menˈteɪ.ʃən/

fistula /ˈfɪs.tʃə.lə/ pl **fistulae**

flame /fleɪm/

flow /fləʊ/

flushing /flʌʃ.ɪŋ/

Foley catheter /ˈfəʊ.liː ˈkæθ.ɪ.tər/

formula /ˈfɔː.mjʊ.lə/

foul /faʊl/

frequency /ˈfriː.kwən.si/

fructose /ˈfrʌktəʊs/

gamma-globulin /gamˈæ.glɒb.jə.lɪˈn/

gastrinoma /gas.trə.ˈnəʊ.mə/

gastroenteropathy /ˌgæs.trəʊˌentəˈrɒpəθɪ/

gauge /geɪdʒ/

gauze /gɔːz/

gavage /gə.ˈvɑːʒ/

Giardia /dʒiː.ˈɑːr.diː.ə/

glomerulonephritis /glɒˌmer.jʊ.ləʊ.nɪˈfraɪ.tɪs/

gravity /ˈgræv.ɪ.tɪ/

haemolytic /ˌhiː.məˈlɪt.ɪk/

heparin /ˈhe.pə.rɪn/
Hirschsprung's disease /ˈhɪrʃ.ˌprʊŋz dɪˈziːz/
hives /haɪvz/
hornet /ˈhɔːnɪt/
hydrochloric acid /ˌhaɪ.drə.klɔː.rɪk ˈæs.ɪd/
hydrostatic /ˌhaɪdrəʊˈstæt.ɪk/
hyperthyroidism /ˌhaɪ.pəˈθaɪ.rɔɪd.ɪzəm/
hypertonic /ˌhaɪ.pərˈtɑː.nik/
hypertrophic /ˌhaɪ.pərˈtrɑf.ɪk/
hypoglobulinemia /ˌhaɪ.pəʊ.glɒb.jə.lɪˈniː.mi.ə/
hypotonic /ˌhaɪ.pəˈtɑː.nik/
IgA /ˌaɪ.dʒiːˈeɪ/ **immunoglobulin** /ɪˌmjuːn.əʊˈglɒb.jə.lɪn/
ignition /ɪgˈnɪʃən/
ignore /ɪgˈnɔːr/
ileum /ˈɪl.i.əm/ pl **ilea**
ileus /ˈɪl.i.əs/
iliac /ˈɪl.i.æk/
ill /ɪl/
illicit /ɪˈlɪs.ɪt/
immature /ˌɪm.əˈtʃʊər/
immunosuppressant /ˌɪm.jə.nəʊ.səˈpres.ᵊnt/
impending /ɪmˈpen.dɪŋ/
implanted /ɪmˈplɑː.nt.ɪd/
impregnate /ˈɪm.preg.neɪt/
inability /ˌɪn.əˈbɪl.ɪ.ti/
inappropriate /ˌɪn.əˈprəʊ.pri.ət/
incomplete /ˌɪn.kəmˈpliːt/
inconsolable /ˌɪn.kənˈsəʊ.lə.bl/
indwelling /ˈɪn.dwel.ɪŋ/
infestation /ˌɪn.fesˈteɪ.ʃən/
infusion /ɪnˈfjuː.ʒən/
ingestion /ɪnˈdʒest.ʃən/
initiate /ɪˈnɪʃ.i.eɪt/
innervation /ˌɪ.nɜːˈveɪ.ʃən/
insensible /ɪnˈsen.sə.bᵊl/
insert /ɪnˈsɜːt/
insufficiency /ˌɪn.səˈfɪʃ.ən.si/
intelligent /ɪnˈtelɪdʒənt/
intermittent /ˌɪn.təˈmɪt.ənt/
interstitial /ˌɪn.təˈstɪ.ʃəl/
intoxication /ɪnˌtɒk.sɪˈkeɪ.ʃən/
intradermally /ˌɪn.trəˈdɜː.məl.i/
intrathoracic /ˌin.trə.thəˈra.sik/
intravenously /ˌɪn.trəˈviː.nəs.li/
ion /ˈaɪ.ɒn/
iso-maltase /aɪ.səʊˈmɔːl.teɪz/
isotonic /aɪ.səʊ ˈtɒn.ɪk/

itching /ˈɪtʃ.ɪŋ/
jellyfish /ˈdʒelɪˌfɪʃ/
jewellery /ˈdʒuː.əl.ri/
judgement /ˈdʒʌdʒ.mənt/
jugular /ˈdʒʌɡ.jə.lər/
ketoacidosis /ˈkiː.təʊˌæ.ɪˈdəʊ.sɪs/
ketosis /kiː.təʊ.sɪs/
label /ˈleɪ.bəl/
lactate /lækˈteɪt/
lactic /ˈlæk.tɪk/ **acid** /ˈæs.ɪd/
laryngeal /ləˈrɪn.dʒi.əl/
laxative /ˈlæk.sə.tɪv/
leak /liːk/
legume /ˈleg.juːm/
lentil /ˈlentɪl/
lidocaine /ˈlaɪdəˌken/
lymphangiectasia /ˌlim.ˌfan.dʒiː.ek.ˈteɪ.ʒiː.ə/
lymphatic /limˈfæ.tik/
maintenance /ˈmeɪn.tɪ.nəns/
majority /məˈdʒɒr.ə.ti/
match /mætʃ/
Ménétrier disease /meɪ.neɪ.triː.eɪˈ dɪˈziːz/
mercury /ˈmɜː.kjʊ.ri/
methanol /ˈmeθ.ə.nɒl/
micro-method /maɪˈkrɒ.ˈmeθ.əd/
minute /maɪˈnjuːt/
motility /ˌməʊ.ˈtil.i.ˈtiː/
narcotize /ˈnɑː.r.kə.ˌtaɪz/
nephrotic /nɪˈfrɒt.ɪk/
net /net/
numb /nʌm/
obligatory /ɒˈblɪɡətərɪ/
occlusion /əˈkluː.ʒən/
occlusive /ɒˈkluː.sɪv/
oliguria /ˌɒl.ɪˈgjʊə.rɪ.ə/
ongoing /ˈɒŋˌɡəʊ.ɪŋ/
organic /ɔːˈɡæn.ɪk/
organic /ɔːˈɡæn.ɪk/ **phosphate** /ˈfɒsfeɪt/
orogastric /ˌəʊ.rəˈɡæst.rɪk/
osmolality /ˌɑːz.məʊ.ˈla.lə.tiː/
osmotic /ɒzˈmɒt.ɪk/
ostomy /ˈɒs.tə.mi/
overfeeding /ˌəʊ.vəˈfiː.dɪŋ/
pancreatic /ˌpæŋ.krɪˈæ.tɪk/
pancreatitis /ˌpæŋ.kri.əˈtaɪ.tɪs/
parasite /ˈpær.ə.saɪt/
parasitic /ˌpær.əˈsɪt.ɪk/

parenteral /pəˈren.tə.rəl/
participation /pɑːˌtɪsɪˈpeɪʃən/
particle /ˈpɑː.tɪ.kl̩/
passage /ˈpæs.ɪdʒ/
percentage /pəˈsen.tɪdʒ/
perioral /ˌper.ɪˈɔː.rəl/
periorbital /ˌper.ɪˈɔːbɪtəl/
permeability /ˌpɜː.mi.əˈbɪl.ɪ.ti/
pertussis /pəˈtʌ.sɪs/
plunger /ˈplʌn.dʒər/
pneumomediastinum /ˌnu.məˌmiː.di.əˈstaɪ.nəm/
pneumonia /njuːˈməʊ.ni.ə/
pore /pɔr/
port /pɔːt/
precaution /prɪˈkɔː.ʃən/
precipitation /prɪˌsɪpɪˈteɪʃən/
pressure /ˈpreʃ.ə/
pulmonary /ˈpʊl.mə.nə.ri/
puncture /ˈpʌŋk.tʃə/
purple /ˈpɜː.pl̩/
pyelonephritis /ˌpaɪ.ə.lə.nɪˈfraɪ.tɪs/
pyloric /paɪˈlɔːr.ik/
random /ˈrændəm/
rating /ˈreɪ.tɪŋ/
reabsorption /riː.əbˈzɔːp.ʃən/
receptor /rɪˈsep.tər/
recurrence /rɪˈkʌr.əns/
recurrent /rɪˈkʌr.ənt/
refrigeration /rɪˌfrɪdʒ.əˈreɪ.ʃən/
reinstitution /riːˌɪn.stɪˈtʃuː.ʃ°n/
rejection /rɪˈdʒek.ʃən/
retrograde /ˈret.rəʊ.greɪd/
rhinitis /raɪˈnaɪtɪs/
rhinorrhoea /raɪ.nəˈri.ə/
roll /rəʊl/
salicylate /səˈlɪs.ə.leɪt/
sample /ˈsɑːm.pl̩/
sanitation /ˌsæn.ɪˈteɪ.ʃən/
seafood /ˈsiː.fuːd/
secretory /ˈsek.rə.tər.i/
secure /sɪˈkjʊə/
seizure /ˈsiː.ʒə/
selective /sɪˈlek.tɪv/
semipermeable /sem.iˈpɜː.mi.ə.bl̩/
separation /ˌsepəˈreɪʃən/
shake /ʃeɪk/ (shook, shaken)
shellfish /ˈʃel.fɪʃ/

short-chain /ʃɔːt tʃeɪn/
Schwachman syndrome /ʃwaːkmæn ˈsɪndrəʊm/
skeletal /ˈskel.ɪ.təl/
smell /smel/
smother /ˈsmʌð.ər/
snake /sneɪk/
sneezing /sniːz.ɪŋ/
sorbitol /səʊrˈbiˌtol/
spare /ˈspeə/
specimen /ˈspes.ə.mɪn/
sphincter /ˈsfɪŋk.tər/
starvation /staːˈveɪˌʃən/
stenosis /steˈnəʊ.sɪs/
stigmata /stɪgˈmaːtə/
straining /streɪn.ɪŋ/
stream /striːm/
stretch /stretʃ/
stridor /straɪd.ər/
subclavian /sʌbˈkleɪv.ɪ.ən/
subcutaneously /ˌsʌb.kjʊˈteɪ.ni.əs.li/
sucrase /ˈsuːkreɪz/
suprapubic /ˌsuː.prəˈpjuː.bɪk/
susceptible /səˈsep.tɪ.bl̩/
suspension /səˈspenˌʃən/
syrup /ˈsɪr.əp/
tend to /tend/
tension /ˈtenˌʃən/
tetanus /ˈtet.ən.əs/
tetany /ˈtet.ən.i/
thickness /ˈθɪk.nəs/
thoracic /θəˌræs.ɪk/
threat /θret/
thymic /ˈθaɪ mɪk/
treat /triːt/
tube /tjuːb/
tubular /ˈtjuː.bjʊ.lər/
tunnel /ˈtʌn.əl/
ultrafiltration /ˈʌl.trə.fɪlˈtreɪˌʃən/
unclamp /ʌnˈklæmp/
underlying /ˌʌn.dəˈlaɪ.ɪŋ/
unused /ʌnˈjuːzd/
uremic /ˌjʊə ˈriː.mɪk/
urethra /jʊəˈriː.θrə/
urethritis /ˌjʊə.riːˈθraɪ.tɪs/
urosepsis /jʊə.rəʊˈsep.sɪs/
urticaria /ˌɔː.tɪˈkeə.ri.ə/
vasopressor /ˌveɪzəʊˈpresər/

venom /ˈvenəm/
vesicoureteral /ˈves.ɪ.kə jʊr.əˈter.əl/
vessel /ˈves.əl/
victim /ˈvɪk.tɪm/
viscous /ˈvɪs.kəs/
volume /ˈvɒl.juːm/
voluntarily /ˈvɒl.ən.tər.i.li/
wheat /wiːt/
wheeze /wiːz/
Wiskott-Aldrich syndrome /wɪsˈkɒt-ɔːlˈdrɪch ˈsɪndrəʊm/

The child with disturbance of oxygen and carbon dioxide exchange; Causes of cough; The child with respiratory dysfunction; The child with gastrointestinal dysfunction

Text 1
Causes of cough
Inflammatory disorders:
- asthma, infections

Lung disease:
- cystic fibrosis, bronchiolitis, retained foreign body, congenital malformations

Focal or anatomic lesions
Psychogenic or habit cough
Postnasal drip and/or sinusitis

Cough assessment
Onset and duration
Type — dry, hacking, moist, barking, brassy, paroxysmal (a sudden attack, outburst, or intensification of symptoms)

Progress — better, worse, unchanged, persistent

Pattern — daytime, night time, both, different intensity with time or activity

Associated symptoms — sore throat, dyspnoea, pain and its location

Secretions — sputum presence, consistency, colour, frequency, evidence of swallowing sputum, postnasal drip

Signs of respiratory failure
Cardinal signs:
- restlessness, increase in respiratory effort, tachypnoea, tachycardia, diaphoresis

Early but less obvious signs.
- mood changes, such as euphoria or depression
- headache
- altered depth and pattern of respirations
- hypertension
- exertional dyspnoea
- anorexia, increased cardiac output and renal output
- central nervous system symptoms (decreased efficiency, impaired judgement, anxiety, confusion, restlessness, irritability, depressed level of consciousness)
- flaring nares
- chest wall retractions
- expiratory grunt
- wheezing and/or prolonged expiration
- absent or decreased breath sounds

Signs of more severe hypoxia
- hypotension or hypertension
- dimness of vision
- somnolence
- stupor
- coma
- dyspnoea
- depressed respirations/agonal respirations
- bradycardia
- cyanosis, peripheral of central
- apnoea

Nursing observations for the child with respiratory failure
Visual inspection of **skin colour** to estimate level of arterial O_2 saturation

Observation of **respiratory effort** or distress — nasal flaring, grunting, gasping, retraction, agonal

Observation of diaphragmatic movement, lung expansion, and the use of accessory muscles — depth, symmetry, inspiration/expiration ratio

Auscultation of thorax to assess:
- breath sounds — presence, intensity, quality, symmetry,
- abnormal sounds — stridor, wheezes, crackles, rubs, crepitation, increase or decrease in sounds

- tube placement and need for endotracheal suction when child is intubated

Exercise 1
Answer the following questions. Prepare short talks and/or dialogues on these topics

1. What do you know about causes of cough and cough assessment?
2. Describe signs of respiratory failure.
3. Speak about nursing observations for the child with respiratory failure.

Exercise 2
Match the column A with the column B. Try to learn the expressions and/or sentences by heart.

A

1. The major functions of the respiratory tract are...
2. Several anatomic features predispose infants and young children to airway obstruction and atelectasis: ...
3. Gas exchange depends on the amount and composition of gases inhaled, thickness of the alveolar wall, ...
4. The amount of O_2 that diffuses into the blood depends on a pressure gradient between alveolar air and capillary blood, ...
5. Defence mechanisms of the respiratory tract include the lymphatic system, mucus secretion, ciliary action, epiglottis, cough reflex, ...
6. Complete assessment of respiratory function involves detailed history, physical examination, pulmonary function tests, ...
7. Pulse oximetry is a noninvasive method of determining the O_2 saturation in the blood. ...
8. Improvement in respiratory function may be accomplished with measures such as ...

B

a. ... *adequacy of circulation to the alveoli, and substances within the alveoli that prevent their inflation of gas exchange.*
b. ... *there is less alveolar surface for gas exchange; narrowly branching peripheral airways become easily obstructed; and lack of collateral pathways inhibits ventilation beyond obstructed units.*
c. .... *radiography, and blood gas determination.*

d. ... O_2 therapy, positioning, humidification, aerosol therapy, and artificial ventilation; O_2 for administration must always be humidified.

e. ... radiography, and blood gas determination.

f. ... the total functional surface area of the alveolocapillary membrane, minute volume, and alveolar ventilation.

g. ... One limitation of the technology is that it does not identify dangerously high O_2 levels.

h. ... to distribute air and exchange gases to supply cells with oxygen (O_2) and to remove carbon dioxide (CO_2).

i. ... tracheobronchial dynamics, body position changes, and humoral defences.

Exercise 3
Fill in the missing words. Choose the correct ones.

1. Chest _____ is useful for patients with increased _____ _____ but is contraindicated for some.	a sputum production b physiotherapy
2. Implications for possible intubation include airway _____, respiratory _____, pulmonary toilet, neuromuscular compromise and/or _____, and hypoxaemia.	a arrest, b obstruction c paralysis
3. Respiratory _____ is defined as the inability of the respiratory system to maintain _____ oxygenation of the blood, with or without CO_2 _____.	a adequate b failure c retention
4. Management of respiratory failure is to _____ O_2, maintain _____, apply appropriate therapy, and _____ complications.	a ventilation b provide c anticipate
5. Endotracheal and tracheostomy _____ involves premeasured _____ of the catheter, application of suction for 3 to 4 seconds then _____ the catheter, and _____ O_2 before and after suctioning.	a supplemental b withdrawing c suctioning d insertion

6. _____ of the endotracheal and tracheostomy tube is life-threatening; therefore _____ for replacing a tube must always be __ _____.	a at hand b equipment c Occlusion
7. _____ cardiopulmonary resuscitation (CPR) includes 1 minute of _____ ___ _____ before summoning emergency help.	a ventilations and compressions b Paediatric
8. Two essentials for CPR are to support the patient's _____ and to apply forceful, but not traumatic, _____ _____.	a sternal pressure b spine
9. The Heimlich manoeuvre is reserved for children for whom _____ is witnessed or strongly suspected. A combination of _____ _____ and _____ _____ is used for infants with obstructed airways.	a back blows b aspiration c chest thrusts

Translation 1

1. Causes of cough are: inflammatory disorders, lung disease, focal or anatomic lesions, psychogenic or habit cough, postnasal drip and/or sinusitis. 2. Cough assessment includes: onset and duration, type, progress, pattern, associated symptoms, and secretions. 3. Signs of respiratory failure are: restlessness, increase in respiratory effort, tachypnoea, tachycardia, diaphoresis, mood changes, such as euphoria or depression, headache, altered depth and pattern of respirations, hypertension, and exertional dyspnoea. 4. Other signs include: anorexia, increased cardiac output and renal output, central nervous system symptoms, flaring nares, chest wall retractions, expiratory grunt, wheezing and/or prolonged expiration, and absent or decreased breath sounds. 5. Signs of more severe hypoxia are: hypotension or hypertension, dimness of vision, somnolence, stupor, coma, dyspnoea, depressed respirations/agonal respirations, bradycardia, cyanosis, peripheral of central apnoea. 6. Nursing observations for the child with respiratory failure include: visual inspection of skin colour, observation of respiratory effort or distress — nasal flaring, grunting, gasping, retraction, agonal, observation of diaphragmatic movement, lung expansion, and the use of accessory muscles — depth, symmetry, inspiration/expiration ratio. 7. Auscultation of thorax may assess: presence, intensity, quality, symmetry of breath sounds, stridor, wheezes, crackles, rubs, crepitation, increase or decrease in sounds, and tube placement.

Text 2
The child with respiratory dysfunction
Signs and symptoms associated with respiratory infections in infants and small children

Fever
- May be absent in newborn infants
- Greatest at ages 6 months to 3 years (temperature may reach 39.5°C to 40.5°C even with mild infections)
- Often appears as first sign of infection
- May be listless and irritable or somewhat euphoric and more active than normal, temporarily; some children talk with unaccustomed rapidity.
- Tendency to develop high temperatures with infection in certain families
- may precipitate febrile seizures.
- febrile seizures uncommon after 3 or 4 years of age.

Meningism
Meningeal signs without infection of the meninges
Occurs with abrupt onset of fever
Accompanied by:
- headache
- pain and stiffness in the back and neck
- presence of Kernig and Brudzinski signs

Subsides as the temperature drops.

Anorexia
- Common with most childhood illnesses
- Frequently the initial evidence of illness
- Almost invariably accompanies acute infection in small children
- Persists to a greater or lesser degree throughout febrile stage of illness; often extends into convalescence

Vomiting
- Small children vomit readily with illness
- A clue to the onset of infection
- May precede other signs by several hours
- Usually short lived, but may persist during the illness

Diarrhoea

- Usually mild, transient diarrhoea but may become severe
- Often accompanies respiratory infections, especially viral infections
- Is frequent cause of dehydration

Abdominal pain

- Common complaint
- Sometimes indistinguishable from pain of appendicitis
- Mesenteric lymphadenitis may be cause
- Muscle spasm from vomiting may be a factor, especially in nervous, tense children

Nasal blockage

- Small nasal passages of infants easily blocked by mucosal swelling and exudation
- Can interfere with respiration and feeding in infants
- May contribute to the development of otitis media and sinusitis

Nasal discharge

- Frequently accompanies respiratory infections
- May be thin and watery (rhinorrhoea) or thick and purulent
- Depends on the type and/or stage of infection
- Associated with itching
- May irritate upper lip and skin surrounding the nose

Cough

- Common feature of respiratory disease
- May be evident only during the acute phase
- May persist several months after a disease

Respiratory sounds

- Sounds associated with respiratory disease: cough, hoarseness, grunting, stridor, wheezing.
- Auscultation: wheezing, crackles, absence of sound

Sore throat

Frequent complaint of older children

Young children (unable to describe symptoms) may not complain even when highly inflamed

- often, child will refuse to take oral fluids or solids

- elastic nature of the tissues in young children may cause less pressure on nerve endings

Early evidence of respiratory complications

Parents are instructed to notify the health professionals if any of the following are noted:

- evidence of earache
- respirations faster than 50 to 60 per minute
- fever over 101F chloride concentration
- listlessness
- increasing irritability with or without fever
- persistent cough 2 days or more
- wheezing
- crying
- refusal to eat
- restlessness and poor sleep patterns

General signs of pneumonia

Fever: usually quite high

Respiratory:
- cough, unproductive to productive with whitish sputum
- tachypnoea
- breath sounds: rhonchi or fine crackles
- dullness with percussion
- chest pain
- retractions
- nasal flaring
- pallor to cyanosis (depends on severity)

Chest x-ray film: diffuse or patchy infiltration, with peri-bronchial distribution
Behaviour: irritable, restless, lethargic
Gastrointestinal: anorexia, vomiting, diarrhoea, abdominal pain

Triggers tending to precipitate and/or aggravate asthmatic exacerbations
Allergens
- Outdoor: trees, shrubs, weeds, grasses, moulds, pollens, air pollution, spores

- Indoor: dust and/or dust mites, mould, cockroach antigen

Irritants: tobacco smoke, wood smoke, odours, sprays

Exposure to occupational **chemicals**

Exercise, cold air, changes in weather or temperature

Environmental change: moving to new home, starting new school, etc.

Colds and **infections**

Animals: cats, dogs, rodents, horses

Medications: aspirin, nonsteroidal anti-inflammatory (NSAIDs), antibiotics, beta blockers

Strong **emotions**: fear, anger, laughing, crying

Conditions: gastroesophageal reflux, tracheoesophageal fistula

Food **additives**: sulphite preservatives

Foods: nuts, milk, dairy products

Endocrine factors: menses, pregnancy, thyroid disease

Conditions that may mimic asthma

Obstruction involving large airways

Foreign body in trachea, bronchus, or oesophagus

Vascular rings

Laryngotracheomalacia

Enlarged **lymph nodes**

Tumour laryngeal webs

Tracheostenosis or bronchostenosis

Vocal cord paralysis

Obstruction involving both large and small airways

Bronchiolitis: viral or obliterative

Cystic fibrosis

Bronchopulmonary dysplasia

Aspiration from swallowing dysfunction; gastroesophageal reflux, tracheoesophageal fistula

Pulmonary oedema

Acute inflammation of the airways

Family home care
"Allergy proofing" the home
- Keep humidity between 40% and 50%; use dehumidifier if available. Have carpets cleaned professionally frequently or remove them, including carpeting on concrete. Avoid vacuuming carpets, which sends allergens into the air, although it does remove waste particles of dust mite. If available, use **central vacuum cleaner** with collecting bag outside of home or use cleaner filters. Use **chemical** agents to kill mites or alter antigens in house. Keep child away from treated areas during and several hours after chemical application.
- If possible, use an **air-cleaning** device, such as electrostatic precipitator in child's room. Have air and heat ducts professionally cleaned annually; change or clean filters monthly. Use foam rubber mattress and pillows, and synthetic blankets. **Launder** blankets and sheets in hot water. Store nothing under bed, keep closets and storage areas uncluttered. Use washable shades rather than blinds or curtains.
- Use child's room for sleeping, not playing. **Remove** from room unnecessary furniture, rugs, stuffed or real animals, toys, books, **upholstered furniture**, plants, aquariums, wall hangings etc. Cover or replace upholstered furniture; avoid rattan or wicker furniture. Cover walls with washable paint or wallpaper.

- Limit child's **exposure to animals**. Change child's clothes after playing outdoors; wash hair nightly if outside and pollen count is high. Keep child indoors while lawn is being mowed, bushes/trees are being trimmed, or pollen count is high. Keep windows and doors closed during pollen season; use air conditioner if available. Cover heating vents with filter material (e. g., cheesecloth) to prevent circulation of dust, especially when heat is turned on after summer.
- Use smooth cotton or synthetic fabrics for bedcovers, curtains, and scatter rugs and launder weekly. Wet mop bare floors weekly. **Wet dust and clean** room weekly; child should not be present during housecleaning activities. Limit or avoid child's exposure to tobacco and wood smoke. **Avoid odours or sprays** (e. g., perfumes, talcum powder, room deodorizers, fresh paint). Avoid cellar (basement) as play area and use dehumidifier in damp cellar. Clean showers and tile areas, spray with **antimould agent** (e. g., Lysol). Keep vaporizers and air conditioners clean and free of mould.

Use a peak expiratory flow meter
- Before each use, make sure the sliding marker on arrow on the PEFM is at the bottom of the numbered scale.
- Stand up straight.
- Remove gum or any food from the mouth.
- Close your lips tightly around the mouthpiece. Be sure to keep your tongue away from the mouthpiece.
- Blow out as hard and as quickly as you can, a "fast hard puff."
- Note the number by the marker on the numbered scale.
- Repeat entire routine three times.
- Record the highest of the three readings, not the average.
- Measure your peak respiratory flow rate (PEFR) close to the same time and same way each day (i.e., morning and evening; before and/ or 15 minutes after taking medication).
- Keep a chart of your PEFRs.

Use of a metered-dose inhaler
Steps for checking how much medicine is in the canister

- If the canister is new, it is full
- If the canister has been used repeatedly, it might be empty (check product label to see how many inhalations should be in each canister)

- To check how much medicine is left in the canister, put the canister (not the mouthpiece) in a cup of water.
- If the canister sinks to the bottom, it is full.
- If the canister floats sideways on the surface, it is empty

Steps for using the inhaler
- Remove the cap and hold inhaler upright.
- Shake the inhaler
- Tilt the head back slightly and breathe out
- With the inhaler in an upright position, insert the mouthpiece:
- about 3 to 4 cm from the mouth or
- into an aero-chamber or
- into the mouth, forming an airtight seal between the lips and the mouthpiece
- At the end of a normal expiration, depress the top of the inhaler canister firmly to release the medication (into either the aero-chamber or the mouth), and breathe in slowly (about 3-5 seconds). Relax the pressure on the top of the canister.
- Hold the breath for at least 5 to 10 seconds to allow the aerosol medication to reach deeply into the lungs.
- Remove the inhaler and breathe out slowly through the nose.
- Wait 1 minute between puffs (if additional one is needed).
- To determine if child is using an inhaler properly, have child use the device in front of a mirror. If vapour does not appear on the mirror, the inhaler is being used correctly.

Exercise 4
Answer the following questions. Prepare short talks and/or dialogues on these topics

1. Describe signs and symptoms associated with respiratory infections in infants and small children.
2. What can you say about early evidence of respiratory complications?
3. Characterize general signs of pneumonia.
4. Which are triggers tending to precipitate and/or aggravate asthmatic exacerbations?
5. Which conditions may mimic asthma?
6. Speak about obstruction involving both large and small airways.
7. Characterize "allergy proofing" the home.
8. How to use a peak expiratory flow meter?
9. How to use of a metered-dose inhaler?

10. What are steps for checking how much medicine is in the canister?
11. Describe steps for using the inhaler.

Exercise 5
Match the column A with the column B. Try to learn the expressions and/or sentences by heart.

A

1. Acute infection of the respiratory tract …
2. The incidence and severity of respiratory tract infections …
3. Symptoms of respiratory tract infections include fever, febrile convulsions, anorexia, vomiting, diarrhoea, abdominal pain, …
4. Common respiratory tract infections of childhood …
5. Severe bleeding from the tonsil site can occur …
6. Factors that predispose children to otitis media are the shape and position of the Eustachian tubes, …
7. The most common upper respiratory infections are categorized as …
8. Epiglottitis is a medical emergency and is characterized by …

B

a. *… are influenced by the infectious agent involved, the child's age, and the child's natural defences.*
b. *… include acute nasopharyngitis, acute pharyngitis, influenza, tonsillitis, and otitis media.*
c. *… nasal blockage and discharge, wheezing, cough, respiratory sounds, and presence or absence of sore throat.*
d. *… croup syndromes, which include acute laryngotracheobronchitis, acute spasmodic laryngitis, and acute epiglottitis*
e. *…. is the most common cause of illness in infancy and childhood*
f. *… high fever, toxic appearance, and difficulty swallowing.*
g. *… underdeveloped cartilage lining, abundant pharyngeal lymphoid tissue, immature humoral defence mechanisms, and the recumbent position (in infants)*
h. *… within 6 hours after surgery or 5 to 10 days after tonsillectomy.*

Exercise 6
Fill in the missing words. Choose the correct ones.

1. The primary _____ _____ in the care of children with croup is _____ for signs of respiratory embarrassment and _____ ___ laryngeal obstruction.	a relief of b nursing function c observation
2. _____ _____ conditions constitute ____ _____ of respiratory problems in children and are usually viral in nature (excluding _____ _____ aspiration).	a the majority b foreign body c Lower airway
3. Common infections of the lower airway include bacterial _____, asthmatic _____, _____, and pneumonia.	a bronchiolitis b bronchitis c tracheitis
4. _____ are generally classified either __ _____ (lobar, bronchial, or interstitial) or by _____ _____ (viruses, bacteria, mycoplasmas, or associated with foreign bodies).	a by site b etiologic agent c Pneumonias
5. _____ of uncomplicated _____ and _____ _____ is symptomatic in otherwise healthy infants.	a viral pneumonia b bronchiolitis c Management
6. In _____, resistance to the bacillus can be _____ by heredity, sex, age, stress states, poor nutrition, intercurrent infection, and _____ with therapy.	a noncompliance b altered c tuberculosis
7. Signs of _____ include inability to speak, _____ _____, and _____ level of activity.	a decreased b colour change c choking
8. Inhaled _____ are rarely coughed up _____; therefore, they must be removed by direct _____ or bronchoscopy.	a spontaneously b objects c laryngoscopy

9. Inducing a child to vomit is _____ in the event of hydrocarbon _____ because of the danger of hydrocarbon _____.	a ingestion b contraindicated c aspiration
10. Asthma is now thought to occur mostly because of _____ to environmental substances that trigger a complex _____ _____, therefore an important _____ of therapy is elimination of environmental allergens, or triggers.	a allergic response b component c hypersensitivity
11. Asthma can be _____ by a variety of agents and is characterized by _____, oedema of the bronchial mucosa, and increased bronchial _____ _____, which can result in the classic manifestations of cough, dyspnoea, and _____.	a bronchospasm b mucus secretion c wheeze d triggered
12. The mainstays of treating _____ include use of _____, anti-inflammatory agents, _____, and rest.	a bronchodilators b oxygen c asthma
13. _____ _____ is the most frequently occurring _____ disease of white children	a Cystic fibrosis b inherited
14. Diagnosis of cystic fibrosis is based on _____ _____, absence of _____ _____, chronic pulmonary involvement, and an abnormally high sweat _____ _____, with the pilocarpine (or sweat test) being the most commonly used diagnostic test.	a pancreatic enzymes b chloride concentration c family history

Translation 2

1. Signs and symptoms associated with respiratory infections in infants and small children include: fever, meningism, anorexia, vomiting, diarrhoea, abdominal pain, nasal blockage, nasal discharge, cough, respiratory sounds, and sore throat. 2. Parents are instructed to notify the health professionals if any of the following are noted: earache, fast respirations, fever, listlessness, increasing irritability, persistent cough, wheezing, crying, refusal to eat, restlessness and poor sleep patterns. 3. General signs of pneumonia are: high fever, cough, tachypnoea, rhonchi or fine crackles, dullness with percussion, chest pain, retractions, nasal flaring, pallor to cyanosis, irritable behaviour, anorexia, vomiting, diarrhoea, and abdominal pain. 4. Triggers tending to precipitate and/or aggravate asthmatic exacerbations are: allergens,

irritants, occupational chemicals, exercise, cold air, changes in weather or temperature, colds and infections, animals, medications, strong emotions, food additives, foods, or endocrine factors. 5. Conditions that may mimic asthma include: obstruction involving large airways, foreign body in trachea, bronchus, or oesophagus, vascular rings, laryngo-tracheomalacia, enlarged lymph nodes, tumour, trachea-stenosis or broncho-stenosis, and vocal cord paralysis. 6. Obstruction of both large and small airways involve: bronchiolitis, cystic fibrosis, bronchopulmonary dysplasia, aspiration, pulmonary oedema, and acute inflammation of the airways. 7. Have carpets cleaned professionally frequently or remove them, including carpeting on concrete. 8. Use chemical agents to kill mites or alter antigens in house. 9. If possible, use an air-cleaning device, such as electrostatic precipitator in child's room. 10. Use foam rubber mattress and pillows, and synthetic blankets and launder blankets and sheets in hot water.

Exercise 7
Match the column A with the column B. Try to learn the expressions and/or sentences by heart.

A

1. Remove from room unnecessary furniture, rugs, keep child indoors while lawn is being mowed, ...
2. Use smooth cotton or synthetic fabrics ...
3. Limit or avoid child's exposure to tobacco and wood smoke ...
4. Clean showers and tile areas, ...
5. Before each use of a peak expiratory flow meter, ...
6. Measure your peak respiratory flow rate (PEFR) ...
7. These are steps for checking how much medicine is in the canister ...
8. If the canister is new, ...
9. Steps for using the inhaler are: at the end of a normal expiration, depress the top of the inhaler canister firmly to release the medication (into either the aero chamber or the mouth), ...
10. To determine if child is using an inhaler properly, have child use the device in front of a mirror; ...
11. Asthma can be triggered by a variety of agents and is characterized ...
12. Diagnosis of cystic fibrosis is based on family history, absence of pancreatic enzymes, chronic pulmonary involvement, ...

B

a. ... *bushes/trees are being trimmed, or pollen count is high*

b. ... *and avoid odours or sprays (e. g., perfumes, talcum powder, room deodorizers, fresh paint).*

c. ... *spray with antimould agent.*

d. ... *close to the same time and same way each day.*

e. ... *a metered-dose inhaler: to check how much medicine is left in the canister, put the canister (not the mouthpiece) in a cup of water.*

f. ... *by bronchospasm, oedema of the bronchial mucosa, and increased bronchial mucus secretion, which can result in the classic manifestations of cough, dyspnoea, and wheeze.*

g. ... *if vapour does not appear on the mirror, the inhaler is being used correctly.*

h. ... *and an abnormally high sweat chloride concentration, with the pilocarpine (or sweat test) being the most commonly used diagnostic test.*

i. ... *and breathe in slowly (about 3-5 seconds), then relax the pressure on the top of the canister.*

j. ... *it is full and if the canister floats sideways on the surface, it is empty.*

k. ... *make sure the sliding marker on arrow on the PEFM is at the bottom of the numbered scale.*

l. ... *for bedcovers, curtains, and scatter rugs and launder weekly.*

Text 3
The child with gastrointestinal dysfunction
Functions of the gastrointestinal tract

- process and absorb nutrients necessary to maintain metabolic processes and to support growth and development
- perform an excretory function for both digestive residue and other waste products that pour into the intestine from the blood or are excreted in the bile
- provide detoxification while other routes of elimination (kidneys, liver, skin) are still immature
- participate in maintaining fluid and electrolyte balance in infancy

Clinical manifestations of gastrointestinal dysfunction in children

Failure to thrive — deceleration from established growth pattern or consistently bellow the 5th percentile for height and weight on standard growth charts; sometimes accompanied by developmental delays.

Spitting up or regurgitation — passive transfer of gastric contents into the oesophagus or mouth.

Vomiting — forceful ejection of gastric contents; involves a complex process under central nervous system control that causes salivation, pallor, sweating, and tachycardia; usually accompanied by nausea. **Projectile vomiting**, vomiting accompanied by vigorous peristaltic waves and typically associated with pyloric stenosis or pylorospasm.

Nausea — unpleasant sensation vaguely referred to the throat or abdomen with an inclination to vomit

Constipation — passage of firm or hard stools or infrequent passage of stool with associated symptoms such as difficulty expelling the stools, blood-streaked stools, and abdominal discomfort

Encopresis — overflow of incontinent stool causing soiling often due to faecal retention or impaction

Diarrhoea — increase in the number of stools with an increased water content as a result of alterations of water and electrolyte transport by the GI tract; may be acute or chronic

Hypoactive, hyperactive, or absent bowel sounds – evidence of intestinal motility problems that may be caused by inflammation or obstruction.

Abdominal distention — protuberant contour of the abdomen that may be caused by delayed gastric emptying, accumulation of gas or stool, inflammation, or obstruction

Abdominal pain — pain associated with the abdomen that may be localized or diffuse, acute or chronic; often caused by inflammation, obstruction, or haemorrhage

Gastrointestinal bleeding — may be from an upper or lower GI source and may be acute or chronic

Haematemesis — vomiting of bright red blood denatured blood that results from bleeding in the upper GI tract or from swallowed blood from the nose or oropharynx

Haematochezia — passage of bright red blood per rectum, usually indicating lower GI tract bleeding

Melaena — passage of dark-coloured, "tarry" stools due to denatured blood, suggesting upper GI tract bleeding or bleeding from the right colon

Jaundice — yellow colouration of the skin and sclerae associated with liver dysfunction

Dysphagia — difficulty swallowing caused by abnormalities in the neuromuscular function of the pharynx or upper oesophageal sphincter or by disorders of the oesophagus

Dysfunctional swallowing — impaired swallowing due to central nervous system defects or structural defects of the oral cavity, pharynx, or oesophagus; can cause feeding problems or aspiration

Fever — common manifestation of illness in children with GI disorders; usually associated with dehydration, infection, or inflammation

Emergency treatment
Foreign body ingestion
  Seek medical treatment immediately if:
  • Any sharp or large object or a battery was ingested.
  • There are signs that the object may have been aspirated (i.e., coughing, choking, inability to speak, or difficulty breathing)
  • There are signs of GI perforation (i.e., chest or abdominal pain, evidence of bleeding in vomitus, stool, haematocrit, or vital signs).
  • There are signs that the object may be lodged in the oesophagus (i.e., increased salivation, drooling, gagging, or difficulty swallowing)
  • There are signs that the object may be lodged in the pharynx (i.e., discomfort in the throat or chest — more likely with a fish or chicken bone or large piece of meat).

  Seek medical advice even if the object is smooth and small (usually less than the size of a coin).
  If no treatment is advised, check the stool for passage of the object; do not give laxatives.

High-fibre foods
Bread, grains
  Whole-grain bread or rolls, whole-grain cereals, bran, pancakes, waffles, and muffins with fruit or bran, unrefined (brown) rice

Vegetables
Raw vegetables, especially broccoli, cabbage, carrots, cauliflower, celery, lettuce, and spinach

Cooked vegetables, such as those listed above, and asparagus, beans, Brussels sprouts, corn, potatoes, rhubarb, squash, string beans, and turnips

Fruits
Prunes, raisins, or other drain fruits

Raw fruits, especially those with skins or seeds, other than ripe banana or avocado

Miscellaneous
Legumes (beans), popcorn, nuts, seeds

High-fibre snack and bars

Atraumatic care
Palpating the abdomen for abdominal care
Because children associate the stethoscope with listening, use the bell piece for initial palpation of the abdomen for tenderness. Children usually endure pressure from the stethoscope that they would not tolerate from a probing hand. Follow with manual palpation, using a gentle touch without lifting the hand from the abdomen while observing the child's face for signs of discomfort.

Ask the child to lift the heels and drop them to the floor two or three times, to hop on one foot, or to puff out or pull in the abdomen to check for tenderness without more painful probing.

Abdominal circumference measurements
To reduce any stress to the acutely ill child when frequent measurements of abdominal circumference are needed, leave the tape measure in place beneath the child. Measure the abdomen at the same time that vital signs are taken to avoid frequently disturbing the child.

Exercise 8
Answer the following questions. Prepare short talks and/or dialogues on these topics

1. What are functions of the gastrointestinal tract?
2. Describe clinical manifestations of gastrointestinal dysfunction in children.
3. Characterize emergency treatment in foreign body ingestion.

4. Speak about high-fibre foods.
5. What is meant by atraumatic care?

Exercise 9
Study the following summary and then interpret basic information in English.

1. The essential functions of the GI system are to process and absorb nutrients necessary to maintain metabolic processes and support growth and development, to perform excretory functions, to provide detoxification, and to maintain fluid and electrolyte balance.
2. Digestion is the catabolism of foodstuffs (water, vitamins, minerals, carbohydrates, proteins and fats) from their original complex form to simple, assimilable nutrients.
3. The small intestine is the principal absorptive site in the GI system.
4. Most ingested foreign bodies pass through the alimentary tract without difficulty. Those lodged in the oesophagus or objects with sharp edges require further evaluation.
5. Constipation is usually managed by diet therapy and measures to keep the bowel relatively empty of stool.
6. Hirschsprung disease requires surgical removal of a-ganglionic segments of bowel.
7. Nursing care of gastroesophageal reflux is aimed primarily at instructing caregivers regarding home care feeding and positioning, and caring for the child undergoing surgical intervention.
8. Although the cause of appendicitis is poorly understood, it is commonly a result of obstruction of the lumen, often by a fecalith. Common signs and symptoms are colicky abdominal pain, guarding of the abdomen, and fever.
9. Meckel diverticulum is a congenital malformation of the GI tract characterized by rectal bleeding.
10. Inflammatory bowel disease refers to ulcerative colitis and Crohn disease. Chronic diarrhoea and growth abnormalities are common features.

Exercise 10
Fill in the missing words. Choose the correct ones.

1. Management of inflammatory _____ _____ includes nutritional support, sulfasalazine, corticosteroids or other _____ drugs, antibiotics, and general _____ _____. Surgical _____ of inflamed bowel may be necessary.	a immunosuppressive
	b supportive therapy
	c removal
	d bowel disease

2. _____ _____ are poorly understood, but a likely cause is interference with the normal _____ _____ of the _____ _____.	a mucosal lining b Peptic ulcers c protective mechanisms
3. General signs of __ _____ include abdominal pain, nausea and vomiting, abdominal _____, and a decline in the amount of excreted _____.	a distention b stool c GI obstruction
4. Hypertrophic _____ _____ is characterized by _____ vomiting without loss of appetite, dehydration, and _____ _____. Therapy is surgical pyloromyotomy.	a projectile b pyloric stenosis c metabolic alkalosis
5. _____ is a cause of intestinal obstruction during infancy. _____ is either nonsurgical hydrostatic reduction or _____ _____	a surgical reduction b Treatment c Intussusception
6. _____ syndromes are disorders associated with some degree of _____ _____ and/or absorption. They include digestive defects, absorptive defects, and _____ _____.	a impaired digestion b anatomic defects c Malabsorption
7. The prognosis for children with _____ _____ _____ improved dramatically as a result of advances in _____ ___ _____ nutritional support, which is the primary therapy for this _____. Home care is an important component of these children's quality of life.	a short bowel syndrome b condition c parenteral and enteral
8. Celiac disease is characterized by an intolerance for _____. The major role of the nurse in the management of _____ _____ is helping the parents and child _____ __ diet therapy.	a adhere to b gluten c celiac disease
9. GI bleeding may be _____ __ _____ GI tract bleeding, and initial management should include assessment of the _____ of bleeding and restoration of _____ _____.	a haemodynamic stability b magnitude c upper or lower
10. _____ _____ is caused by at least _____ _____ __ _____ hepatitis A virus, hepatitis B virus, hepatitis C virus, hepatitis D virus, and hepatitis E virus.	a five types or virus b Viral hepatitis

11. Hepatitis A virus is spread by the _____-_____ route, whereas hepatitis B and C viruses are transmitted primarily by the _____ _____. The single most effective measure in prevention and control of hepatitis in any setting is _____.	a faecal-oral b parenteral route c handwashing
12. Universal _____ against hepatitis B virus is _____ for all newborns.	a immunization b recommended
13. _____ _____ offers hope to children with ____-_____ liver disease.	a Liver transplantation b end-stage

Translation 3

1. Functions of the gastrointestinal tract are: process and absorb nutrients, perform an excretory function, provide detoxification, maintain fluid and electrolyte balance. 2. Clinical manifestations of gastrointestinal dysfunction in children are: failure to thrive, spitting up or regurgitation, vomiting, nausea, constipation, encopresis, diarrhoea, hypoactive, hyperactive, or absent bowel sounds, abdominal distention, abdominal pain, gastrointestinal bleeding, jaundice, dysphagia, dysfunctional swallowing, and fever. 3. In foreign body ingestion look for: any object, if there are signs that the object may have been aspirated (i.e., coughing, choking, inability to speak, or difficulty breathing), there are signs of GI perforation, or there are signs that the object may be lodged in the oesophagus (i.e., increased salivation, drooling, gagging, or difficulty swallowing).

Exercise 11
Match the column A with the column B. Try to learn the expressions and/or sentences by heart.

A

1. If no treatment is advised, ...
2. High-fibre foods are e.g.: bread, grains (whole-grain bread or rolls, whole-grain cereals, bran, unrefined (brown) rice; ...
3. In palpating the abdomen for abdominal care, use the bell piece of the stethoscope ....
4. Follow with manual palpation ...
5. In abdominal circumference measurements measure the abdomen ....

B

a.   *... while observing the child's face for signs of discomfort.*

b.   *... raw vegetables, especially broccoli, cabbage, carrots, cauliflower, celery, lettuce, and spinach and cooked vegetables, beans, Brussels sprouts, corn, potatoes, rhubarb, squash, string beans, and turnips, legumes (beans), popcorn, nuts, seeds, prunes, raisins, or other drain fruits.*

c.   *... check the stool for passage of the object; do not give laxatives.*

d.   *... at the same time that vital signs are taken to avoid frequently disturbing the child.*

e.   *... for initial palpation of the abdomen for tenderness.*

Key 17
Exercise 2
1h; 2b; 3a; 4f; 5i; 6c; 7g; 8d

Exercise 3
1 b, a; 2 b, a, c; 3 b, a, c; 4 b, a, c; 5 d, c, b, a; 6 c, b, a; 7 b, a; 8 b, a; 9 b, a, c

Exercise 5
1e; 2a; 3c; 4b; 5h; 6g; 7d; 8f;

Exercise 6
1b,c,a; 2c,a,b; 3c,b,a; 4c,a,b; 5c,b,a; 6c,b,a; 7c,b,a; 8b,a,c; 9b,a,c; 10c,a,b; 11d,a,b,c; 12c,a,b; 13a,b; 14c,a,b

Exercise 7
1a; 2l; 3b; 4c; 5k; 6d; 7e; 8j; 9i; 10g; 11f; 12h

Exercise 10
1d,a,b,c; 2b,c,a; 3c,a,b; 4b,a,c; 5c,b,a; 6c,a,b; 7a,c,b; 8b,c,a; 9c,b,a; 10b,a; 11a,b,c; 12a,b; 13a,b

Exercise 11
1c; 2b; 3e; 4a; 5d

VOCABULARY 17

abrupt /əˈbrʌpt/
accessory /əkˈses.ər.i/
additive /ˈæd.ɪ.tɪv/
adhere /ədˈhɪər/
aero-chamber /eərəˈtʃeɪm.bə/
a-ganglionic /eɪˈ.gæŋ.gli.ən.ɪk/
aggravate /ˈæg.rə.veɪt/
airtight /ˈeə.taɪt/ vzduchotěsný
alter /ˈɒl.tər/
alteration /ˌɒl.təˈreɪ.ʃən/
altered /ˈɒl.tərd/
alveolus /ˌæl.viˈəʊ.ləs/ pl alveoli
antigen /ˈæn.tɪ.dʒən/
anti-inflammatory /ˌæn.ti.ɪnˈflæm.ə.tər.i/
antimould /ˌæn.ti.məʊld/
appendicitis /əˌpen.dɪˈsaɪ.tɪs/
aquarium /əˈkwe.ə.rɪ.əm/
arrest /əˈrest/
arrow /ˈær.əʊ/
artificial /ˌɑː.tɪˈfɪʃ.əl/
asparagus /əˈspær.ə.gəs/
aspirate /ˈæs.pɪ.rət/
assimilable /əˈsi.mə.lə.bəl/
at /æt/ **hand** /hænd/
auscultation /ˌɔː.skəlˈteɪ.ʃən/
average /ˈæv.ər.ɪdʒ/
balance /ˈbæl.əns/
bar /bɑː/
battery /ˈbæt.ər.i/
bedcover /ˈbed.ˌkə.vər/
bell /bel/
beta /ˈbiː.tə/ **blockers** /blɒk.ərs/ bile /baɪl/
blind /blaɪnd/
blockage /ˈblɒk.ɪdʒ/
blood-streaked /blʌd striːkt/
bran /bræn/
branch /brɑːntʃ/
brassy /ˈbrɑː.si/ **cough** /kɒf/
bronchial /ˈbrɒŋ.ki.əl/
bronchiolitis /ˈbrɒŋ.ki.əˈla.ɪ.tɪs/
bronchitis /brɒŋˈkaɪ.tɪs/
bronchodilator /ˈbrɒŋ.kə.daɪˈleɪ.tər/
bronchopulmonary /ˈbrɒŋ.kəˈpʊl.mə.ner.i/
bronchoscopy /brɒn.ˈkɒ.skə.piː/
bronchostenosis /ˌbrɒŋ.kəʊ.steˈnəʊ.sɪs/

bronchus /ˈbrɒŋ.kəs/ pl **bronchi** /ˈbrɒŋ.kaɪ/

Brudzinski sign /bruː.dʒinˈskiː saɪn/

Brussels /ˈbrʌsəlz/ **sprouts** /spraʊts/

canister /ˈkæn.ɪ.stər/

cap /kæp/

carpeting /ˈkɑː.pɪ.tɪŋ/

cartilage /ˈkɑː.təl.ɪdʒ/

catabolism /kəˈta.bə.ˌli.zəm/

celiac /ˈsiː.li:.ˌak/

cellar /ˈsel.ər/

cheesecloth /ˈtʃiː.z.ˌklɒθ/

choke /tʃəʊk/

ciliary /ˈsɪ.lɪ:.ˌər.iː/

circumference /səˈkʌm.fər.əns/

closet /ˈklɒzɪt/

cockroach /ˈkɒk.ˌrəʊtʃ/

coin /kɔɪn/

colicky /ˈkɒl.ɪ.ki/

collateral /kəˈlæt.ər.əl/

complaint /kəmˈpleɪnt/

concrete /ˈkɒŋ.kriːt/

consistency /kənˈsɪs.tənt .si/

constipation /ˌkɒnt .stɪˈpeɪ.ʃən/

contour /ˈkɒn.tɔːr/

convalescence /ˌkɒn.vəˈles.əns/

crackle /ˈkræk.l̩/

crepitation /ˌkrep.ɪˈteɪ.ʃən/

croup /kruːp/

damp /dæmp/

dangerously /ˈdeɪn.dʒər.əs.li/

deceleration / diːˌseləˈreɪ.ʃən/

defence /dɪˈfent s/

dehumidifier /ˌdiː.hjuːˈmɪd.ɪ.faɪ.ər/

deodorizer /diːˈəʊdə.ˌraɪzə/

detoxification /diːˌtɒksəfɪˈkeɪʃən/

diaphoresis /ˌdaɪ.ə.fəˈriː.sɪs/

diaphragmatic /ˌdaɪə.fræɡˈmæt.ɪk/

digestion /daɪˈdʒes.tʃən/

dimness /ˈdim.nəs/

drip /drɪp/

drool /druːl/

dullness /ˈdʌl.nəs/

dysphagia /dɪsˈfeɪ.dʒi.ə/

earache /ˈɪə.reɪk/

ejection /ɪˈdʒekt.ʃən/

electrochemical /ɪˌlek.trəʊˈkem.ɪ.kəl/ **gradient** /ˈɡreɪ.di.ənt/

electrostatic /iˌlek.trəʊˈstæt.ɪk/

embarrassment /ɪmˈbærəsmənt/

encopresis /ˌenˌkɑːpˈriː.səs pl **encopreses** /ˌsiːz/

endotracheal /en.dɒ.trəˈkiː.əl/ **tube** /tjuːb/ (**ET tube**)

endure /ɪnˈdjʊər/

epiglottitis /ˌep.ɪ.gləˈtaɪ.tɪs/

estimate /ˈes.tɪ.meɪt/

euphoria /juːˈfɔː.ri.ə/

Eustachian /juːˈsteɪ.ki.ən/ **tube** /tjuːb/

exacerbation /ɪgˌzæs.əˈbeɪ.ʃən/

excretory /ˈek.skrəˌtɔːr.iː/

exertional /ɪgˈzɜː.ʃən.əl/

expel /ɪkˈspel/

exudation /ˌek.sjuːˈdeɪ.ʃən/

fabric /ˈfæb.rɪk/

faecal-oral /ˈfiː.kəl ˈɔː.rəl/

feature /ˈfiː.tʃər/

fecalith /ˈfiː.kəˌlith/

float /fləʊt/

foam /fəʊm/

focal /ˈfəʊ.kəl/

foodstuff /ˈfuːdˌstʌf/

gag /gæg/

gasp /gɑːsp/

gastroesophageal /ˌgæstrəʊˈiːˌsɒfəˈdʒiːəl/

gluten /ˈgluː.tⁿn/

grunt /grʌnt/

guard /gɑːd/

hacking /ˈhæk.ɪŋ/ **cough** /kɒf/

haematemesis /ˌhiː.məˈte.mɪ.sɪs/

haematochezia /ˌhiː.məˈtəʊ.kiː.ziː.æ/

haematocrit /hiː.məˈtə.krɪt/

hanging /ˈhæŋ.ɪŋ/

heel /hiːl/

Heimlich manoeuvre /ˈhaɪm.lɪk məˌnuː.vər/

hoarseness /hɔːsnɪs/

humidification /hjʊˌmi.də.fəˈkeɪ.ʃən/

humidity /hjuːˈmɪd.ɪ.ti/

humoral /ˈhjʊ.mə.rə/

hydrocarbon /ˌhaɪ.drəʊ ˈkɑː.bən/

identify /aɪˈden.tɪ.faɪ/

immunosuppressive /ˌɪm.jə.nəʊ.səˈpres.ɪv/

impaction /ɪmˈpæk.ʃən/

impaired /ɪmˈpeəd/

inclination /ˌɪnklɪˈneɪʃən/

indistinguishable /ˌɪndɪˈstɪŋgwɪʃəbəl/

infiltration /ˌɪn.fɪlˈtreɪ.ʃən/

inflation /ɪnˈfleɪ.ʃən/

inhaler /ɪnˈheɪ.lər/
inherit /ɪnˈher.ɪt/
inhibit /ɪnˈhɪb.ɪt/
intensification /ɪnˌtensɪfɪˈkeɪʃən/
intercurrent /ˌɪn.təˈkʌr.ᵊnt/
interference /ˌɪn.təˈfɪə.rəns/
invariably /ɪnˈveə.ri.ə.bli/
involvement /ɪnˈvɒlv.mənt/
Kernig sign /ˈker.nig saɪn/
laryngitis /ˌlær.ɪnˈdʒaɪ.tɪs/
laryngoscopy /ˌlærɪŋˈgɒ.skə.pi/
laryngotracheobronchitis /læˈrɪŋ.gəˌtreɪ.kɪ.ə.brəŋˈkaɪ.tɪs/
laryngo-tracheomalacia /ləˈrin. dʒəˌtreɪ.ki:.əʊ.məˈleɪ.ʃ.i:.ə/
launder /ˈlɔːndə/
lining /ˈlaɪn.ɪŋ/
listless /ˈlɪst.ləs/
lobar /ˈləʊ.bəʳ/
lodge /lɒdʒ/
lumen /ˈlu.mən/ pl **lumina**
lymph /lɪmf/ **node** /nəʊd/
lymphadenitis /ˌlim.ˌfa.dəˈnaɪ.təs/
lymphoid /ˈlɪm. fɔɪd/
magnitude /ˈmægnɪˌtjuːd/
mainstay /meɪnˌsteɪ/
mattress /ˈmæt.rəs/
Meckel /ˈmek.əl/ **diverticulum** /ˌdaɪ.və.tɪk.jʊ.ləm/ pl **diverticula**
melaena /məˈliːn.ə/
membrane /ˈmem.breɪn/
meningismus /ˌmen.ən.ˈdʒiz.məs/
mesenteric /ˌmes.enˈter.ɪk/
mite /maɪt/
mouthpiece /ˈmaʊθ.piːs/
mow /məʊ/
mucosa /mjuːˈkəʊ.sə/
mucosal /mjuːˈkəʊ.səl/
mycoplasma /ˌmaɪ.kəʊˈplæz.mə/
nasopharyngitis /ˈneɪ.zəˌfær.ɪnˈdʒaɪ.tɪs/
nature /ˈneɪ.tʃər/
nonsteroidal /ˌnɑːn.stəˈrɔːi.dᵊl/
notify /ˈnəʊ.tɪ.faɪ/
nutrient /ˈnjuː.tri.ənt/
obliterative /əˈblɪt.ᵊr.eɪt.ɪv/
oesophagus /ɪˈsɒf.ə.gəs/
outburst /ˈaʊt.bɜːst/
pallor /ˈpæl.ər/
palpation /pælˈpeɪ.ʃən/
paralysis /pəˈræl.ə.sɪs/ pl **paralyses**

paroxysmal /ˈpær.ɒk.sɪz.məl/
patch /pætʃ/
pathway /ˈpɑː.θ.weɪ/
pattern /ˈpæt.ən/
perforation /pɜː.fərˈeɪ.ʃən/
peristaltic /ˌper.ə.ˈstɔː.l.tik/
pillow /ˈpɪl.əʊ/
pilocarpine /ˌpaɪ.lə.ˈkɑː.rˌpiːn/
pollen /ˈpɒl.ən/
postnasal /ˈpəʊst.ˈneɪ.zᵒl/
pour /pɔːr/
precede /prɪˈsiːd/
precipitate /prɪˈsɪp.ɪ.teɪt/
precipitator /prɪˌsɪp.ɪˈteɪ.təʳ/
preservative /prɪˈzɜː.vətɪv/
principal /ˈprɪnt.sɪ.pəl/
probe /prəʊb/
projectile /prəˈdʒek.taɪl/
proof /pruːf/
protective /prəˈtek.tɪv/
protuberant /prəˈtjuː.bərənt/
prune /pruːn/
psychogenic /ˌsaɪ.kəʊˈdʒɛ.nɪk/
puff /ˈpʌf/
pull /pʊl/ **in** /ɪn/
purulent /ˈpjʊə.rʊ.lənt/
pyloric /paɪ.ˈlɔː.r.ik/
pyloromyotomy /ˌpaɪlɔːrˈmaɪə.tə.mɪ/
pyloro-spasm /paɪ.ˈləʊr.əˌspaz.əm/
raisin /ˈreɪzən/
rapid /ˈræpɪd/
rattan /ræˈtæn/
recumbent /rɪˈkʌm.bənt/
residue /ˈrez.ɪ.djuː/
retention /rɪˈtenʃən/
rhonchus /ˈrɒŋkəs/ pl **rhonchi** /ˈrɒŋ.kaɪ/
rhubarb /ˈruː.bɑːb/
ring /rɪŋ/
rodent /ˈrəʊ.dənt/
rub /rʌb/
rubber /ˈrʌbə/
rug /rʌg/
salivation /ˈsæl.ɪ.veɪˌʃən/
saturation /ˌsæt.jʊˈreɪˌʃən/
scatter /ˈskæt.ər/
secretion /sɪˈkriːˌʃən/
seed /siːd/

segment /ˈseg.mənt/

sensation /senˈseɪ.ʃən/

shade /ʃeɪd/

sharp /ʃɑːp/

sheet /ʃiːt/

shrub /ʃrʌb/

sideways /ˈsaɪdˌweɪz/

sink /sɪŋk/

sinusitis /ˌsaɪˌnəˈsaɪ.tɪs/

slide /slaɪd/ (slid, slid)

somnolence /ˈsɒm.nəl.əns/

spasmodic /spæzˈmɒd.ɪk/

spit /spɪt/ **up** /ʌp/

spore /spɔːr/

sputum /ˈspjuː.təm/ pl **sputa**

sternal /ˈstɜː.nəl/

stethoscope /ˈsteθ.ə.skəʊp/

stiffness /ˈstɪf.nəs/

storage /ˈstɔː.rɪdʒ/

string /strɪŋ/ **bean** /biːn/

stupor /ˈstjuː.pər/

suction /ˈsʌk.ʃən/

sulfasalazine /sulfaː.sal.aː.ziːn/

sulfite /ˈsʌl.faɪt/

summon /ˈsʌm.ən/

supplemental /ˌsʌp.lɪˈmen.təl/

suspected /səˈspek.tɪd/

swallow /ˈswɒl.əʊ/

talcum powder /ˈtælkəmˈpaʊdə/

tarry /ˈtær.i/

temporarily /ˈtem.pər.er.ɪ.li/

tenderness /ˈten.də.nəs/

thrive /θraɪv/

thyroid /ˈθaɪə.rɔɪd/

tile /taɪl/

trachea-stenosis /træk.iˈɒ.stɪˈnəʊ.sɪs/

tracheitis /treɪ.kiː.aɪˈtis/

tracheoesophageal /treɪˈkiː.əʊ.iˌsɒfəˈdʒiːəl/

tracheostomy /ˌtræk.iˈɒst.ə.mi/

transient /ˈtræn.zi.ənt/

trigger /ˈtrɪg.ər/

trim /trɪm/

turnip /ˈtɜː.nɪp/

unaccustomed /ˌʌnəˈkʌstəmd/

uncluttered /ʌnˈklʌtəd/

unrefined /ˌʌn.rɪˈfaɪnd/

upholstered /ʌpˈhəʊlstəd/

upright /ˈʌp.raɪt/
vague /veɪg/
vaporizer /ˈveɪpəˌraɪzər/
vent /vent/
ventilation /ˌven.tɪˈleɪ.ʃən/
vocal /ˈvəʊkəl/ cords /kɔːdz/
wallpaper /ˈwɔːlˌpeɪpə/
wave /weɪv/
wicker /ˈwɪkə/
withdraw /wɪðˈdrɔː/
witness /ˈwɪt.nəs/
Word Index

A

abandonment /əˈbæn.dən.mənt/
abduction /æbˈdʌk.ʃən/
aberrant /æˈber.ənt/
aberration /ˌæb.əˈreɪ.ʃən/
abortion /əˈbɔː.ʃən/
abrasion /əˈbreɪ.ʒən/
abrupt /əˈbrʌpt/
absence /ˈæb.səns/
abuse /əˈbjuːz/
abusive /əˈbjuː.sɪv/
accelerate /ækˈse.ləˌreɪt/
accentuation /ækˈsent.ʃʊ.eɪ.ʃən/
accept /əkˈsept/
acceptance /əkˈsep.təns/
access /ˈæk.ses/
accessibility /əkˌses.əˈbɪl.ɪ.ti/
accessible /əkˈses.ə.bļ/
accessory /əkˈses.ər.i/
accident /ˈæk.sɪ.dənt/
acclaim /əˈkleɪm/
accountability /əˌkaʊn.təˈbɪl.ɪ.tɪ/
accretion /əˈkriː.ʃən/
accummulation /əˌkjuːmjʊˈleɪ.ʃən/
accumulate /əˈkjuː.mjʊ.leɪt/
accumulation /əˌkjuːmjʊˈleɪ.ʃən/
accurate /ˈæk.jʊ.rət/
acetabulum /ˌæ.sɪˈtæb.jə.ləm/ pl acetabula
acetate /ˈæsɪˌteɪt/
acetic /əˈsiː.tɪk/ acid /ˈæsɪd/
acetone /ˈæs.ɪ.təʊn/
acidification /əˌsɪd.ɪ.fɪˈkeɪ.ʃᵊn/
acidophil /ˈæsɪdəʊˌfɪl/
acidosis /ˌæs.ɪˈdəʊ.sɪs/

506

acquainted /əˈk.weɪn.tɪd/

acquire /əˈkwaɪər/

acquired /əˌkwaɪ.əd/

acquired /əˌkwaɪ.əd/

acquisition /æk.wɪˈzɪ.ʃən/

acrocyanosis /ˌækrəʊˌsaɪəˈnəʊ.sɪs/

acromion /əˈkrəʊ.mi.ən/ pl acromia /əˈkrəʊ.mi.ə/

acyclovir /əˈsaɪkləʊvɪr/

adaptability /əˌdæp.təˈbɪl.ɪ.tɪ/

adaptation /ˌæd.əpˈteɪ.ʃən/

adapter /əˈdæp.tər/

added /ˈædɪd/

addictive /əˈdɪk.tɪv/

Addison /ædˈɪ.sən/ disease /dɪˈziːz/

addition /əˈdɪʃ.ən/

additional /əˈdɪʃ.ən.əl/

additive /ˈæd.ɪ.tɪv/

adduct /ædˈdʌkt/

adduction /əˈdəkt.ʃən/

adenoectomy /ad.en.əʊm.ek.tə.mi/

adenoid /ˈædɪˌnɔɪd/

adenoidectomy /ˈædɪˌnɔɪd.ek.tə.mi/

adenotonsillar /ˌædɪnəʊ.tɒn.sələ/

adenovirus /ˈæd.ɪ.nəʊˌvaɪə.rəs/

adequacy /ˈæd.ə.kwə.si/

adhere /ədˈhɪər/

adherence /ədˈhɪə.rənt s/

adhesion /ədˈhiː.ʒən/

adhesive /ədˈhiː.sɪv/

Adison disease /æd.ə.sən dɪˈziːz/

adjacent /əˈdʒeɪ.sənt/

adjust /əˈdʒʌst/

adjustment /əˈdʒʌst.mənt/

adjuvant /ˈædʒəvənt/

administer /ədˈmɪn.ɪ.stər/

admired /ədˈmaɪ.əd/

admission /ədˈmɪʃ.ən/

adopt /əˈdɒpt/

adrenal /əˈdriː.nəl/

adrenaline /əˈdren.əl.ɪn/

adrenocortical /ædˌriː.nəˈkɒ.ti.kəl/

adrenoleukodystrophy /əˌdriːnəʊˈluːkəʊˈdɪstrəfɪ/

adulthood /ˈæd.ʌlt.hʊd/

advance /ədˈvɑːnt s/

advanced /ədˈvɑːnst/

advancement /ədˈvɑːnsmənt/

advantage /ədˈvɑːn.tɪdʒ/

adventuresome /əd'ventʃəsəm/
adverse /'æd.vɜːs/
adversely /'æd.vɜː.sli/
advisable /əd'vaɪ.zə.bl̩/
advise /əd'vaɪz/
advocacy /'æd.və.kə.si/
advocated /'æd.və͵keɪt.ɪd/
aerochamber /eərə'tʃeɪm.bə/
aerosol /'eərə͵sɒl/
aetiology /͵iː.ti'ɒl.ə.dʒi/
affect /ə'fekt/
affection /ə'fek͵ʃən/
affective /ə'fektɪv/ **disorder** /dɪs'ɔːdə/
affluence /'æfluəns/
afford /ə'fɔːd/
agammaglobulinemia /eɪ.gam'æ.glɒb.jə.lɪ'niː.mi.ə/
aganglionic /eɪ'.gæŋ.gli.ən.ɪk/
agenesis /eɪ'dʒenɪs.ɪs/
aggravate /'æg.rə.veɪt/
agitation /͵ædʒ.ɪ'teɪ.ʃən/
agonal /'əg.əʊ.nəl/
agreeable /ə'grɪəbəl/
agreement /ə'griː.mənt/
aim /eɪm/ **at** /æt/
airtight /'eə.taɪt/
airway /'eə.weɪ/
alarm /ə'lɑːm/
albumin /'æl.bjʊ.mɪn/
alert /ə'lɜːt/
alertness /ə'lɜːt.nəs/
alienated /͵eɪl.jə'neɪ.təd/
align /ə'laɪn/
alignment /ə'laɪn.mənt/
alimentary /͵æli.men'tə.ri/
alimentation /͵æli.men'teɪ.ʃən/
alkalosis /͵ælkə'ləʊ.sɪs/
alkylating /͵ælkə'leɪtɪŋ/
allele /ə'liːl/
allergen /'æl.ə.dʒən/
allogeneic /'æləʊdʒɪ.neɪɪk/
allogeneic /'æləʊdʒɪ.neɪɪk/
alopecia /͵ə'.lə'.piː͵ʃiː.ə/
Alpers disease /al'perz dɪ'ziːz/
alpha-fetoprotein /'ælfə͵fiːtə.'prəʊ.tiːn/
alter /'ɒl.tər/
alteration /͵ɒl.tə'reɪ.ʃən/
altered /'ɒl.tərd/

alternate /ˈɒl.tə.neɪt/
alternative /ɒlˈtɜː.nə.tɪv/
alternatively /ɒlˈtɜː.nə.tɪv.li/
altitude /ˈæl.tɪ.tjuːd/
alveolus /ˌæl.viˈəʊ.ləs/ pl **alveoli**
ambient /ˈæm.bi.ənt/
ambiguous /æmˈbɪgjʊəs/
ambulatory /ˌæm.bjəˈleɪ.tər.i/
ameliorate /əˈmiː.ljəˌreɪt/
amenorrhoea /ˌeɪ.men.əˈriː.ə/
amicable /ˈæm.ɪk.ə.bəl/
aminoaciduria /əˌmiː.nəʊ.ˌæ.sɪd.ju.əˌriə/
ammonium chloride /əˈməʊ.ni.əm ˈklɔː.raɪd/
amniocentesis /ˌæm.ni.əʊ.senˈtiː.sɪs/
amniotic /ˌæm.niˈɒt.ɪk/
amphetamine /æmˈfetəˌmiːn/
amplify /ˈæm.plɪ.faɪ/
amyloidosis /ˌa.məl.ɔː.i.ˈdəʊ.sɪs/
anaemia /əˈniː.mi.ə/
anaesthesia /ˌænɪsˈθiː.zɪə/
analogue /ˈænəˌlɒg/
anaphylaxis /ˌæn.ə.fɪˈlæk.sɪs/
anchor /ˈæŋ.kər/
androgen /ænˈdrɒ.dʒən/
anencephaly /æn.en.ˈse.fə.liː/
aneurysm /ˌæn.jʊə.rɪ.zəm/
anger /ˈæŋ.gər/
angiocapillary /ˌæn.dʒiˈə kəˈpɪl.ər.i/
angioedema /ˌæn.ˌdʒɪˈdiː.m.ə/
angiofibroma /anˈdʒiː.əʊ.faɪ.brəʊˈmæ/
angiomyolipoma /anˈdʒiː.əʊ.lɪmˈfəʊmə/
angle /ˈæŋgəl/
animate /ˈæn.ɪ.mət/
annually /ˈænjʊəlɪ/
annular /ˈænjʊələr/
anomaly /əˈnɒm.ə.li/
anorectal /æn.əʊ.ˈrek.təl/
anoxia /ænˈɒk.si.ə/
ant /ænt/ mravenec
antagonise /ænˈtægəˌnaɪz/
antecedent /ˌæntɪˈsiː.dənt/
antenatal /ˌæn.tiˈneɪ.təl/
anterior /ænˈtɪə.ri.ər/
anteversion /ænˈtɪ.vɜːʃən/
anti /ˈæntɪ/
anticipate /ænˈtɪs.ɪ.peɪt/
anticoagulant /ˌæn.ti.kəʊˈæg.jʊ.lənt/

anticonvulsant /ˌæn.ti.kənˈvʌl.sənt/
antidiuretic /ˌæn.tiˌdaɪ.jʊˈret.ɪk/
antifungal /æn.tɪˈfʌŋ.gəl/
antigen /ˈæn.tɪ.dʒən/
antihistamine /ˌæn.tiˈhɪs.tə.mɪːn/
antiinflammatory /ˌæn.ti.ɪnˈflæm.ə.tər.i/
antimicrobial /ˌæn.ti.ˈmaɪ.krəʊ.baɪ.əl/
antimould /ˌæn.ti.məʊld/
antipseudomonal /ˌæntɪˌsuːˈdə.məʊˈnəl/
antipyretic /ˈæn.tɪpaɪəˈret.ɪk/
antiretroviral /æn.tiˌret.rəʊˈvaɪə.rəl/
antiserum /æn.tiˌsɪə.rəm/ pl antisera
antistreptolysin /ˌæntɪˌstreptəˈlaɪ.sɪn/
anus /ˈeɪ.nəs/
anxiety /æŋˈzaɪ.ə.ti/
aortic /eɪˈɔː.tɪk/ valve /vælv/
aplasia /əˈpleɪ.zɪə/
aplastic /əˈplæs.tɪk/
apnoea /ˈæp.ni.ə/
apparent /əˈpær.ənt/
apparently /əˈpær.ənt.li/
appeal /əˈpiːl/
appearance /əˈpɪə.rənt s/
appendage /əˈpen.dɪdʒ/
appendicitis /əˌpen.dɪˈsaɪ.tɪs/
appliance /əˈplaɪ.əns/
applicable /əˈplɪk.ə.bļ/
apply /əˈplaɪ/
appreciate /əˈpriː.ʃi.eɪt/
apprehension /ˌæp.rɪˈhen.ʃən/
apprehensive /ˌæp.rɪˈhen.sɪv/
appropriate /əˈprəʊ.pri.ət/
approval /əˈpruː.vəl/
aquagenic /ˈækwədʒənɪk/
aquarium /əˈkwe.ə.rɪ.əm/
aqueduct /ˈækwɪˌdʌkt/
arch /ɑːtʃ/
argue /ˈɑːg.juː/
argumentative /ˌɑːgjʊˈmen.tə.tɪv/
arise /əˈraɪz/ (arose, arisen)
arousability /əˈraʊz.ə.bɪl.ɪ.ti/
arousal /əˈraʊzəl/
aroused /əˈraʊzd/
arrangement /əˈreɪndʒ.mənt/
array /əˈreɪ/
arrest /əˈrest/
arrow /ˈær.əʊ/

arsenic /ˈɑː.sən.ɪk/
arterial /ɑːˈtɪə.ri.əl/
arteriosus /ɑː.tɪə.riːˈəʊ.səs/
arteriovenous /ɑː.tɪə.ri.əʊˈviː.nəs/
arthralgia /ɑːˈθræl.dʒɪ.ə/
artificial /ˌɑː.tɪˈfɪʃ.əl/
artificially /ˌɑː.tɪˌfɪʃ.iˈæl.ɪ/
Ascaris /ˈæs.kə.rɪs/
ascend /əˈsend/
ascertain /ˌæs.əˈteɪn/
ashamed /əˈʃeɪmd/
asparagus /əˈspær.ə.gəs/
aspect /ˈæs.pekt/
aspergillosis /æˌspɔːdʒɪˈləʊ.sɪs/
aspirate /ˈæs.pɪ.rət/
aspiration /ˌæspɪˈreɪʃən/
assay /aˈseɪ/
assert /əˈsɜːt/
assess /əˈses/
assign /əˈsaɪn/
assimilable /əˈsi.mə.lə.bəl/
assistance /əˈsɪs.tənt s/
assume /əˈsjuːm/
assumption /əˈsʌmp.ʃən/
assurance /əˈʃʊərəns/
assure /əˈʃɔːr/
asymmetry /eɪˈsɪm.ə.tri/
asymptomatic /əˌsɪmp.təˈmæt.ɪk/
asystolic /ˌæsɪsˈtɒlɪk/
at /æt/ **ease** /iːz/
at /æt/ **hand** /hænd/ po ruce
ataxia /əˈtæk.si.ə/
atelectasis /ˌætəˈlek.tə.sɪs/
atonic /ˌeɪˈtɒ.nik/
atopic /əˈtɒp.ɪk/ **eczema** /ˈek.sɪ .mə/
atraumatic /ˈeɪ.trə.ˈmat.ik/
atresia /əˈtriː.ʃə/
atrial /ˈeɪ.tri.əl/
atrioventricular /ˌaːtrɪ.ə.venˈtrɪk.jə.lər/
atrophy /ˈæt.rə.fi/
attachment /əˈtætʃ.mənt/
attain /əˈteɪn/
attempt /əˈtempt/
attend /əˈtend/
attendant /əˈten.dənt/
attendee /əˌtenˈdiː/
attention /əˈten.t ʃən/ **span** /spæn/

attentive /əˈten.tɪv/
attentively /əˈten.tɪv.li/
attitude /ˈæt.ɪ.tjuːd/
attract /əˈtrækt/
attributable /əˈtrɪ.bjʊt.ə.bəl/
attribute /ˈæt.rɪ.bjuːt/
audiologist /ˈɔːdɪˈ ɒ.lə.dʒist/
audiology /ˈɔːdɪˈɑː.lədʒɪ/
audiometry /ˌɔːdɪˈɒmɪtrɪ/
auditory / ˈɔːdɪtərɪ/
augmentation /ˌɔːgmenˈteɪʃən/
auricle /ˈɔːrɪkəl/
auricular /ɔːˈrɪkjʊlə/
auscultation /ˌɔː.skəlˈteɪʃən/
authoritarian /ɔːˌθɒrɪˈteərɪən/
authoritative /ɔːˈθɒrɪtətɪv/
autoimmune /ˈɔː.təʊ.ɪˈmjuːn/
autoinjector /ˌɔː.təʊ.ɪnˈɪndʒektˀr/
autologous /ɔːˈtɒl.ə.gəs/
autosome /ˈɔː.tə.ˌsəʊm/
availability /əˌveɪ.ləˈbɪl.ɪ.ti/
avascular /əˈvæskjʊlə/
average /ˈæv.ər.ɪdʒ/
aversion /əˈvɜːʃən/
avoid /əˈvɔɪd/
avoidance /əˈvɔɪ.dəns/
awake /əˈweɪk/
awaken /əˈweɪ.kən/
awareness /əˈweə.nəs/
away /əˈweɪ/
awkward /ˈɔː.kwəd/
axilla /ækˈsɪl.ə/ pl axillae
axillary /æˈksɪl.ər.i/
azotemic /ˌaɪ.zəʊ.tiː.mik/

B
babble /ˈbæbəl/
Babinski's /bəˈbin.skiː z/ reflex /ˈriː.fleks/
bacteriuria /bækˈtɪə.riˈjʊə.ri.ə/
balance /ˈbæl.əns/
balanitis /ˌbal.ə.ˈnaɪ.təs/
balanoposthitis /ˌbæləˈnəʊ.pɒsˈθaɪ.tɪs/
Balloon /bəˈluːn/
ban /bæn/
band /bænd/
bandage /ˈbæn.dɪdʒ/
bang /bæŋ/
bar /bɑː/

bark /bɑːk/
barrel /ˈbær.əl/
Bartonella henselae /bɑhr,təʊ.nelˈæ henˈse.liː/
bartonellosis /ˈbɑːtᵊn.eəʊ.sɪs/
bat /bæt/
battery /ˈbæt.ər.i/
beak /biːk/
beam /biːm/
Beckwith /ˈbek.wəth/ **syndrome** /ˈsɪn.drəʊm/
bedbug /ˈbedˌbʌg/
bedcover /ˈbed.ˌkə.vər/
bed-wetting /ˈbedˌwet.iŋ/
beef /biːf/
belch /beltʃ/
belief /bɪˈliːf/
bell /bel/
Bell palsy /ˈpɔːl.zi/
belligerent /bəˈlɪdʒ.ər.ənt/
bellows /ˈbeləʊz/
belt /belt/
bending /bend.ɪŋ/
benign /bɪˈnaɪn/
benzylpenicillin /ben.zɪlˌpen.əˈsɪl.ɪn/
bereavement /bɪˈriːvmənt/
beta /ˈbiː.tə/ **blockers** /blɒk.ərs/
beverage /ˈbev.ər.ɪdʒ/
beware /bɪˈweə/
bewilderment /bɪˈwɪldəmənt/
biased /ˈbaɪ.əst/
bifurcate /ˈbaɪ.fə.keɪt/
bilateral /baɪˈlæt.ər.əl/
bile /baɪl/
bile /baɪl/ **duct** /dʌkt/
biliary /ˈbɪl.i.ər.i/
bilirubin /ˌbɪl.ɪˈruː.bɪn/
binge /bɪndʒ/
biosynthesis /ˌbaɪ.əʊ.ˈsɪn.θə.sɪs/
biphasic /baɪˈfeɪz.ɪk/
bipolar disorder /baɪˈpəʊ.lə dɪˌsɔː.dər/
birthmark /ˈbɜːθˌmɑːk/
biting /ˈbaɪ.tɪŋ/
bladder /ˈblæd.ər/
blade /bleɪd/
blame /bleɪm/
blanch /blɑːntʃ/
blank /blæŋk/
blanket /ˈblæŋ.kɪt/

blast /ˌblæst/ **cell** /sel/
blepharitis /ˌblef.əˈraɪ.təs/
blind /blaɪnd/
blindfold /ˈblaɪnd.fəʊld/
blindness /ˈblaɪnd.nɪs/
blink /blɪŋk/
blister /ˈblɪs.tər/
blockage /ˈblɒk.ɪdʒ/
blood /blʌd/ **count** /kaʊnt/
blood /blʌd/ **vessel** /ˈves.əl/
blood-stained /blʌd steɪnd/
blotchy /blɒtʃ.i/
Blount /blunt/ **disease** /dɪˈziːz/
blueberry /ˈbluːbərɪ/
blunt / blʌnt/
blurred /blɜːd/
blush /blʌʃ/
boast /bəʊst/
bob /bɒb/
boggy /ˈbɒgɪ/
bolus /bəʊ.ləs/
bond /bɒnd/
bone /bəʊn/ **marrow** /ˈmær.əʊ/
booster /ˈbuː.stər/
border /bɔː.dər/
borderline /ˈbɔːr.dər.laɪ n/ **personality** /ˌpɜː.sənˈæl.ə.ti/ **disorder BPD** /dɪsˈɔːdə/
Bordetella /bəʊ.də.tel.æ/ *pertussis* /pəˈtʌs.ɪs/
bored /bɔːd/
boredom /ˈbɔːdəm/
bossy /ˈbɒsɪ/
bother /ˈbɒðə/
botulism /ˈbɒt.jʊ.lɪ.zəm/
bounce /baʊns/
boundary /ˈbaʊn.dər.i/
bout /baʊt/
bowel /ˈbaʊ.əl/ **habit** /ˈhæbɪt/
bowel /ˈbaʊ.əl/ **movement** /ˈmuː.v.mənt/
bowing /ˈbəʊɪŋ/
bowling /ˈbəʊlɪŋ/
brace /breɪs/
brachial /ˈbreɪ.ki.əl/
bracing /ˈbreɪ.sɪŋ/
bradycardia /ˌbræd.ɪˈkaːdi.ə/
brainstem /ˈbreɪn.stem/
bran /bræn/
branch /brɑːntʃ/
brand /brænd/

brassy /ˈbrɑː.si/ **cough** /kɒf/
Brazelton /breɪˈzel.tɒn/ **scale** /ˈskeɪl/
breakage /ˈbreɪ.kɪdʒ/
breakdown /ˈbreɪk.daʊn/
breathless /ˈbreθ.lɪs/
breathlessness /ˈbreθlɪs.nɪs/
breech /briːtʃ/
breech /briːtʃ/ **delivery** /dɪˈlɪv.ər.i/
bridge /brɪdʒ/
bring /brɪŋ/ **up** /ʌp/
broad /brɔːd/
broccoli /ˈbrɒk.əl.i/
broil /brɔɪl/
bronchial /ˈbrɒŋ.ki.əl/
bronchiectasis /ˌbrɒŋ.kɪˈɛktə.sɪs/
bronchiolitis /ˈbrɒŋ.ki.əˈla.ɪ.tɪs/
bronchitis /brɒŋˈkaɪ.tɪs/
bronchodilator /ˈbrɒŋ.kə.daɪˈleɪ.tər/
bronchopulmonary /ˈbrɒŋ.kəˈpʊl.mə.ner.i/
bronchoscopy /brɒnˈkɒ.skə.piː/
bronchostenosis /ˌbrɒŋ.kəʊ.steˈnəʊ.sɪs/
bronchovesicular /ˈbrɒŋ.kə.vəˈsɪk.jə.lər/
bronchus /ˈbrɒŋ.kəs/ pl **bronchi** /ˈbrɒŋ.kaɪ/
brow /braʊ/
Brucella /bruːsɪˈlləo/
Brudzinski sign /bruː.dʒinˈskiː saɪn/
bruising /ˈbruː.zɪŋ/
bruit /bruːt/
Brussels /ˈbrʌsəlz/ **sprouts** /spraʊts/
buccal /ˈbʌk.əl/
bud /bʌd/
buffer /ˈbʌf.ər/
bug /bʌg/ **bursting** /ˈbɜːstɪŋ/
bulb /bʌlb/ **syringe** /sɪˈrɪndʒ/
bulging /ˈbʌl.dʒɪŋ/
bulky /ˈbʌl.ki/
bulla /bulˈæ/ pl. **bullae** /iː/
bulletproof /ˈbʊl.ɪt.pruːf/
bullous /ˈbʊ.ləs/
bullying /ˈbʊlɪɪŋ/
bump /ˈbʌmp/
bumper /ˈbʌm.pər/
bunk /bʌŋk/
burette /bjʊˈret/
Burkholderia cepacia /burk.hol.derˈiː.æ siːpeɪˈʃiː.æ/
burn /bɜːn/
burrow /ˈbʌrəʊ/

butterfly /ˈbʌt.ə.flaɪ/
buttock /ˈbʌt.ək/
bypass /ˈbaɪ.pɑːs/

C
caesarean section /sɪˌzeə.ri.ənˈsek.ʃən/
calcification /ˌkæl.sɪ.fɪˈkeɪ.ʃən/
calcium /ˈkæl.si.əm/ **gluconate** /ˈgluː.kə.ˌneɪt/
calibrate /ˈkælɪˌbreɪt/
caliper /ˈkælɪpə/
callus /ˈkæl.əs/
calming /kɑːm.ɪŋ/
calyx pl /ˈkeɪ.lɪks/ **calyces**
Candida /ˈkændɪdə/
candidiasis /ˌkan.də.ˈdaɪ.ə.səs/ pl. **candidiases** /ˌkan.də.ˈdaɪ.ə.ˌsiːz/
canister /ˈkæn.ɪ.stər/
cannabis /ˈkænəbɪs/
cannula /ˈkæn.jʊ.lə/ pl **cannulae**
canthus, /ˈkan.θəs/ pl **canthi** /ˈkan.ˌθaɪ/
cap /kæp/
capillary /kəˈpɪl.ər.i/ **refill** /ˈriː.fɪl/
capital /ˈkæpɪtəl/
capsule /ˈkæp.sjuːl/
caput /ˈkeɪp.ˌuːt/
carbon /ˈkɑː.bən/ **dioxide** /daɪˈɒk.saɪd/
carbon monoxide /ˌkɑː.bən.məˈnɒk.saɪd/
carcinoma /ˌkɑːsɪˈnəʊmə/
cardiomegaly /ˌkɑː.r.diəˈmeg.ə.laɪ/
carditis /kɑːˈdaɪ.tɪs/
caregiver /ˈkeəˌgɪv.ər/
caregiving /ˈkeəˌgɪvɪŋ/
carnitine /karˈni.tiːn/
carpeting /ˈkɑː.pɪ.tɪŋ/
carriage /ˈkær.ɪdʒ/
carrier /ˈkær.i.ər/
carry /ˈkær.i/ **out** /aʊt/
cartilage /ˈkɑː.təl.ɪdʒ/
cartridge /ˈkɑː.trɪdʒ/
case /keɪs/
casein /ˈkeɪ.ˌsiːn/
cashews /ˈkæʃuː/
cast /kɑːst/
catabolic /ˌkætəˈbɒl.ɪk/
catabolism /kə.ˈta.bə.ˌli.zəm/
catering /ˈkeɪtərɪŋ/
catheter /ˈkæθ.ɪ.tər/
Caucasian /kɔːˈkeɪ.ʒən/

causal /ˈkɔːzəl/
causative /ˈkɔː.zə.tɪv/
cautiously /ˈkɔː.ʃəs.li/
cavernous /ˈkævənəs/
cease /siːs/
celiac /ˈsiː.liː.ˌak/
cell /sel/
cellar /ˈsel.ər/
cellular /ˈsel.jʊ.lər/
cement /sɪˈment/
central /ˈsen.trəl/
central /ˈsen.trəl/ **venous** /ˈviː.nəs/ **line** /laɪn/
cephalalgia /ˌsefəˈlældʒɪə/
cephalhaematoma /ˌsefəlˌhiːməˈtəʊmə/
cereal /ˈsɪə.ri.əl/
cerebellar /ˌser.ə.ˈbe.lər/
cerebellitis /serˈe.bel.aɪˈtɪs/
cerebral /ˈser.ɪ.brəl/
cerebral /ˈser.ɪ.brəl/ **artery** /ˈɑː.təri/
cerebral /ˈser.ɪ.brəl/ **infarction** /ɪnˈfɑːk.ʃən/
cerebrospinal /ˌser.əbrəˈspaɪ.nəl/
ceroid /ˈsɪərəɪd/
ceruloplasmin /seˌruˈləʊ.plazˈmin/
cessation /sesˈeɪʃən/
chalazion /kəˈleɪ.ziː.ən/ pl **chalazia** /ziːə/
chalky-white /ˈtʃɔːkɪ waɪt/
challenge /ˈtʃæl.ɪndʒ/
chaotic /keɪˈɒtɪk/
chaperone /ˈʃæp.ə.rəʊn/
chart /tʃɑːt/
check /tʃek/
checklist /ˈtʃek.lɪst/
cheesecloth /ˈtʃiːzˌklɒθ/
chemoreceptor /ˌkiː.məʊ.rɪˈsep.tər/
chest /tʃest/
chest piece /tʃest.piːs/
chew /tʃuː/
Cheyne-Stokes /cheɪn.iː.ˌstəʊks/ **respirations** /ˌrespəˈreɪʃənz/
Chiary /kiːahrˈiː/ **syndrome** /ˈsɪndrəʊm/
chickenpox /ˈtʃɪk.ɪn.pɒks/
chief /tʃif/
chignon /ˈʃiːnjɒn/
child /tʃaɪld/ **rearing** /rɪər.ɪŋ/
childbearing /ˈtʃaɪldˌbeə.rɪŋ/
chill /tʃɪl/
chin-lift /tʃɪn lɪft/
chipped /ˈtʃɪpt/

chlamydia /kləm.iˈde.ə/ pl **chlamydiae**
choana /ˈkəʊ.ə.nə/
choke /tʃəʊk/
cholangitis /kəˈlændʒaɪ.tɪs/
cholestasis /ˈkɒləˈsteɪ.sɪs/
cholinergic /ˌkəʊlɪˈnɜːdʒɪk/
chorea /koˈrɪə/
chores /tʃɔːz/
chorionic /ˈkɔːr.ɪ.ən.ɪk/
chromosome /ˈkrəʊmə.səʊm/
chux /tʃʌks/
ciliary /ˈsɪ.lɪː.ˌər.iː/
circuit /ˈsɜː.kɪt/
circum- /ˈsɜː.kəm/
circumcision /ˌsɜː.kəmˈsɪ.ʒən/
circumference /səˈkʌm.fər.əns/
circumferential /səˈkʌm.fər.ən.ʃəl/
circumscribe /ˌsɜː.kəmˈskraɪb/
citrate /ˈsaɪ.treɪt/
clammy /ˈklæm.i/
clarify /ˈklær.ɪ.faɪ/
clarity /ˈklær.ɪ.ti/
clasp /klɑːsp/
clavicle /ˈklæv.ɪ.kl̩/
clearance /klɪər.əns/
clearing /ˈklɪə.rɪŋ/
cleft /kleft/ **lip** /lɪp/
cleft /kleft/ **palate** /ˈpæl.ət/
clergy /ˈklɜː.dʒɪ/
cling /klɪŋ/
cling film /ˈklɪŋ.fɪlm/
clonic /ˈkləʊ.nɪk/
closely /ˈkləʊ.sli/
closeness /kləʊsnɪs/
closet /ˈklɒzɪt/
closure /ˈkləʊ.ʒə/
cloth /klɒθ/
cloudy /ˈklaʊ.di/
club foot /klʌb.fʊt/
clue /kluː/
clumsiness /ˈklʌm.zi.nəs/
clunk /klʌŋk/
cluster headache /ˈklʌs.tərˌhed.eɪk/
coagulation /kəʊˈæg.jʊ.leɪ.ʃən/
coagulopathy /kəʊˌæg.juˈlɒ.pə.θi/
coalition /ˌkəʊəˈlɪʃən/
coarse /kɔːs/

coated /ˈkəʊ.tɪd/
cocaine /kəˈkeɪn/
cockroach /ˈkɒkˌrəʊtʃ/
co-exist /ˌkəʊɪgˈzɪst/
coexistent /ˌkəʊɪgˈzɪstənt/
cognition /kɒgˈnɪʃ.ən/
cognitive /ˈkɒg.nɪ.tɪv/
cohesive /kəʊˈhiːsɪv/
coin /kɔɪn/
coincide /ˌkəʊɪnˈsaɪd/
colic /ˈkɒl.ɪk/
colicky /ˈkɒl.ɪ.ki/
colitis /kəˈlɪ.tɪs/
collaboration /kəˌlæb.əˈreɪʃən/
collateral /kəˈlæt.ər.əl/
colloidal /ˈkɒ.lɒ.ɪd.əl/
colloquial /kəˈləʊkwɪəl/
coloboma /ˌkə.l.əˈbəʊ.mə/
colon /ˈkəʊ.lɒn/
coma /ˈkəʊ.mə/
comb /koʊm/
comedo /ˈkɑː.mə.ˌdəʊ/ pl comedones /niːz/
comedon /ˈkʌm.daʊn/
comfort /ˈkʌm.fət/
comforting /ˈkʌm.fə.tɪŋ/
commence /kəˈmens/
comment /ˈkɒm.ent/
commercial /kəˈmɜːʃəl/
commitment /kəˈmɪt.mənt/
committed /kəˈmɪ.tɪd/
compare /kəmˈpeər/
comparison /kəmˈpær.ɪ.sən/
compartment /kəmˈpɑːt.mənt/
compatibility /kəmˌpætəˈbɪlɪtɪ/
compatible /kəmˈpæt.ɪ.bl̩/
compensate /ˈkɒm.pən.seɪt/
compete /kəmˈpiːt/
competence /ˈkɒm.pɪ.tənt s/
complaint /kəmˈpleɪnt/
complement /ˈkɒm.plɪ.ment/
complex /kɒm.pleks/
compliance /kəmˈplaɪ.ənt s/
complimentary /ˌkɒmplɪˈmen.tə.rɪ/
comply /kəmˈplaɪ/ with /wɪð/
composition /ˌkɒm.pəˈzɪʃ.ən/
comprehend /ˌkɒm.prɪˈhend/
comprehensive /ˌkɒm.prɪˈhen.sɪv/

compress /kəmˈpres/
compression /kɒm.ˈpreʃˌen/
comprise /kəmˈpraɪz/
compromise /ˈkɒmprəˌmaɪz/
concave /ˈkɒnkeɪv/
conceal /kənˈsiːl/
concentration /ˌkɒn.sənˈtreɪ.ʃən/
concept /ˈkɒn.sept/
conception /kənˈsep.ʃən/
concern /kənˈsɜːn/
conclusion /kənˈkluː.ˌʒən/
concomitant /kənˈkɒ.mɪ.tənt/
concrete /ˈkɒŋ.kriːt/
condom /ˈkɒn.dɒm/
conduct /kənˈdʌkt/
conductive /kənˈdʌk.tɪv/
confident /ˈkɒn.fɪ.dənt/
confidential /ˌkɒn.fɪˈden.tʃəl/
confidentiality /ˌkɒn.fɪ.den.tʃiˈæl.ɪ.ti/
configuration /kənˌfɪg.əˈreɪ.ʃən/
confined /kənˈfaɪnd/
confirmatory /kənˈfɜː.mə.tər.i/
confluent /kənˈfluː.ənt/
conform /kənˈfɔːm/
conformity /kənˈfɔːm.ɪ.tɪ/
confrontation /ˌkɒnfrʌnˈteɪʃən/
confused /kənˈfjuːzd/
confusion /kənˈfjuː.ʒən/
congenital /kənˈdʒen.ɪ.təl/
congruent /ˈkɒŋgrʊənt/
conization /kəʊnɪ.zəɪˈʃən/
conjugate /kənˈdʒʌ.gət/
conjugated /ˈkɒn.dʒə.geɪt.ɪd/
conjunction /kənˈdʒʌŋk.ʃən/
conjunctiva /ˌkɒn.dʒʌŋkˈtaɪ.və/ pl **conjunctivae**
conjunctival /ˌkɒn.dʒʌŋkˈtaɪ.vəl/ **sac** /sæk/
conjunctivitis /kənˌdʒʌŋk.tɪˈvaɪ.tɪs/
connective tissue /kəˌnek.tɪvˈtɪʃ.uː/
consciousness /ˈkɒn.ʃəs.nəs/
consent /kənˈsent/
consequence /ˈkɒn.sɪ.kwəns/
consequential /ˌkɒnsɪˈkwen.ʃəl/
considerable /kənˈsɪd.ər.ə.bļ/
consistency /kənˈsɪs.tənt .si/
consistent /kənˈsɪs.tənt/ **with** /wɪð/
consistently /kənˈsɪs.tənt.li/
consolability /kənˈsəʊl.əˈbɪlɪtɪ/

520

consonant /ˈkɒnsənənt/
constipation /ˌkɒnt.stɪˈpeɪ.ʃən/
constitute /ˈkɒn.stɪ.tjuːt/
constraint /kənˈstreɪnt/
constrict /kənˈstrɪkt/
constriction /kənˈstrɪk.ʃən/
contagiosum /kənˈteɪdʒɪəsəm/
contagious /kənˈteɪ.dʒəs/
contamination /kənˌtæm.ɪˈneɪ.ʃən/
contemporary /kənˈtem.prə.rɪ/
continuation /kənˌtɪnjʊˈeɪʃən/
continue /kənˈtɪn.juː/
continuous /kənˈtɪn.ju.əs/
contour /ˈkɒn.tɔːr/
contraception /ˌkɒntrəˈsepʃən/
contraction /kənˈtræk.ʃən/
contraindicate /ˌkɒn.trəˈɪn.dɪ.keɪt/
contraindication /ˌkɒn.trəˌɪn.dɪˈkeɪ.ʃən/
contralateral /ˌkɒn.trəˈlæt.ər.əl/
contribute /kənˈtrɪb.juːt/
controversy /ˈkɒntrəˌvɜːsɪ/
convalescence /ˌkɒn.vəˈles.əns/
convalescent /ˌkɒnvəˈles.ənt/
convection /kənˈvek.ʃən/
conventional /kənˈvent.ʃən.əl/
conversely /kɒnˈvɜːslɪ/
conversion /kənˈvɔː.ʃən/
convince /kənˈvɪns/
convulsion /kənˈvʌl.ʃən/
convulsive /kənˈvʌl.sɪv/
coo /kuː/
cool /kuːl/
cooling /ˈkuː.lɪŋ/
cope /kəʊp/
coping /kəʊp.ɪŋ/
copper /ˈkɒp.ər/
cord /kɔːd/
cordial /ˈkɔːdɪəl/
core /kɔːr/
cornea /ˈkɔːnɪə/ pl **corneae**
corpora /ˈkɔːpər.ə/ **carvenosa** /ˈkæv.ən.əʊs ə/ **clitoridis** /klɪˈtɒr.ɪ.dɪs/
corporal /ˈkɔːpər.əl/
corpus /ˈkɔː.pəs/ pl **corpora** /ˈkɔː.pər.ə/
correct /kəˈrekt/
correctable /kəˈrekt.ə.bļ/
correlate /ˈkɒrɪˌleɪt/
corticospinal /ˌkɔːtɪkəʊˈspaɪnəl/

corticosteroid /ˌkɔːtɪ.kəʊ'stɪə.rɔɪd/

coryza /kə'raɪ.zə/

costal /'kɒs.təl/

cotton /'kɒt.ən/

coughing /kɒf.ɪŋ/

counselling /'kaʊnt.səl.ɪŋ/

counterproductive /ˌkaʊn.tə.prə'dʌk.tɪv/

couple /'kʌp.l̩/

course /kɔːs/

court /kɔːt/

cover /'kʌv.ə/

coverage /'kʌv.ər.ɪdʒ/

cracked /krækt/

crackle /'kræk.l̩/

cradle /'kreɪ.dəl/ **cap** /'kap/

cramp /kræmp/

cranial /'kreɪ.ni.əl/

craniopharyngioma /'kreɪ.ni.əʊ.fəˌrin.dʒiː.ˈəʊ.mə/

cranky /'kræŋkɪ/

crawl /krɔːl/

crayon /'kreɪən/

create /kriː'eɪt/

creep /kriːp/

cremaster /ˌkriːməs'ter/ **muscle** /'mʌs.l̩/

cremasteric /ˌkriːməs'ter.ɪk/

crepitation /ˌkrep.ɪ'teɪˌʃən/

crest /krest/

crippling /'krɪp.lɪŋ/

crop /krɒp/

cross /krɒs/

cross-country /'krɒsˌkʌntrɪ/ **running** /'rʌnɪŋ/

cross-eyed /krɒs. aɪd/

crossing /'krɒs.ɪŋ/

cross-match /krɒs mætʃ/

cross-section /krɒs.'sekˌʃən/

croup /kruːp/

crucial /'kruːˌʃəl/

crude /kruːd/

cruel /'kruːəl/

cruelty /'kruːəltɪ/

crumb /krʌm/

crush /krʌʃ/

crust /krʌst/

crusted /'krʌs.tɪd/

crutch /krʌtʃ/

cube /kjuːb/

cubital /kjuːbət.əl/

cuddle /ˈkʌd.l̩/
cue /kjuː/
cuff /kʌf/
culminate /ˈkʌl.mɪ.neɪt/
cumulative /ˈkjuː.mjʊ.lə.tɪv/
cup /kʌp/
curative /ˈkjʊərətɪv/
curd /kɜːd/
curiosity /ˌkjʊərɪˈɒsɪtɪ/
curvature /ˈkɜː.və.tʃər/
cushion /ˈkʊʃ.ən/
cutaneous /kjuːˈteɪ.ni.əs/
cutting /ˈkʌt.ɪŋ/
cyanosis /ˌsaɪəˈnəʊ.sɪs/
cyberbullying /ˈsaɪbə ˈbʊlɪɪŋ/
cyst /sɪst/
cystic fibrosis /ˌsɪs.tɪk.faɪˈbrəʊ.sɪs/
cystine /sɪs.tɪn/
cystinosis /ˈsɪstɪ.nəʊ.sɪs/
cystitis /sɪˈstaɪ.tɪs/
cytomegalovirus /ˌsaɪ.təʊ.ˌmeg.ə.lə.ˈvaɪ.rəs/
cytopathy /ˌsaɪtɒpəθɪ/
cytotoxic /ˌsaɪ.təʊˈtɒk.sɪk/

D
dacryocystitis /ˈdæk.ˌkrɪəʊ.sɪs.taɪ.tis/
dactylitis /ˈdæktɪ.laɪ.tɪs/
dam /dæm/
damp /dæmp/
dangerously /ˈdeɪn.dʒər.əs.li/
darkness /ˈdɑːknɪs/
dart /dɑːt/
day-care /ˈdeɪˌkeə/
daydream /ˈdeɪ.driːm/
deafness /ˈdef.nəs/
deal /dɪəl/ **with** /wɪð/
debilitate /dɪˈbɪl.ɪ.teɪt/
deceive /dɪˈsiːv/
deceleration /ˌdiːˌseləˈreɪ.ʃən/
deceptively /dɪˈseptɪvlɪ/
decision /dɪˈsɪʒ.ən/
decline /dɪˈklaɪn/
decompression /ˌdi.kəmˈpre.ʃən/
decrease /dɪˈkriːs/
deep /diːp/
defecate /ˈdef.ə.keɪt/
defective /dɪˈfek.tɪv/

defence /dɪˈfent s/
defiance /dɪˈfaɪəns/
defiant /dɪˈfaɪənt/
deficiency /dɪˈfɪʃ.ən.si/
deficit /ˈdef.ɪ.sɪt/
deformity /dɪˈfɔː.mɪ.ti/
degenerative /dɪˈdʒen.ər.ə.tɪv/
dehumidifier /ˌdiː.hjuːˈmɪd.ɪ.faɪ.ər/
delay / dɪˈleɪ/
deliberate /dɪˈlɪb.ər.ət/
deliberately /dɪˈlɪb.ər.ət.li/
delirious /dɪˈlɪr.ɪəs/
delirium /dɪˈlɪrɪ.əm/
delivery /dɪˈlɪv.ər.i/
delusional /dɪˈluː.ʒən.əl/
demanding /dɪˈmɑːn.dɪŋ/
dementia /dɪˈmenʃə/
dendritic /denˈdrɪ.tɪk/
dengue /ˈdeŋgɪ/ fever /ˈfiːvə/
denial /dɪˈnaɪ.əl/
dense /dens/
dental /ˈden.təl/
dentistry /ˈdentɪstrɪ/
dentition /denˈtɪʃ.ən/
denude /dɪˈnjuːd/
deny /dɪˈnaɪ/
deodorizer /diːˈəʊdəˌraɪzə/
depart /dɪˈpɑːt/
dependence /dɪˈpen.dənt s/
dependency /dɪˈpen.dənt .si/
dependent /dɪˈpen.dənt/
depigmented /deˈpɪg.mənt.ɪd/
depleted /dɪˈpliː.tɪd/
depletion /dɪˈpliː.ʃən/
deposition /ˌdep.əˈzɪʃ.ən/
depress /dɪˈpres/
depressant /dɪˈpres.ənt/
depressed /dɪˈprest/
deprivation /ˌdep.rɪˈveɪ.ʃən/
depth /depθ/
derangement /dɪˈreɪndʒd.mənt/
derivative /dɪˈrɪvətɪv/
dermatitis /ˌdɜːməˈtaɪ.tɪs/
dermatomyositis /ˌdər.mə.təʊˌmaɪ.əˈsaɪ.təs/
dermatophyte /ˌdər.ˈma.təˌfaɪt/
dermis /ˈdɜː.mɪs/
desaturation /dɪˈsætʃərˈeɪʃən/

desirable /dɪˈzaɪə.rə.bl̩/
desire /dɪˈzaɪər/
despair /dɪˈspeər/
desquamate /ˈdeskwəˈmeɪt/
desquamation /ˌdeskwəˈmeɪ.ʃən/
destroy /dɪˈstrɔɪ/
destruction /dɪˈstrʌk.ʃən/
detached /dɪˈtætʃt/
detect /dɪˈtekt/
detection /dɪˈtek.ʃən/
detergent /dɪˈtɜː.dʒənt/
deteriorate /dɪˈtɪə.ri.ə.reɪt/
deterioration /dɪˌtɪə.ri.əˈreɪ.ʃən/
determinant /dɪˈtɜː.mɪ.nənt/
determine /dɪˈtɜː.mɪn/
deterrant /dɪˈter.ənt/
detoxification /diːˌtɒksəfɪˈkeɪʃən/
detrimental /ˌdet.rɪˈmen.təl/
detrusor /dɪˈtruːzə/
devastating /ˈdev.ə.steɪ.tɪŋ/
deviation /ˌdiːvɪˈeɪʃən/
dexterity /dekˈster.ə.ti/
dextrose /ˈdek.strəʊs/
diabetes /ˌdaɪəˈbiː.ti:z/ **insipidus** /ɪn.sɪpˈɪ.dəs/
diamine /ˌdɪˈeɪ.miːn/
diamond /ˈdaɪəmənd/
Diamond-Blackfan anaemia /ˈdaɪəmənd blakˈfan əˈniːmi.ə/
diaper /ˈdaɪəpə/
diaper /ˈdaɪəpə/ **rash** /ræʃ/
diaphoresis /ˌdaɪ.ə.fəˈriː.sɪs/
diaphragm /ˈdaɪ.ə.fræm/
diaphragmatic /ˌdaɪə.frægˈmæt.ɪk/
diathesis /daɪˈæθɪsɪs/
dictatorial /ˌdɪktəˈtɔːrɪəl/
differ /ˈdɪf.ər/
differential /ˌdɪf.əˈren.tʃəl/
differentiate /ˌdɪfəˈrenʃieɪt/
differentiation /ˌdɪf.ər.en.ʃiˈeɪ.ʃən/
diffuse /dɪˈfjuːz/
digestion /daɪˈdʒes.tʃən/
digit /ˈdɪdʒ.ɪt/
dignity /ˈdɪg.nɪ.ti/
dilatation /ˌdɪl.əˈteɪ.ʃən/
dilute /daɪˈluːt/
dimness /ˈdim.nəs/
dip /dɪp/
diphtheria /dɪfˈθəɪr.i.ə/

dipstick /ˈdɪpˌstɪk/
disability /ˌdɪs.əˈbɪl.ɪ.ti/
disadvantage /ˌdɪs.ədˈvɑːn.tɪdʒ/
disagree /ˌdɪs.əˈgriː/
disappear /ˌdɪs.əˈpɪər/
disapproval /ˌdɪs.əˈpruː.vəl/
disaster /dɪˈzɑː.stər/
discard /dɪˈskɑːd/
discharge /dɪsˈtʃɑːdʒ/
discipline /ˈdɪsɪplɪn/
discitis /dɪsˈkaɪ.tɪs/
disclose /dɪsˈkləʊz/
discolouration /dɪsˌkʌləˈreɪʃən/
disconnected /ˌdɪs.kəˈnek.tɪd/
discord /ˈdɪs.kɔːd/
discordant /dɪsˈkɔːdənt/
discouragement /dɪˈskʌr.ɪdʒ.mənt/
discovery /dɪˈskʌvəri/
discredit /dɪsˈkredɪt/
discrete /dɪsˈkriːt/
discrimination /dɪˌskrɪm.ɪˈneɪ.ʃən/
disengage /ˌdɪsɪnˈgeɪdʒ/
disfigure /dɪsˈfɪgə/
disgust /dɪsˈgʌst/
dishormonogenesis /dɪs hɔːˈməʊ.nəˈdʒen.ə.sɪs/
disinterested /dɪˈsɪn.trə.stɪd/
dislike /dɪsˈlaɪk/
dislocation /ˌdɪs.ləˈkeɪ.ʃən/
disobedience /ˌdɪsəˈbiː.dɪəns/
disobey /ˌdɪsəˈbeɪ/
disorder /dɪˈsɔː.dər/
displaced /dɪˈspleɪst/
displasia /dɪsˈpleɪzɪə/
disposable /dɪˈspəʊ.zə.bəl/
disrupt /dɪsˈrʌpt/
disruption /dɪsˈrʌp.ʃən/
disseminate /dɪˈsem.ɪ.neɪt/
disseminated /dɪˈsem.ɪ.neɪt.ɪd/
dissemination /dɪˌsem.əˈneɪ.ʃən/
dissociative /dɪˈsəʊ.ʃi.eɪt.ɪv/
dissolve /dɪˈzɒlv/
distal /ˈdɪs.təl/
distention /dɪˈsten.ʃən/
distort /dɪˈstɔːt/
distortion /dɪ ˈstɔː.ʃən/
distract /dɪˈs.trækt/
distractibility /dɪˌstræktəˈbɪl.ə.ti/

distraught /dɪˈstrɔːt/
disturb /dɪˈstɜːb/
disturbance /dɪˈstɜː.bəns/
diuretic /ˌdaɪ.jʊˈret.ɪk/
diversity /daɪˈvɜː.sɪ.ti/
diverticulum /ˌdaɪ.vəˌtɪk.jʊ.ləm/ pl **diverticula**
divorce /dɪˈvɔːs/
dizziness /ˈdɪz.ɪ.nəs/
dizzy /ˈdɪzɪ/
DNAse B, deoxyribonuclease / diːˌɒksɪˌraɪbəʊˈnjuːklɪeɪz/
doll /dɒl/
dominant /ˈdɒm.ɪ.nənt/
dominate /ˈdɒmɪˌneɪt/
donor /ˈdəʊ.nər/
doom /duːm/
dorsiflexion /ˌdɔːsɪˈflekʃən/
dorsum /ˈdɔː.səm/ pl **dorsa**
dosage /ˈdəʊ.sɪdʒ/
double /ˈdʌb.l̩/
double-bunk /ˈdʌbəl bʌŋk/
downgrade /ˈdaʊn.ˌɡreɪd/
drain /dreɪn/
drainage /ˈdreɪ.nɪdʒ/
draught /drɑːft/
drawing /ˈdrɔː.ɪŋ/
dreaming /driːmɪŋ/
dressing /ˈdres.ɪŋ/
drip /drɪp/
drool /druːl/
drop /drɒp/
droplet /ˈdrɒp.lət/
drowning /ˈdraʊn.ɪŋ/
drowsiness /ˈdraʊ.zɪ.nəs/
dryness /draɪnɪs/
Duchenne /dɑːˈʃen/ **muscular** /ˈmə.skjə.lər/ **dystrophy** /ˈdi.strə.fiː/
duct /dʌkt/
ductus arteriosus /ˈdək.təs.ɑːrˌtir.iːˈəʊ.səs/
dull /dʌl/
dullness /ˈdʌl.nəs/
durable /ˈdjʊərəbəl/
dural /ˈdjʊə.rəl/
dwelling /ˈdwel.ɪŋ/
dye /daɪ/
dysaesthesia /dɪsəsˈθiːzɪə/
dysentery /ˈdɪs.ənˌter.i/
dysfunction /dɪsˈfʌŋk.ʃən/
dysgenesis /ˌdis.ˈdʒe.nə.səs/

dyskinesia /ˌdɪs.kaɪˈniː.zɪ.ə/
dysmorphia /dɪsˈmɔːfɪə/
dysmorphic /dis.ˈmɔːr.fik/
dysmotility /dɪsˈməʊ.tɪl.ɪ.tɪ/
dysphagia /dɪsˈfeɪ.dʒi.ə/
dysplasia /dɪsˈpleɪ.zi.ə/
dyspnoea /dɪs.pniː.ə/
dystonia /dɪsˈtəʊnɪə/
dystrophia /dɪˈstrəʊfɪə/
dystrophy /ˈdɪs.trə.fi/
dysuria /dɪˈsju.ə.riə/

E

earache /ˈɪə.reɪk/
eardrum /ˈɪə.drʌm/
ease /iːz/
ecchymosis /ˌeki.ˈməʊ.sɪs/ pl **ecchymoses** /ˌe.ki.ˈməʊ.ˌsiːz/
ecstasy /ˈekstəsɪ/
ectodermal /ˌektəʊˈdɜːməl/
ectopic /ekˌtɒp.ɪk/
eczema /ˈek.sɪ.mə/
eczematous /ekˈsem.ə.təs/
edge /edʒ/
educate /ˈedjʊˌkeɪt/
education /ˌedjʊˈkeɪʃən/
efficiently /ɪˈfɪʃ.ənt.li/
egocentric /ˌiːgəʊˈsentrɪk/
Eisenmenger syndrome /aɪˈzen.men.ˈger ˈsɪn.drəʊm/
ejection /ɪˈdʒektˌʃən/
elbow /ˈelbəʊ/
electrochemical /ɪˌlek.trəʊˈkem.ɪ.kəl/ **gradient** /ˈgreɪ.di.ənt/
electrode /ɪˈlekˌtroʊd/
electrolyte /ɪˈlek.trə.laɪt/
electrostatic /iˌlek.trəʊˈstæt.ɪk/
element /ˈelɪmənt/
elevation /ˌel.ɪˈveɪ.ʃn/
elicit /ɪˈlɪs.ɪt/
eliminate /ɪˈlɪm.ɪ.neɪt/
elimination /ɪˌlɪm.ɪˈneɪ.ʃən/
elixir /ɪˈlɪk.sɪər/
embarrassed /ɪmˈbær.əst/
embarrassment /ɪmˈbær.əs.mənt/
embolus /ˈem.bə.ləs/ pl **emboli**
embrace /ɪmˈbreɪs/
embroiled /ɪmˈbrɔɪld/
embryonic /ˌembrɪˈɒnɪk/
emerge /ɪˈmɜːdʒ/

emergence /ɪˈmɜːdʒəns/

emesis /eˈmɪ.sɪs/

emission /ɪˈmɪʃən/

emit /ɪˈmɪt/

emollient /ɪˈmɒljənt/

emotional /ɪˈməʊ.ʃən.əl/

empathy /empəθɪ/

emphasize /ˈem.fə.saɪz/

empower /ɪmˈpaʊər/

encapsulate /ɪnˈkæp.sjʊ.leɪt/

encephalitis /ˌen.kef.əˈlaɪ.tɪs/

encephalocele /in.ˈsef.ə.ləʊ.ˌsi:l/

encephalomyelitis /enˌsefələʊˌmaɪəˈlaɪtɪs/

encephalopathic /enˌsefələˈpæθɪk/

encephalopathy /enˌsef.əˈlɒp.ə.θi/

encompass /ɪnˈkʌm.pəs/

encopresis /ˌenˌkɑːp.ˈriː.səs pl encopreses /ˌsiːz/

encounter /ɪnˈkaʊn.tə/

encouragement /ɪnˈkʌr.ɪdʒ.mənt/

endemic /enˈdem.ɪk/

endoscopy /enˈdɒskəpɪ/

endothelial /ˌendəʊˈθiːlɪəl/

endotracheal /en.dɒ.trəˈkiː.əl/

endotracheal /en.dɒ.trəˈkiː.əl/ tube /tjuːb/ (ET tube)

endure /ɪnˈdjʊər/

enforce /ɪnˈfɔːs/

engage /ɪnˈgeɪdʒ/

engender /ɪnˈdʒendə/

enhance /ɪnˈhɑːns/

enlarge /ɪnˈlɑːdʒ/

enlargement /ɪnˈlɑːdʒ.mənt/

enormous /ɪˈnɔː.məs/

ensue /ɪnˈsjuː/

ensure /ɪnˈʃɔːr/

entail /ɪnˈteɪl/

Entamoeba /ˌentəˈmiːbə/ histolytica /ˌhɪs.təˈlɪ.tɪ.kə/

enteral /ˈen.tə.rəl/

enteric /enˈtər.ɪk/

enteritis /ˌen.təˈraɪ.təs/

enterocolitis /ˌen.tə.rəʊ.kə.ˈlaɪ.təs/

enterovirus /ˌɛn.tə.roʊˈvaɪ.rəs/

enthusiasm /ɪnˈθjuː.zi.æz.ᵊm/

entire /ɪnˈtaɪə/

entirely /ɪnˈtaɪə.li/

entrapment /ɪnˈtræp.mənt/

enucleation /ɪˈnjʊklɪˈeiʃⁿn/

enuresis /ˌen.jʊəˈriː.sɪs/

envelope /ɪnˈveləp/
environmental /ɪnˌvaɪə.rən.ˈmen.təl/
eosinophil /ˌiːəʊˈsɪnə.fɪl/
eosinophylic /ˌiː.əˈsɪn.ə.fɪl.ɪk/
epicanthal /ˌe.pə.ˈkan.thəl/
epidermis /ˌep.ɪˈdɜː.mɪs/ epidermis, pokožka
epidermolysis /ˌep.ə.ˌdər.ˈmɑː.l.ə.səs/ pl **epidermolyses** /ˌsiː.z/
epidural /ˌep.ɪˈdjʊə.rəl/
epiglottitis /ˌep.ɪ.ɡləˈtaɪ.tɪs/
epinephrine /ˌepɪˈnef.riːn/
epiphysis /əˈpɪf.ɪ.sɪs/
epistaxis /ˌe.pɪ.ˈstæk.sɪs/
Epstein /ˈep.ˌstaɪn/ **pearls** /pər.ə.lz/
Epstein-Barr /ˈep.ˌstaɪn bɑː/ **virus** /ˈvaɪrəs/
epulis /əˈpjʊ.ləs/
equality /ɪˈkwɒl.ɪ.ti/
equation /ɪˈkweɪʒən/
equilibrium /ˌiːkwɪˈlɪbrɪəm/
eradication /ɪˌrædiˈkeɪ.ʃən/
Erb palsy /erb ˈpɔːl.zi/
erectile /ɪˈrek.taɪl/
erosion /ɪˈrəʊ.ʒən/
erosive /ɪˈrəʊ.ʒɪv/
erratic /ɪˈræt.ɪk/
error /ˈer.ər/
erythema /ˌer.ɪˈθiː.mə/
erythematous /ˌer.ɪ.ˈθiː.mə.təs/
erythroblastopenia /e.riθˈrəʊ.blasˈtəʊ.piːˈniː.æ/
erythrocyte /ɪˈrɪθ.rəʊ.saɪt/
erythropoietin /eˌrɪθ.rəˈpɒɪ.ə.tɪn/
escalate /ˈes.kə.leɪt/
escape /ɪˈskeɪp/
eschar /ˈɛskɑː/
escharotomy /ˌes.kɑːˈrɒt.ə.mɪ/
essential /ɪˈsen.ʃəl/
establish /ɪˈstæb.lɪʃ/
esterase /es.tə.ˌreɪs/
estimate /ˈes.tɪ.meɪt
estimated /ˈes.tɪ.meɪt.ɪd/
ethanol /ˈeθ.ə.nɒl/
ethylene /ˈeθ.ɪ.liːn/
ethylene /ˈeθ.ɪ.liːn/ **glycol** /ˈɡlaɪ.kɒl/
etiologic /ˌiː.tiː.ə.ˈlɑː.ə.dʒik/ **agent** /ˈeɪ.dʒᵊnt/
euphoria /juːˈfɔː.ri.ə/
Eustachian /juːˈsteɪ.ki.ən/ **tube** /tjuːb/
evaluate /ɪˈvæl.ju.eɪt/
evaporative /ɪˈvæp.ər.eɪ.tɪv/

event /ɪˈvent/
evident /ˈev.ɪ.dənt/
evoke /ɪˈvəʊk/
evolve /ɪˈvɒlv/
Ewing /juˈing/ sarcoma /sɑːˈkəʊ.mə/
exacerbate /ɪɡˈzæs.ə.beɪt/
exacerbation /ɪɡˌzæs.əˈbeɪ.ʃən/
exaggerated /ɪɡˈzædʒ.ə.reɪ.tɪd/
exception /ɪkˈsep.ʃən/
excessive /ekˈses.ɪv/
excessively /ɪkˈsesɪvlɪ/
exchange /ɪksˈtʃeɪndʒ/
excision /ˌekˈsi.ʃən/
excite /ɪkˈsaɪt/
excitement /ɪkˈsaɪt.mənt/
exclusion /ɪkˈskluːʒən/
exclusive /ɪkˈskluːsɪv/
excoriate /ɪkˈskɔːrɪˌeɪt/
excrete /ɪkˈskriːt/
excretion /ɪkˈskriː.ʃən/
excretory /ˈek.skrə.ˌtɔːr.iː/
excuse /ɪkˈskjuːz/
exercise /ˈeksəˌsaɪz/
exerciser /ˈek.sər.ˌsaɪ.zər/
exert /ɪɡˈzɜːt/
exertion /ɪɡˈzɜː.ʃən/
exertional /ɪɡˈzɜː.ʃən.əl/
exfoliative /eksˈfeʊlɪˌeɪ.tɪv/
exhausted /ɪɡˈzɔː.stɪd/
exhaustion /ɪɡˈzɔːs.tʃən/
exhibitionism /ˌeksɪˈbɪʃəˌnɪzəm/
exogenous /ekˈsɑdʒ.ə.nəs/
expand /ɪkˈspænd/
expectation /ˌek.spekˈteɪ.ʃən/
expectorate /ɪkˈspek.tər.eɪt/
expel /ɪkˈspel/
expenditure /ɪkˈspendɪtʃə/
experience /ɪkˈspɪə.ri.ənts/
expiration /ˌek.spəˈreɪ.ʃən/
expiratory /ˌɪk.spɪr.ə.tər.i/
exploitation /ˌek.splɔɪˈteɪ.ʃən/
explorative /ek.spləˈrə.tɪv/
exploratory /ɪkˈsplɒrətərɪ/
explore /ɪkˈsplɔːr/
explosive /ɪkˈspləʊ.sɪv/
exposure /ɪkˈspəʊ.ʒə/
express /ɪkˈspres/

expressivity /ˌek.ˌspreˈsi.və.tiː/
expulsion /ɪkˈspʌl.ʃən/
exquisite /ɪkˈskwɪzɪt/
extended /ɪkˈsten.dɪd/
extensive /ɪkˈsten.sɪv/
extensor /ɪkˈsten.sər/
extent /ɪkˈstent/
extradural /ˈek.strəˈdjʊr.əl/
extraneous /ɪkˈstreɪnɪəs/
extraordinary /ɪkˈstrɔːdənrɪ/
extrapyramidal /ˌek.strə.pəˈra.mə.dᵊl/
extrauterine /ˌek.strəˈjʊ.tə.rən/
extremely /ɪkˈstriːm.li/
extremity /ɪkˈstrem.ɪ.ti/
extrusion /ɪk.ˈstrʊ.ʒən/
exuberance /ɪgˈzjuː.bər.əns/
exudate /ɪgˈzjuːdəɪt/
exudation /ˌek.sjuːˈdəɪ.ʃən/

F
fabric /ˈfæb.rɪk/
fabricate /ˈfæbrɪˌkeɪt/
face /feɪs/
facies /ˈfeɪ.ʃɪˌiːz/
facilitate /fəˈsɪl.ɪ.teɪt/
facility /fəˈsɪl.ɪ.ti/
fade /feɪd/
faecal /ˈfiː.kəl/
faecal-oral /ˈfiː.kəl ˈɔː.rəl/
fail /feɪl/
failing /ˈfeɪ.lɪŋ/
failure /ˈfeɪ.ljər/
faint /feɪnt/
fall /ˈfɔːl/ **asleep** /əˈsliːp/
fall /ˈfɔːl/ **out**
falsely /ˈfɒl.sli/
fan /fæn/
Fanconi /faːn.kəʊˈniː/ **anaemia** /əˈniː.mi.ə/
Fanconi syndrome /faːn.kəʊˈniː ˈsɪn.drəʊm/
farming /ˈfɑːmɪŋ/
fasciitis /ˈfeɪʃ.ɪaɪ.tɪs/
fasciotomy /ˈfæʃ.i.ɒ.tə.mi/
fashion /ˈfæʃ.ən/
fatal /ˈfeɪ.təl/
fatigue /fəˈtiːg/
favourable /ˈfeɪ.vər.ə.bl/
favouritism /ˈfeɪvərɪˌtɪzəm/

fearful /ˈfɪə.fəl/
feature /ˈfiː.tʃər/
febrile /ˈfiː.braɪl/
fecalith /ˈfiː.kə.ˌlith/
feeding /ˌfiː.dɪŋ/
feign /feɪn/
femoral /ˈfem.ər.əl/
femoral /ˈfem.ər.əl/ **head** /hed/
femur /ˈfiː.mər/ pl **femora**
fermentation /ˌfɜr.menˈteɪ.ʃən/
ferritin /ˈfer.ə.tən/
fertility /ˌfəˈtɪl.ɪ.ti/
fervent /ˈfɜːvənt/
fibroma /faɪˈbrəʊmə/
fibrous /ˈfaɪbrəs/
fidelity /fɪˈdel.ə.ti/
fidgety /ˈfɪdʒ.ɪ.ti/
fight /faɪt/
finally /ˈfaɪ.nə.li/
fine /faɪn/
finger /ˈfɪŋ.gə/ **cot** /ˈkɑːt/
fissure /ˈfɪʃ.ər/
fistula /ˈfɪs.tʃə.lə/ pl **fistulae**
fit in /fɪt ɪn/
fix /fɪks/
flaccid /ˈflæksɪd/
flake /fleɪk/
flaky /ˈfleɪkɪ/
flame /fleɪm/
flame-shaped /fleɪm ʃeɪpt/
flatulence /ˈflæt.jʊ.lənts/
flea /fliː/
flection /ˈflek.ʃən/
flee /fliː/
flesh /fleʃ/
flexed /flekst/
flexion /flek.ʃən/
flexor /ˈflek.sər/
flexure /ˈflek.ʃər/
flick /flɪk/
flicker /ˈflɪkə/
flit /flɪt/
float /fləʊt/
floppy /ˈflɒp.i/
flow /fləʊ/
fluctuate /ˈflʌk.tju.eɪt/
fluid /ˈfluː.ɪd/

flulike /fluː.laɪk/
fluoride /ˈflʊə.raɪd/
flushed /flʌʃt/
flushing /flʌʃ.ɪŋ/
foam /fəʊm/
focal /ˈfəʊ.kəl/
foetal /ˈfiː.təl/
fold /fəʊld/
folding /fəʊldɪŋ/
Foley catheter /ˈfəʊ.li ˈkæθ.ɪ.tər/
folic /ˈfəʊ.lik/ **acid** /ˈæs.ɪd/
follicle /ˈfɒl.ɪ.kl̩/
follow-up /ˈfɒl.əʊ.ʌp/
fontanelle /ˌfɒn.təˈnel/
foodstuff /ˈfuːdˌstʌf/
foramen /fəˈreɪ.mən/ pl **foramina**
force /fɔːs/
force-feeding /fɔːs ˌfiː.dɪŋ/
forceps /ˈfɔː.seps/
forearm /ˈfɔː.rɑːm/
forefoot /ˈfɔːˌfʊt/
foreskin /ˈfɔːˌskɪn/
forgetfulness /fəˈget.fʊl.nɪs/
forgiveness /fəˈgɪvnɪs/
formula /ˈfɔː.mjʊ.lə/
fortified /ˈfɔː.tɪˌfaɪd/
fossa /ˈfɒs.ə/ pl **fossae** /fɒs.iː/
foster /ˈfɒstə/
foul /faʊl/
foundation /faʊnˈdeɪ.ʃən/
fragile /ˈfrædʒ.aɪl/
frame /freɪm/
frankly /ˈfræŋklɪ/
fray /freɪ/
freckle /ˈfrekəl/
frequency /ˈfriː.kwən.si/
friction /ˈfrɪk.ʃən/
frictional /ˈfrɪk.ʃᵊn.ᵊl/
fried /fraɪd/
Friedreich ataxia /əˈtæk.si.ə/
frightened /ˈfraɪ.tənd/
frightening /ˈfraɪtnɪŋ/
frontal /ˈfrʌn.təl/
frontonasal /ˈfrʌntə ˈneɪzəl/
frown /fraʊn/
fructose /ˈfrʌktəʊs/
frustration /frʌsˈtreɪ.ʃən/

fully /ˈfʊl.i/
fulminant /ˈfʊl.mɪ.nənt/
fume /fjuːm/
fundus /ˈfʌn.dəs/ pl **fundi**
fungal /ˈfʌŋ.gəl/
fungus /ˈfʌŋ.gəs/ (pl **fungi**)
furrowed /ˈfʌrəʊd/
fusion /ˈfjuː.ʒən/
fussiness /ˈfə.siː.nəs/
fussy /ˈfʌsɪ/

G
G6PD, Glucose-6-phosphate dehydrogenase /gluˈkəʊs fosfəɪt diːˈhaɪ.drɒdʒˈen.eɪs/
deficiency /dɪˈfɪʃ.ən.si/
gag /gæg/
gait /geɪt/
Galactosemia /gəˌlæktəˈsiː.mɪə/
gallstone /ˈgɔːl.stəʊn/
gamete /ˈgæmiːt/
gamma /ˈgæmə/
gammaglobulin /gamˈæ.glɒb.jə.lɪˈn/
ganglion pl **ganglia** /ˈgæŋ.gli.ə/
ganglioneuroma /ˈgæŋglɪəʊnjʊˈrəʊmə/
garment /ˈgɑːmənt/
gasp /gɑːsp/
gastrinoma /gas.trəˈnəʊ.mə/
gastroenteropathy /ˌgæs.trəʊˌentəˈrɒpəθɪ/
gastroesophageal /ˌgæstrəʊˈiːˌsɒfəˈdʒiːəl/
gastroschisis /ˌgæs.trəʊˌs.kə.səs/
gastrostomy /gæsˈtrə.stə.mi/
gather /ˈgæð.ər/
gauge /geɪdʒ/
gauze /gɔːz/
gavage /gəˈvɑːʒ/
gaze /geɪz/
gear /gɪə/
gender /ˈdʒen.dər/
gene /dʒiːn/
generalized /ˈdʒenrəˌlaɪzd/
genitourinary /ˌdʒen.ɪ.təʊˈjʊə.rɪ.nər,i/
gentle /ˈdʒen.tlˌ/
germinal /ˈdʒɜː.mə.nᵊl/
gestational /dʒesˈteɪ.ʃən.əl/
get /get/ **off** /ɒf/
ghost /gəʊst/
Giardia /dʒiːˈɑːr.diː.ə/
gingival /dʒɪnˈdʒaɪ.vəl/

gingivostomatitis /ˈdʒɪn.dʒɪ.vəˈstəʊməˈtaɪ.tɪs/
give /ɡɪv/ **up** /ʌp/
glandular /ˈɡlæn.djʊ.lər/
glans /ɡlænz/
glioma /ɡlaɪˈəʊmə/
glomerular /ɡlɒˈmərʊlə/
glomerulonephritis /ɡlɒˌmer.jʊ.ləʊ.nɪˈfraɪ.tɪs/
glucocorticoid /ɡluːkəˈkɔːtɪ.kɒ.ɪd/ glukokortikoid, hormon kůry nadledvin
glucose /ˈɡluːkəʊz/ **meter** /ˈmiːtə/ glukoměr
Glucose-6-phosphate dehydrogenase (G6PD) /ɡluˈkəʊs fosfəɪt diːˈhaɪ.drodʒˈenˌeɪs/ **deficiency** /dɪˈfɪʃ.ənt .si/
Glucose-6-phosphate dehydrogenase /ɡluˈkəʊs fosfəɪt diːˈhaɪ.drodʒˈenˌeɪs/
glue /ɡluː/
gluten /ˈɡluː.tᵊn/
glycosaminoglycan /ɡlaɪkəʊs.ə.miːˈnəʊ.ɡlaɪˈkæn/
glycosuria /ˌɡlaɪkəʊˈsjʊərɪə/
gonad /ˈɡɒnæd/
gonadal /ˈɡɒnædᵊl/
gonorrhoea /ˌɡɒn.əˈriː.ə/
gossip /ˈɡɒsɪp/
govern /ˈɡʌv.ən/
grade /ɡreɪd/
graduation /ˌɡrædjʊˈeɪʃən/
granulocyte /ˌɡræn.jəˈlə.saɪt/
granuloma /ˌɡræn.jəˈləʊ.mə/
granulomatous /ˌɡrænjʊˈlɒm.ə.təs/
grasp /ɡrɑːsp/
gratification /ˌɡræt.ɪ.fɪˈkeɪ.ʃən/
gravity /ˈɡræv.ɪ.ti/
greasy /ɡriːs.i/
grimace /ˈɡrɪ.məs/
grind /ɡraɪnd/ **(ground, ground)**
gross /ɡrəʊs/ **national** /ˈnæʃənəl/ **income** /ˈɪnkʌm/
growth /ɡrəʊθ/
grunt /ɡrʌnt/
guaiacol /ˈɡwaɪ.ˌakel/
guard /ɡɑːd/
guardrail /ˈɡɑːdˌreɪl/
guesswork /ˈɡesˌwɜːk/
guidance /ˈɡaɪ.dəns/
Guillain-Barré /ɡiˈjæn bəˈrei/ **syndrome** /ˈsɪndrəʊm/
guilt /ɡɪlt/
gum /ɡʌm/
gun /ɡʌn/

H
habit /ˈhæb.ɪt/

habitual /həˈbɪtjʊəl/
habituation /həˌbɪtʃ.uˈeɪ.ʃᵊn/
hacking /ˈhæk.ɪŋ/ **cough** /kɒf/
haemangioma /ˌhiːmˌænˌdʒɪˈəʊ.mə/
haematemesis /ˌhiː.məˈte.mɪ.sɪs/
haematochezia /ˌhiː.məˈtəʊ.kiː.zi.æ/
haematocrit /hiː.məˈtə.krɪt/
haematoma pl **haematomata** /ˌhiː.məˈtəʊ.mə/
haematuria /ˌhiː.mə.tˈjʊə.ri.ə/
haemoccult test /ˈhiː.mə.ˌkəlt test/
haemodialysis /ˌhiː.məʊ.daɪˈæl.ə.sɪs/
haemoglobinopathy ˌhiːməʊɡləʊbɪˈnɒpəθɪ/
haemolysis /ˌhiː.məˈlɪ.sɪs/
haemolytic /ˌhiː.məˈlɪt.ɪk/
haemophagocytosis /ˈhiːməˌfæɡə.saɪˈtəʊ.sɪs/
haemophilia /ˌhiː.məˈfɪl.i.ə/
Haemophilus /hiː.ˈmɑː.fə.ləs/
haemopoiesis /ˌhiːməʊpɔˈiːsɪs/
haemorrhage /ˈhem.ər.ɪdʒ/
hailed /heɪld/
hallmark /ˈhɔːl.mɑːk/
hallucinogenic /həˌluːsɪnəʊˈdʒenɪk/
halt /hɔːlt/
hamartoma /hæmˈærˈtəʊˈmə/
hammer /ˈhæm.ər/
hand /hænd/
handhold /ˈhændˌhəʊld/
handicap /ˈhændɪˌkæp/
handle /ˈhæn.dəl/
hanging /ˈhæŋ.ɪŋ/
harbour /ˈhɑːbə/
hard /hɑːd/ **palate** /ˈpæl.ət/
hardship /ˈhɑːdʃɪp/
harm /hɑːm/
harmless /ˈhɑːm.ləs/
harvest /ˈhɑː.vɪst/
hasten /ˈheɪ.sən/
have butterflies /ˈbʌt.ə.flaɪ/ **in one's stomach**
hay /heɪ/ **fever** /ˈfiː.vər/
healer /ˈhiːlə/
hearing /ˈhɪə.rɪŋ/ **loss** /lɒs/
heartbeat /ˈhɑːt.biːt/
hearty /ˈhɑː.ti/
heel /hiːl/
Heimlich manoeuvre /ˈhaɪm.lɪk məˌnuː.vər/
hemangioma /ˌhiː.ˌman.dʒiː.ˈəʊ.mə/
hematopoietic /hi.ˌma.tə.pɔː.i.ˈe.tik/

hemiplegia /ˌhæm.ɪˈpliː.dʒi.ə/
hemiplegic /ˌhe.mi.ˈpliː.dʒik/
hemofiltration /ˈhiː.mə.fɪlˈtreɪ.ʃən/
Henoch-Schönlein purpura /ˈhen.ək ˌʃœn.laɪn ˈpər.pjə.rə/
heparin /ˈhe.pə.rɪn/
hepatocellular /hɪˈpætəˈseljʊlə/
hepatomegaly /ˌhɛp.ə.toʊˈmɛg.ə.li/
herald /ˈher.əld/
hereditary /həˈred.ɪ.tər.i/
heredity /həˈred.ə.ti/
hernia /ˈhɜːnɪə/
herniation /ˌhɜː.niˈeɪ.ʃən/
heroin /ˈherəʊɪn/
herpangina /ˈhɜːpænˈdʒaɪ.nə/
herpes /ˈhɜː.piːz/
herpes /ˈhɜː.piːz/ **simplex** /ˈsɪm.pleks/
herpetic /həˈpetɪk/
herpetic /hɜːˈpetɪk/ **whitlow** /ˈwɪtləʊ/
hesitancy /ˈhez.ɪ.tən.si/
Hib, /ˈhib/ *Haemophilus* /ˌhiːmˈhiːməʊˌfɪləs/ *influenzae* /ɪnˌflʊ.ˈen.zə/
hiccough /ˈhɪk.ʌp/
highlight /ˈhaɪ.laɪt/
hiking /ˈhaɪ.kɪŋ/
hinged /ˈhɪndʒd/
Hirschsprung's disease /ˈhirʃˌprʊŋz dɪˈziːz/
hirsutism /ˈhər.sə.ˌti.zəm/
histiocyte /ˈhɪstɪəˌsaɪt/
histiocytosis /ˈhɪstɪəˌsaɪtəʊ.sis/
histological /ˌhɪstəˈlɒdʒɪkˀl/
hives /haɪvz/
hoarseness /ˈhɔːsnɪs/
Hodgkin /ˈhɒdʒkɪn/ **lymphoma** /lɪmˈfəʊ.mə/
holding /ˈhoʊl.dɪŋ/
holophrastic /ˌhəʊ.lə.ˈfra.stik/
homelessness /ˈhəʊm.ləs.nəs/
homicidal /ˌhɒm.ɪˈsaɪ.dəl/
homicide /ˈhɒm.ɪ.saɪd/
homogeneous /ˌhəʊməˈdʒiːnɪəs/
hopeless /ˈhəʊp.ləs/
hordeolum /hɔː.r.ˈdiː.ə.ləm/ pl **hordeola** /-lə/
horn /hɔːn/
hornet /ˈhɔːnɪt/
horny /ˈhɔːnɪ/
horror /ˈhɒrə/
hostile /ˈhɒs.taɪl/
household /ˈhaʊs.həʊld/ **chores** /tʃɔːz/
housing /ˈhaʊ.zɪŋ/

hum /hʌm/

human /ˈhjuː.mən/ **papilloma virus** /ˌpa.pə.ˈləʊ.mə.ˈvaɪə.rəs/

humidification/hjʊ.ˌmi.də.fə.ˈkeɪ.ʃən/

humidified /hjuːˈmɪd.ɪ.faɪd/

humidity /hjuːˈmɪd.ɪ.ti/

humoral /ˈhjʊ.mə.rə/

Huntington's disease /ˈhʌn.tɪŋ.tənz dɪˌzi:z/

hydrocarbon /ˌhaɪ.drəʊ ˈkɑː.bən/

hydrocele /ˈhaɪdrəʊˌsi:l/

hydrocephalic /ˌhaɪdrəʊseˈfælɪk/

hydrocephalus /ˌhaɪ.drəˈsef.ə.ləs/

hydrochloric acid /ˌhaɪ.drə.klɔː.rɪk ˈæs.ɪd/

hydrops /haɪdrɒps/

hydrostatic /ˌhaɪdrəʊˈstæt.ɪk/

hymen /ˈhaɪmen/

hymenotomy /ˈhaɪmen.ɒtəmɪ/

hyperammonemia /ˌhaɪ.pə.ˌram.ə.ˈniː.miː.ə/

hypercapnia /ˌhaɪ.pə.kæp.niə/

hyperchloremia /ˈhaɪ.pər.klɔːri.miː.ə/

hypercyanotic /ˌhaɪ.pə.ˌsaɪə.n ɒtik/

hyperextensible /ˌhaɪ.pə.rikˈstens.əbəl/

hyperglycemia /ˌhaɪ.pər.glaɪ.ˈsiː.miː.ə/

hyperinflation /ˌhaɪpəɪnˈfleɪʃən/

hyperinsulinaemia /ˌhaɪ.pə.ˌrin.sə.lə.ˈniː.miː.ə/

hyperkalaemia /ˈhaɪ.pər.kæˈliː.mɪ.ə/

hypermobility /ˌhaɪ.pə.ˌməʊ.ˈbi.lə.ti:/

hypernatraemia /ˌhaɪ.pə.neɪ.ˈtriː.miː.ə/

hyperparathyroidism /ˌhaɪ.pə.ˌpær.əˈθaɪ.rɔɪd.ism/

hyperpnoea /ˌhaɪ.pəˈpni.ə/

hypersplenism /ˌhaɪpəˈspliːnɪzəm/

hyperthyroidism /ˌhaɪ.pəˈθaɪ.rɔɪd.ɪzəm/

hypertonia /ˌhaɪ.pəˈtəʊ.niə/

hypertonic /ˌhaɪ.pər.ˈtɑː.nik/

hypertrophic /ˌhɑɪ.pərˈtrɑf.ɪk/

hypertrophy /haɪˈpɜː.trə.fi/

hyperventilation /ˌhaɪ.pəˌven.tɪˈleɪ.ʃən/

hypha /ˈhaɪfə/ pl **hyphae** /ˈhaɪfi:/

hypnic /hɪpnɪk/

hypoalbuminemia /ˌhaɪpəʊˈælbjʊmɪniːmɪə/

hypocalcaemia /ˌhaɪ.pəʊ.kælˈsiː.mi.ə/

hypocalcaemic/ˌhaɪ.pəʊ.ˌkal.ˈsiː..mik/

hypocapnia /ˌhaɪ.pəʊˈkæp.nɪ.ə/

hypochondriacal /ˌhaɪ.pə.kən.ˈdraɪ.ə.kəl/

hypochromic /ˈhaɪpəˈkrəm.ɪk/

hypoglobulinemia / ˌhaɪ.pəʊ.glɒb.jə.lɪˈniː.miː.ə/

hypoglycaemia /ˌhaɪ.pəʊ ˌglaɪˈsiː.miː.ə/

hypomagnesaemia /ˌhaɪ.pəʊ.ˌmæg.nəˈsiː.miː.ə/

hyponatremia /ˌhaɪ.pəʊˈnetriːmɪ.ə/
hypoplasia /ˌhaɪ.pəʊ.ˈpleɪ.ʒə/
hypoplastic /ˌhaɪ.pəʊ.ˈpla.stik/
hyporeflexia /ˌhaɪ.pəʊˈ.riː.ˈflek.siː.ə/
hyposplenism /ˈhaɪ.pəʊ ˈspliː.nɪzm/
hypotension /ˌhaɪ.pəʊˈten.ʃən/
hypothalamus /ˌhaɪ.pəʊˈθæl.ə.məs/
hypothyroidism /ˌhaɪ.pəʊˈθaɪ.rɔɪd.ɪsm/
hypotonia /ˌhaɪpəʊˈtəʊ.niə/
hypotonic /ˌhaɪ.pə.ˈtɑː.nik/
hypoventilation /ˌhaɪ.pəʊˌven.tɪˈleɪ.ʃən/
hypovolaemia /ˌhaɪ.pəʊ.vəˈliː.mɪ.ə/
hypoxaemia /ˌhai.pɒkˈsiː.mi.ə/
hypoxic /haɪˈpɒk.sɪk/
hypoxic-ischaemic /haɪˈpɒk.sɪk ɪsˈkiː.mɪk/ **IgA** /ˌaɪ.dʒiː.ˈeɪ/

I

ictal /ˈɪktəl/
identification /aɪˌden.tɪ.fɪˈkeɪ.ʃən/
identify /aɪˈden.tɪ.faɪ/
IgA /ˌaɪ.dʒiː.ˈeɪ/ **immunoglobulin** /ɪˌmjuːn.əʊˈglɒb.jə.lɪn/
ignition /ɪɡˈnɪʃən/
ignore /ɪɡˈnɔːr/
ileum /ˈɪl.i.əm/ pl **ilea**
ileus /ˈɪl.i.əs/
iliac /ˈɪl.i.æk/
ill /ɪl/
illicit /ɪˈlɪs.ɪt/
imaginative /ɪˈmædʒɪnətɪv/
imagine /ɪˈmædʒ.ɪn/
imbalance /ˌɪmˈbæl.ənts/
imitate /ˈɪm.ɪ.teɪt/
immature /ˌɪm.əˈtʃʊər/
immaturity /ˌɪm.əˈtʃʊə.rɪ.ti/
immunodeficiency /ˌɪm.jʊ.nəʊ.dɪˈfɪʃ.ənt.si/
immunoglobulin /ɪˌmjuːn.əʊˈglɒb.jə.lɪn/
immunoglobulin E /ɪˌmjuːn.əʊˈglɒb.jə.lɪn/
immunologic /ɪm.jə.nəˈlɒdʒ.ɪ.k/
immunomodulator /ˌi.mjə.nəʊ.ˈmɒdjʊˌleɪt.tər/
immunosuppressant /ˌɪm.jə.nəʊ.səˈpres.ᵊnt/
immunosuppressive /ˌɪm.jə.nəʊ.səˈpres.ɪv/
immunotherapy /ˌɪm.jə.nəʊˈθe.rə.pi/
impact /ˈɪm.pækt/
impaction /ɪmˈpæk.ʃən/
impaired /ɪmˈpeəd/
impairment /ɪmˈpeərˌmənt/
impending /ɪmˈpen.dɪŋ/

imperative /ɪmˈper.ə.tɪv/
imperforate /ɪmˈpɜːfərɪt/
impetigo /ˌɪm.pəˈtaɪ.ɡəʊ/
implanted /ɪmˈplɑːnt.ɪd/
implement /ˈɪm.plɪ.ment/
implementation /ˌɪm.plɪ.menˈteɪ.ʃən/
implication /ˌɪm.plɪˈkeɪ.ʃən/
impose /ɪmˈpəʊz/
impossible /ɪmˈpɒsəbəl/
impotence /ˈɪm.pə.təns/
impregnate /ˈɪm.preg.neɪt/
impression /ɪmˈpreʃ.ən/
improve /imˈpruːv/
improvement /ɪmˈpruːv.mənt/
in /ɪn/ **particular** /pəˈtɪk.jʊ.lər/
in situ /ɪn ˈsɪt.juː/
in spite of /spaɪt/
in utero /in.juːˈtər.əʊ/
inability /ˌɪn.əˈbɪl.ɪ.ti/
inaccurate /ɪnˈækjʊrɪt/
inactive /ɪnˈæk.tɪv/
inadvertently /ˌɪn.ədˈvɜː.tənt.li/
inanimate /ɪˈnæn.ɪ.mət/
inappropriate /ˌɪn.əˈprəʊ.pri.ət/
inattentive /ˌɪnəˈtentɪv/
inborn /ˈɪnˈbɔːn/
incarceration /ɪnˌkɑːsəˈreɪʃən/
incense /ˈɪn.sens/
incentive /ɪnˈsentɪv/
incidence /ˈɪn.sɪ.dəns/
incidental ˌɪnsɪˈdentəl/
incidentally /ˌɪnsɪˈdentəlɪ/
incisor /ɪnˈsaɪ.zər/
inclination /ˌɪnklɪˈneɪʃən/
incompatibility /ˌɪn.kəmˌpætəˈbɪlɪtɪ/
incompetence /ɪnˈkɒmpɪtəns/
incomplete /ˌɪn.kəmˈpliːt/
inconsistent /ˌɪn.kənˈsɪs.tənt/
inconsolable /ˌɪn.kənˈsəʊ.lə.bl/
inconvenient /ˌɪnkənˈviːnjənt/
incorrect /ˌɪnkəˈrekt/
indentation /ˌɪn.denˈteɪ.ʃən/
independently /ˌɪn.dɪˈpen.dənt.li/
indeterminate /ˌɪndɪˈtɜːmɪnɪt/
indistinguishable /ˌɪndɪˈstɪŋgwɪʃəbəl/
indrawing /ɪnˈdrɔːɪŋ/
indwelling /ˈɪn.dwel.ɪŋ/

inequality /ˌɪnɪˈkwɒlɪtɪ/
inevitable /ɪnˈevɪt.əbəl/
infancy /ˈɪn.fənt.si/
infantile /ˈɪn.fən.taɪl/
infective /ɪnˈfek.tɪv/
inferior /ɪnˈfɪə.ri.ər/
infertility /ˌɪn.fəˈtɪl.ɪ.ti/
infestation /ˌɪn.fesˈteɪ.ʃən/
infested /ɪnˈfest.ɪd/
infiltration /ˌɪn.fɪlˈtreɪ.ʃən/
inflation /ɪnˈfleɪ.ʃən/
influence /ˈɪn.flʊ.əns/
influenza /ˌɪn.fluˈen.zə/
infrequent /ɪnˈfriː.kwənt/
infusion /ɪnˈfjuː.ʒən/
ingestion /ɪnˈdʒest.ʃən/
inguinal /ˈɪŋ.gwɪ.nəl/
inhaler /ɪnˈheɪ.lər/
inherit /ɪnˈher.ɪt/
inheritance /ɪnˈherɪtəns/
inhibit /ɪnˈhɪb.ɪt/
inhibition /ˌɪn.hɪˈbɪʃ.ən/
inhibitory /ɪnˈhɪb.ɪ.tər.i/
initial /ɪˈnɪʃəl/
initially /ɪˈnɪʃ.əl.i/
initiate /ɪˈnɪʃ.i.eɪt/
innervation /ɪ.nɜːˈveɪ.ʃən/
innocent /ˈɪnəs.ənt/
inoculation /ɪˌnɒk.jʊˈleɪ.ʃən/
inotropes /inˈəʊ.trəʊps/
insect /ˈɪn.sekt/
insecurity /ˌɪn.sɪˈkjʊə.rɪ.ti/
insensible /ɪnˈsen.sə.bᵊl/
insert /ɪnˈsɜːt/
insertion /ɪnˈsɜː.ʃən/
insidious /ɪnˈsɪdɪəs/
insipid /ɪnˈsɪpɪd/
insist /ɪnˈsɪst/
inspection /ɪnˈspek.ʃən/
instruct /ɪnˈstrʌkt/
instrument /ˈɪn.strə.mənt/
insufficiency /ˌin.səˈfɪʃ.ən.siː/
intelligent /ɪnˈtelɪdʒənt/
intended /ɪnˈten.dɪd/
intense /ɪnˈtens/
intensification /ɪnˌtensɪfɪˈkeɪʃən/
intensify /ɪnˈtensɪˌfaɪ/

intent /ɪnˈtent/
intentionally /ɪnˈten.ʃən.əl.i/
inter- /ɪnˈtɜːr/
interact /ˌɪn.təˈrækt/
interaction /ˌɪn.təˈræk.ʃən/
interactive /ˌɪntərˈæktɪv/
interchange /ˌɪn.təˈtʃeɪndʒ/
intercostal /ˌɪn.təˈkɒs.təl/
intercourse /ˈɪntəˌkɔːs/
intercurrent /ˌɪn.təˈkʌr.ənt/
interfere /ˌɪn.təˈfɪər/
interference /ˌɪn.təˈfɪə.rəns/
interferon /ˌɪntəˈfɪə.rɒn/
interferon-gamma /ˌɪn.təˈfɪə.rɒnˈgæm.ə/
intermittent /ˌɪn.təˈmɪt.ənt/
internalize /ɪnˈtɜːnəˌlaɪz/
internally /ɪnˈtɜːnəlɪ/
interrupt /ˌɪn.təˈrʌpt/
interruption /ˌɪn.təˈrʌp.ʃən/
interscapular /ˌɪn.tərˈskæp.jə.lər/
interstitial /ˌɪn.təˈstɪʃ.əl/
intervene /ˌɪn.təˈviːn/
intervention /ˌɪn.təˈven.ʃən/
intervertebral /ˌɪn.tɜːrˈvɜː.tɪ.brəl/ disc /dɪsk/
interviewing /ˈɪntəˌvjuːɪŋ/
intestinal /ˌɪn.ˈtes.tin.əl/
intimacy /ˈɪntɪməsɪ/
intimidation /ɪnˌtɪm.ɪˈdeɪ.ʃən/
in-toeing /ˈɪn.ˈtəʊ.ɪŋ/
intoxication /ɪnˌtɒk.sɪˈkeɪˌʃən/
intraabdominal /ɪn.trə.æbˈdɒm.ɪ.nəl/
intracellular /ˌɪn.trəˈsel.jə.lər/
intracerebral /ˌɪn.trəˈser.ə.brəl/
intracranial /ˌɪn.trəˈkrɪʌ.ni.əl/
intradermally /ˌɪn.trəˈdɜː.məl.i/
intraosseous /ˌɪn.trəˈɒs.i.əs/
intrathoracic /ˌɪn.trə.thəˈra.sik/
intrauterine /ˌɪn.trəˈjuː.tər.aɪn/
intravascular /ˌɪn.trəˈvæs.kjʊ.lər/
intravenously /ˌɪn.trəˈviː.nəs.li/
intraventricular /ɪn.trə.venˈtrɪk.jə.lər/
introitus /ɪntrɔɪtəs/
introvert /ˈɪn.trə.vɜːt/
intrusive /ɪnˈtruː.sɪv/
intubate /ɪnˈtjuː.beɪt/
intussusception /ˌɪn.təs.səsˈsep.ʃən/
inulin /inˈju.lɪn/

invariably /ɪnˈveə.ri.ə.bli/
invasive /ɪnˈveɪ.sɪv/
investigate /ɪnˈves.tɪ.geɪt/
involuntary /ɪnˈvɒləntərɪ/
involvement /ɪnˈvɒlv.mənt/
invulnerability /ɪnˌvʌl.nᵊr.əˈbɪl.ə.ti/
iodine /ˈaɪ.ə.diːn/
ion /ˈaɪ.ɒn/
iris /ˈaɪrɪs/
iron /aɪən/
irradiation /iˌrei.diˈei.ʃən/
irrational /ɪˈræʃ.ən.əl/
irreducible /ˌɪrɪˈdjuːsɪbᵊl/
irregular /ɪˈreg.jə.lər/
irresistibility /ˌɪrɪˌzɪstəˈbɪlɪtɪ/
irreversible /ˌɪr.ɪˈvɜː.sɪ.bl̩/
irritability /ˌɪr.ɪ.təˈbɪl.ɪ.ti/
irritable /ˈɪr.ɪ.tə.bl̩/
ischaemia /ɪˈskiː.mi.ə/
isomaltase /aɪ.səʊˈmɔːl.teɪz/
isotonic /aɪ.səʊ ˈtɒn.ɪk/
issue /ˈɪʃ.uː/
itching /ˈɪtʃ.ɪŋ/
itchy /ˈɪtʃ.i/

J
jagged /ˈdʒæg.ɪd/
jail /dʒeɪl/
jaundice /ˈdʒɔːn.dɪs/
jaw /dʒɔː/
jaw-thrust /dʒɔː θrʌst/ **manoeuvre** /məˈnuː.vər/
jealousy /ˈdʒel.ə.si/
jellyfish /ˈdʒelɪˌfɪʃ/
jerk /dʒɜːk/
jewellery /ˈdʒuː.əl.ri/
jittery /ˈdʒɪ.tə.rɪ/
Jobst spandex /ˈspæn.deks/
judgement /ˈdʒʌdʒ.mənt/
judgemental /dʒʌdʒˈmen.təl/
jugular /ˈdʒʌg.jə.lər/
junction /ˈdʒʌŋk.ʃən/
justifiable /ˈdʒʌstɪˌfaɪəbəl/
juvenile /ˈdʒuː.vɪˌnaɪl/
juvenile /ˈdʒuː.vɪˌnaɪl/ **idiopathic** /ˌɪd.i.əˈpæθ.ɪk/ **arthritis** /ɑːˈθraɪ.tɪs/

K
Kaposi sarcoma /kæpəʊˈziː sɑːˈkəʊmə/

Kawasaki disease /kɑːwəˈsɑːki dɪˌziːz/
keep /kiːp/ **awake** /əˈweɪk/
keratin /ˈker.ət.ɪn/
keratinize /ˈker.ə.təˌnaɪz/
kernicterus /kɜːnˈɪk.tər.əs/
Kernig sign /ˈker.nig saɪn/
ketoacidosis /ˈkiː.təʊˌæ.ɪˈdəʊ.sɪs/
ketone /ˈkiː.təʊn/
ketosis /kiː.təʊ.sɪs/
ketotic /kiːˈtɑː.tik/ **hypoglycaemia** /ˌhaɪ.pəʊ.glaɪˈsiː.mi.ə/
kidnapper /ˈkɪdnæpə/
kidney /ˈkɪd.ni/
kinetic /kɪˈnetɪk/
Koplik spots /kopˈlik spots/
Krabbe leukodystrophy /krabˈiːˌluːkəʊˈdɪstrəfɪ/
Kussmaul /ˈkusˌmaul/ **breathing** /ˈbriːðɪŋ/
kyphosis /kaɪˈfəʊ.sɪs/

L
label /ˈleɪ.bəl/
labial /ˈleɪbɪəl/
lability /leɪˈbi.lə.tiː/
labium /ˈleɪbɪəm/
labour /ˈleɪ.bər/
laboured /ˈleɪ.bəd/
labstick /ləˈbstɪk/
labyrinthitis /ˌlæbərɪnˈθaɪtɪs/
lace /leɪs/
lacrimal /ˈlæk.rɪm.əl/ **sac** /sæk/
lactalbumin /ˌlak.ˌtal.ˈbjʊ.mən/
lactate /lækˈteɪt/
lactation /lækˈteɪ.ʃən/
lactic /ˈlæk.tɪk/ **acid** /ˈæs.ɪd/
Lactobacillus /ˌlæktəʊ.bəˈsɪləs/
lactose /ˈlæk.təʊs/
lag /læg/
lamb /læm/
Langerhans /ˈlæŋəˌhæns/ **cells** /sels/
lanugo /læˈnjuː.gəʊ/
lap /læp/
laparoscopy /ˌlæpəˈrɒskəpɪ/
large /ˌlɑːdʒ/ **bowel** /ˈbaʊ.əl/
laryngeal /ləˈrɪn.dʒi.əl/
laryngitis /ˌlær.ɪnˈdʒaɪ.tɪs/
laryngoscopy /ˌlærɪŋˈgɒ.skə.pi/
laryngotracheobronchitis /læˈrɪŋ.gəˌtreɪ.kɪ.ə.brəŋˈkaɪ.tɪs/
laryngotracheomalacia /ləˈrin. dʒəˌtreɪ.kiː.əʊ.məˈleɪ.ʃi.ə/

lash /læʃ/
lash /læʃ/ **out** /aʊt/
latency /ˈleɪ.tən.si/
laughter /ˈlɑːftə/
launder /ˈlɔːndə/
laxative /ˈlæk.sə.tɪv/
lead /led/
leak /liːk/
lean /liːn/
lecture /ˈlek.tʃə/
legal high /ˌliː.gᵊl ˈhaɪ/
Legg-Calvé-Perthes /ˈleg.ˌkal.ˈveɪ.ˈpər.ˌtiːz/ **disease** /dɪˈziːz/
legume /ˈleg.juːm/
lengthen /ˈleŋkθən/
lentil /ˈlentɪl/
lesion /ˈliː.ʒən/
lethargy /ˈleθ.ə.dʒi/
letter /ˈletə/
leucine /ˈlʊ.ˌsiːn/
leucocyte /ˈljuː.kə.saɪt/
leukodystrophy /ˌluː.kəʊˈdɪstrəfɪ/
leukomalacia /ˈljuː.kə.mə.ˈleɪ.ʃiː.ə/
liaison /liˈeɪ.zɒn/
liberally /ˈlɪbərəlɪ/
licence /ˈlaɪ.sᵊns/
lichenification /laɪ.ˌken.ə.fə.ˈkeɪ.ʃən/
lichenified /laɪ.ˈken.ə.ˌfaɪd/
lid /lɪd/
lidocaine /ˈlaɪdə.ˌken/
lie /laɪ/
life /laɪf/ **expectancy** /ɪkˈspek.tən.si/
life-threatening /ˈlaɪf.ˌθret.ən.ɪŋ/
ligation /lɪˈgeɪ.ʃən/
light /laɪt/
light-headedness /ˌlaɪtˈhed.ɪd.nəs/
limbus /ˈlim.bəs/
limit /ˈlɪm.ɪt/
limiting /ˈlɪm.ɪ.tɪŋ/
limp /lɪmp/
linear /ˈlɪn.i.ər/
lining /ˈlaɪn.ɪŋ/
lipoatrophy /ˈlaɪ.ˌpəʊ.ˈa.trə.fiː/
lipofuscinosis /ˌlɪpəʊfʌskɪˈnəʊsɪs/
lipohypertrophy /ˈlaɪ.ˌpəʊ.haɪˈpɜː.trə.fi/
Lisch nodule /lishˈnɒdjuːl/
listless /ˈlɪst.ləs/
listlessness /ˈlɪstlɪsnɪs/

load /ləʊd/
loaded /ˈləʊdɪd/
lobar /ˈləʊ.bəʳ/
localize /ˈləʊ.kəl.aɪz/
localized /ˈləʊ.kəl.aɪzd/
locate /ləʊˈkeɪt/
lock /lɒk/
locked /lɒkt/
locomotion /ˌləʊkəˈməʊʃən/
locus pl ci /ˈləʊkəs/
lodge /lɒdʒ/
loin /lɔɪn/
loneliness /ˈləʊn.li.nəs/
lonely /ˈləʊnlɪ/
longitudinal /ˌlɒn.dʒɪˈtjuː.dɪ.nəl/
loop /luːp/
loose /luːs/
lose /luːs/ **sight** /saɪt/ **of** /ɒv/
loudness /laʊd.nəs/
louse /laʊs/ pl **lice** /ˈlaɪs/
low pitched /ˌləʊˈpɪtʃt/
Lowe syndrome / ləʊ ˈsɪn.drəʊm/
loyalty /ˈlɔɪ.əl.ti/
lucid /ˈluː.sɪd/
lumbar /ˈlʌm.bər/
lumbar /ˈlʌm.bər/ **punction** /ˈpʌŋk.ʃən/
lumen /ˈlu.mən/ pl **lumina**
lump /lʌmp/
lupus /ˈluː.pəs/
lupus /ˈluː.pəs/ **erythematosus** /ˌer.ə.ˌthiː.mə.ˈtəʊ.səs/
lying /ˈlaɪ.ɪŋ/
lying /ˈlaɪ.ɪŋ/ **about** /əˈbaʊt/
Lyme disease /ˈlaɪm dɪˌziːz/
lymph /lɪmf/
lymph /lɪmf/ **node** /nəʊd/
lymphadenitis /ˌlim.ˌfa.də.ˈnaɪ.təs/
lymphangiectasia /ˌlim.ˌfan.dʒiː.ek.ˈteɪ.ʒiː.ə/
lymphatic /limˈfæ.tik/
lymphoblastic /ˌlɪmfəʊˈblæs.tɪk/
lymphocyte /ˈlim.fə.saɪt/
lymphocytic /ˌlɪɪmfəʊˈsɪtɪk/
lymphocytosis /ˌlɪmfəʊs.aɪˈtəʊ.sɪs/
lymphohistiocytosis /ˌlɪmfəʊˈhɪstɪəˌsaɪtəʊsis/
lymphoid /ˈlɪm.fɔɪd/

M
macrocephaly /ˌmækrəʊ.ˈsef.ə.li/

547

macrolide /ˈmaɪkrəʊl.aɪd/
macrophage /ˈmæk.rəˈfeɪdʒ/
macrovascular /ˈmækrəʊ.væskjʊlə/
macular /ˌmæk.jʊ.lər/
macule /ˈmækjuːl/
maculesvesicular /ˌmæk.jʊ.lə veˈsɪkjʊlə/
maculopapular /ˌmæk.jʊ.lə.pæp.ju.lər/
magical /ˈmædʒ.ɪ.kəl/
magnitude /ˈmæɡnɪˌtjuːd/
magnum /ˈmæɡnəm/
mainstay /meɪnˌsteɪ/
maintain /meɪnˈteɪn/
maintenance /ˈmeɪn.tɪ.nəns/
majority /məˈdʒɒr.ə.ti/
malacia /məˈleɪˌʃɪə/
maladaptive /mæl.əˈdæp.tɪv/
malaise /mælˈeɪz/
malarial /məˈleərɪəl/
maldescent /mæl dɪˈsent/
malformation /ˌmæl.fəˈmeɪ.ʃən/
malnutrition /ˌmæl.njuːˈtrɪ.ʃən/
manage /ˈmæn.ɪdʒ/
manageable /ˈmænɪdʒəbəl/
management /ˈmæn.ɪdʒ.mənt/
manipulation /məˌnɪp.jʊˈleɪˌʃən/
manipulative /məˈnɪpjʊlətɪv/
manoeuvre /məˈnuːvə/
manubrium /məˈnuː.brɪ.əm/
margin /ˈmɑː.dʒɪn/
marginal /ˈmɑːdʒɪn.əl/
marital /ˈmær.ɪ.təl/
mark /mɑːk/
marker /mɑːk.ər/
marking /mɑːk.ɪŋ/
marriage /ˈmær.ɪdʒ/
marrow /ˈmær.əʊ/
martyr /ˈmɑːtə/
mask /mɑːsk/
mass /mæs/
massager /ˈmæsɑːʒə/
mast /mɑːst/ **cell** /sel/
master /ˈmɑː.stər/
mastery /ˈmɑː.stər.i/
mastitis /mæˈstaɪ.tɪs/
mastocyte /mæst.ə.saɪt/
mastoiditis /ˌmæstɔɪˈdaɪ.tɪs/
match /mætʃ/

maternity /mə'tɜː.nə.ti/ **pad** /pæd/
maternity /mə'tɜː.nə.ti/ **ward** /wɔːd/
matter /'mæt.ər/
mattress /'mæt.rəs/
maturation /ˌmæt.jʊəˈreɪ.ʃən/
maturity /məˈtjʊə.rɪ.ti/
maxilla /mæˈksɪ.lə/
maxillary /mæk.sɪl.ə.ri/
mean /miːn/
meaning /'miː.nɪŋ/
meaningful /'miː.nɪŋ.fəl/
measurement /'meʒ.ə.mənt/
meatus /mɪˈeɪtəs/
Meckel /'mek.əl/ **diverticulum** /ˌdaɪ.vəˌtɪk.jʊ.ləm/ pl **diverticula**
meconium /mɪˈkəʊ.nɪ.əm/
mediastimum /ˌmiː.di.əˈstaɪn.əm/
mediastinal /ˌmiː.di.əsˈtaɪ.nəl/
mediated /'miː.di.eɪt.ɪd/
mediator /'miː.di.eɪ.tər/
medulla /meˌdʌl.ə/
medullary /meˌdʌl.ə.ri/
medulloblastoma /mɪˌdʌləʊbæsˈtəʊmə/
meibomian /maɪ.ˈbəʊ.miː.ən/ **gland** /glænd/
melaena /məˈliːn.ə/
membrane /'mem.breɪn/
memory /'mem.ər.i/
menarche /menˈɑː.ki/
Mendelian /men.ˈdiː.liː.ən/ **disorder** /dɪˈsɔː.dər/
Ménétrier disease /meɪ.neɪ.triː.eɪˈ dɪˈziːz/
meningismus /ˌmen.ən.ˈdʒiz.məs/
meningitis /ˌmen.ɪnˈdʒaɪ.tɪs/
meningocele /meˈnɪŋgəʊˌsiːl/
meningoencephalitis /mə.ˌnɪŋ.gəʊ.ən.ˌse.fə.ˈlaɪ.təs/
menorrhagia /ˌmenɔːˈreɪdʒ.ɪə/
mercury /'mɜː.kjʊ.ri/
mesenteric /ˌmes.enˈter.ɪk/
metacarpal /ˌmet.əˈkɑː.pəl/
metal /'met.əl/
metaphysis /ˌmə.ˈtaf.ə.səs/
metastasis /metˈæs.təs.ɪs/
metastatic /ˌmet.əˈstæt.ɪk/
metatarsus /ˌmet.əˈtɑː.səs/
methanol /'meθ.ə.nɒl/
microalbuminuria /'maɪ.krəʊ.al.ˌbjʊ.mə.ˈnjʊər.ɪ.ə/
microangiopathy /ˌmaɪkrəʊˈændʒɪˈɒpəθɪ/
microbial /'maɪ.krəʊ.baɪ.əl/
microbiology /ˌmaɪkrəʊbaɪˈɒlədʒɪ/

microcephalus /ˌmai.krəʊˈse.fəl.əs/
microcephaly /ˌmaɪ.krəʊˈsef.ə.li/
microcytic /ˌmai.krəʊˈsɪt.ɪk/
micrognathia / ˌmaɪ.krəʊ.ˈneɪ.thiː.ə/
microinfarction /ˌmaɪkrə.ɪnˈfɑːk.ʃən/
micromethod /maɪˈkrɒ.ˈmeθ.əd/
micturition /ˌmɪktjʊˈrɪ.ʃən/
middle /ˌmɪd.ļ/
midforehead /ˈmɪd.ˈfɒrɪd/
midline /ˈmɪd.laɪn/
midpoint /ˈmɪd.pɔɪnt/
midshaft /ˈmɪd.ˈʃaft/
midstream /ˌmɪdˈstriːm/
midteens /ˈmɪd.tiːnz/
migrate /maɪˈgreɪt/
migratory /ˈmaɪ.grə.tər.i/
milium /ˈmi.liː.əm/ pl **milia** /ˈmi.liː.ə/
Miller Fisher syndrome /miler fishˈer sɪndrəʊm/
minder /ˈmaɪndə/
mineralocorticoids /ˌmɪn.ə.rəl.əˈkɔː.tɪ.kɒ.ɪdz/
minute /maɪˈnjuːt/
miscarriage /ˈmɪsˌkær.ɪdʒ/
miscellaneous /ˌmɪs.əlˈeɪ.ni.əs/
misery /ˈmɪz.ər.i/
mismatch /ˌmɪsˈmætʃ/
missile /ˈmɪs.aɪl/
mistreat /ˌmɪsˈtriːt/
misunderstood /ˌmɪsʌndəˈstʊd/
mite /maɪt/
mitochondrial /ˌmaɪtəʊˈkɒndrɪəl/
mittens /ˈmɪt.ᵊnz/
mnemonic /nɪˈmɒn.ɪk/
modality /məʊˈdælɪtɪ/
mode /məʊd/
modify /ˈmɒd.ɪ.faɪ/
modulator /ˈmɑː.jə.ˌleɪ.tər/
moisture /ˈmɔɪs.tʃər/
moisturizing /ˈmɔɪstʃəˌraɪzɪŋ/
molar /ˈməʊlə/
molding /ˈməʊl.dɪŋ/
molluscum /mɒˈlʌskəm/ **contagiosum** /kənˈteɪdʒɪəs.əm/
momentary /ˈməʊ.mən.tər.i/
monoarthritis /ˌmɒn.əʊˌɑːˈθraɪ.tɪs/
monospot /ˈmɒnəʊ.spɒt/
monounsaturated /ˌmɒn.əʊ.ʌnˈsætʃ.ᵊr.eɪ.tɪd/
moodiness /ˈmuːdɪnɪs/
moody /ˈmuː.di/

mores /ˈmɔːreɪz/ zvyky, obyčeje
Moro /ˈmɔːr.ˌəʊ/ **reflex** /ˈriː.fleks/
morphogenesis /ˌmɔːr.fə.ˈdʒe.ni.sɪs/
mothering /ˈmʌðərɪŋ/
motility /ˌməʊ.ˈtil.i.ˈtiː/
motor /ˈməʊ.tər/
mottling /ˈmɒt.l̩ɪŋ/
mould /məʊld/
mounted /ˈmaʊn.tɪd/
mouthpiece /ˈmaʊθ.piːs/
movable /ˈmuː.vəbəl/
movement /ˈmuː.v.mənt/
mow /məʊ/
mucocutaneous /mjuː.kəʊ.kjuːˈteɪn.ɪəs/
mucopolysaccaridosis /ˌmjuː.kəʊˌpɒlɪˈsækəˌraɪd əʊsɪs/
mucopurulent /mjuːˈkəʊ ˈpjʊə.rʊ.lənt/
mucosa /mjuːˈkəʊ.sə/
mucosal /mjuːˈkəʊ.səl/
mucositis /mjuːˈkəʊ.saɪ.tɪs/
mucous membrane /ˌmjuː.kəsˈmem.breɪn/
muffin /ˈmʌf.ɪn/
muffled /ˈmʌf.l̩d/
multi /ˈmʌltɪ/
multidisciplinary /ˌmʌl.ti.dɪs.əˈplɪn.ᵊr.i/
multifactorial /ˌməl.tiː.fak.ˈtɔːr.iː.əl/
multiple / ˈmʌl.tɪ.pl̩ /
murmur /ˈmɜː.mər/
muscle /ˈmʌsəl/ **tone** /təʊn/
muscular dystrophy /ˌmʌs.kjʊ.ləˈdɪs.trə.fi/
musculature /ˈmʌs.kjʊ.lə.tʃər/
mutant /ˈmjuːtənt/
mutation /mjuːˈteɪʃən/
mute /mjuːt/
mutilation /ˌmjuː.tɪˈleiˌʃən/
mutual /ˈmjuː.tʃu.əl/
mutuality /ˌmjuːtʃuˈæləti/
muzzle /ˈmʌz.l̩/
myalgia /maɪˈæl.dʒi.ə/
myasthenia /ˌmaɪəˈsθɪːnɪ.ə/ **gravis** /ɡræv.ɪs/
mycobacterium /ˌmaɪkəʊ bækˈtɪərɪəm/
mycoplasma /ˌmaɪ.kəʊ.ˈplæz.mə/
myelodysplasia /ˌmaɪə.ləʊˈdɪsˈpleɪ.zɪə/
myelomeningocele /ˌmaɪ.ə.ləʊ.menˈɪŋ.ɡə.si:l/
myocarditis /ˌmaɪ.əʊ.kɑːdˈaɪ.tɪs/
myoclonic /ˌmaɪəʊˈklɒn.ɪk/
myoclonus /ˌmaɪ.əˈkləʊ.nəs/
myopathy /ˌmɑɪ.oʊˈpə.θi/

myositis /ˌmaɪəʊˈsaɪtɪs/
myotonic /ˌmaɪəˈtɒnɪk/

N

naevus /ˈniː.vəs/ pl **naevi**
nag /næg/
nap /næp/
nape /neɪp/
napkin /ˈnæpkɪn/
narcolepsy /ˈnɑː.kə.lep.si/
narcotize /ˈnɑːr.kə.ˌtaɪz/
narrowing /ˈnær.əʊ.ɪŋ/
nasal /ˈneɪ.zəl/ **flaring** / fleər.ɪŋ/
nasogastric /ˈneɪ.zəˈgæs.trɪk/
nasopharyngitis /ˈneɪ.zəˌfær.ɪnˈdʒaɪ.tɪs/
nature /ˈneɪ.tʃər/
nebulized /ˈneb.jə.laɪzd/
necessitate /nəˈses.ɪ.teɪt/
necrosis /ˈnek.rəʊ.sɪs/
needlestick /ˈniː.dᵊl.ˌstɪk/
negative /ˈneg.ə.tɪv/
neglect /nɪˈglekt/
negotiate /nɪˈgəʊʃɪˌeɪt/
neighbourhood /ˈneɪbəˌhʊd/
neonatorum /ˌniː.ə.nə.ˈtəʊr.əm/
nephritis /nɪˈfraɪ.tɪs/ pl **nephritides**
nephroblastoma /nɪˈfrəʊˌblæsˈtəʊ.mə/
nephrotic /nɪˈfrɒt.ɪk/
net /net/
neural tube /ˈnjʊə.rəl tjuːb/
neuroblastoma /ˌnjʊə.rəʊˈbla.ˈstəʊ.mə/
neurofibrom /ˌnjʊərəʊˈfaɪˈbrəʊmə/
neuroma /njʊˈrəʊ.mə/
neurotoxic /ˌnjʊə.rəʊˈtɒk.sɪk/
neutropenia /njuːtrəˈpiː.nɪə/
neutrophil /njuːtrə.fɪl/
Niemann-Pick disease /niːˈmən pik dɪˈziː.z/
nightmare /ˈnaɪt.meər/
nipple /ˈnɪp.ḷ/
nit /nɪt/
Nitrile /ˈnaɪ.trɪl/
nitrite /ˈnaɪtreɪt/
nitrogen /ˈnaɪ.trə.dʒən/
nocturia /nɒktˈjʊər.ɪ.ə/
node /nəʊd/
nodular /ˈnɒdʒ.ə.ləʳ/
non raised /ˌnɒn reɪzd/

non-blanching /nɒn.blɑːntʃ.ɪŋ/
non-judgemental /ˌnɒn.dʒʌdʒˈmen.təl/
nonpurulent /ˌnɒn.ˈpjʊə.rʊ.lənt/
nonsteroidal /ˌnɑː.n.stəˈrɔːi.dᵊl/
nonthreatening /ˌnɒn.ˈθret.ᵊn.ɪŋ/
nontuberculous /ˌnɒn.tjʊˌbɜːkjʊˈləs/
non-weight /ˌnɒnˈweɪt/
normochromic /ˌnɔːməʊˈkrəm.ɪk/
normocytic /ˌnɔːməʊˈsɪtɪk/
normothermia /ˌnɔːr.məʊ.ˈthər.miə/
nosebleed /ˈnəʊzˌbliːd/
notable /ˈnəʊ.tə.bl̩/
notch /nɒtʃ/
notice /ˈnəʊ.tɪs/
notify /ˈnəʊ.tɪ.faɪ/
notion /ˈnəʊʃən/
nuclear /ˈnjuː.klɪər/
numb /nʌm/
nurse /nɜːs/
nursery /ˈnɜːsrɪ/
nursing /ˈnɜː.sɪŋ/
nurture /ˈnɜːtʃə/
nutrient /ˈnjuː.tri.ənt/
nystagmus /nɪˈstæg.məs/

O
obey /əʊˈbeɪ/
objective /əbˈdʒek.tɪv/
obligatory /ɒˈblɪgətərɪ/
obliterans /əˈblɪtəˌrəns/
obliterate /əˈblɪtəˌreɪt/
obliterative /əˈblɪt.ᵊr.eɪt.ɪv/
obsessional /əbˈseʃənə/
obstacle /ˈɒbstəkəl/
obstetrician /ˌɒb.stəˈtrɪʃ.ən/
obstetrics /ɒbˈstetrɪks/
obviously /ˈɒb.vi.əs.li/
occipital /ɒkˈsɪp.ɪ.təl/
occlusion /əˈkluː.ʒən/
occlusive /ɒˈkluː.sɪv/
occult /əˈkʌlt/
occupant /ˈɒk.jʊ.pənt/
occupational /ˌɒk.jʊˈpeɪ.ʃən.əl/
occur /əˈkɜː/
occurrence /əˈkʌr.ənt s/
oculocerebrorenal /ˌɒkjʊləˌserɪbrəʊˈriːnᵊl/
oculocerebrorenal syndrome /ˌɒkjʊləˌserɪbrəʊˈriːnᵊl ˈsɪn.drəʊm/

odd /ɒd/

odour /ˈəʊ.dər/

oedema /ɪˈdiː.mə/

oesophageal /iːˌsɒfəˈdʒiːəl/

oesophagus /ɪˈsɒf.ə.gəs/

off-duty /ˌɒfˈdʒuː.ti/

offensive /əˈfent.sɪv/

ointment /ˈɔɪnt.mənt/

oliguria /ˌɒl.ɪˈgjʊə.rɪ.ə/

omission /əʊˈmɪʃ.ən/

omit /əʊˈmɪt/

ongoing /ˈɒŋˌgəʊ.ɪŋ/

oophoritis /ˌəʊvə.fəˈraɪ.tɪs/

ooze /uːz/

oozing /uːz,ɪŋ/

opacity /əʊˈpæsɪtɪ/

operational /ˌɒpərˈeɪʃənəl/

ophthalmia /ɑːfˈθal.miː.ə/

ophthalmoplegia /ˌɒf.θælˈmɒ ˈpliː.dʒiː.ə/

opisthotonos /ˌɒpɪsθɒtənəs/

opisthotonus /ˌɒpɪsθɒtə.nəs/

opposition /ˌɒpəˈzɪʃən/

optimise /ˈɒptɪˌmaɪz/

orchidopexy /ˌɔːkɪˈdopəksɪ/

orchitis /ˈɔːkaɪ.tɪs/

orderly /ˈɔːdəl.i/

organic /ɔːˈgæn.ɪk/

origin /ˈɒr.ɪ.dʒɪn/

orogastric /ˌəʊ.rəˈgæst.rɪk/

orthodontist /ˌɔːθəˈdɒntɪst/

orthostatic /ˌɔːθəˈstæt.ɪk/

osmolality /ˌɑːz.məʊ.ˈla.lə.tiː/

osmotic /ɒzˈmɒt.ɪk/

osteoblast /ˈɒstɪəʊˌblæst/

osteochondritis /ˌɒstɪ.əˌkɑːn.ˈdraɪt.əs/

osteodystrophy /ˌɒstɪəʊ.dɪˈstrəʊ.fɪ/

osteogenesis /ˌɒstɪəˈdʒen.ə.sɪs/ imperfecta /ˌim.pərˈfek.tə/

osteoid /ˌɒstɪˌɔid/

osteoma /ˌɒstɪ.ˈəʊ.mə/

osteomyelitis /ˌɒs.ti.əʊ.maɪ.əˈlaɪ.tɪs/

osteopenia /ˌɒstɪəʊˈpiːnə/

osteotomy /ˌɒstɪˈɒtəmɪ/

ostomy /ˈɒs.tə.mi/

otitis /əʊˈtaɪ.tɪs/ media /ˈmiːdɪə/

otoacoustics /ˌəʊ.təʊ.əˈkuː.stɪks/

outbreak /ˈaʊtˌbreɪk/

outburst /ˈaʊt.bɜːst/

outcome /ˈaʊt.kʌm/
outgoing /ˈaʊt.gəʊɪŋ/
outline /ˈaʊt.laɪn/
outpatient /ˈaʊt.peɪ.ʃənt/
outstretched /ˌaʊtˈstretʃt/
outweigh /ˌaʊtˈweɪ/
oval /ˈəʊ.vəl/
overall /ˌəʊ.vəˈrɔːl/
overcome /ˌəʊ.vəˈkʌm/
overcorrection /ˌəʊ.və.kəˈrek.ʃ°n/
overfeeding /ˌəʊ.vəˈfiː.dɪŋ/
overgrowth /ˌəʊ.və.grəʊθ/
overheating /ˌəʊvəˈhiː.tɪŋ/
overinvolved /ˌəʊ.və.ɪnˈvɒlvd/
overload /ˌəʊ.vəˈləʊd/
overlying /ˌəʊ.vəlˈaɪ.ɪŋ/
overnight /ˌəʊ.vəˈnaɪt/
oversee /ˌəʊ.vəˈsiː/
overstepping /ˌəʊ.vəstep.ɪŋ/
overt /əʊˈvɜːt/
over-tiredness /ˌəʊ.vəˈtaɪədnɪs/
overuse /ˌəʊ.vəˈjuːz/
overview /ˈəʊ.və.vjuː/
overwhelm /ˌəʊ.vəˈwelm/
overwhelming /ˌəʊ.vəˈwel.mɪŋ/
overwrought /ˌəʊvəˈrɔːt/
owing to /ˈəʊ.ɪŋ ˌtuː/

P
pace /peɪs/
pacifier /ˈpæs.ɪ.faɪ.ər/
pad /pæd/
paediatrician /ˌpiː.dɪəˈtrɪ.ʃən/
pain-coping /peɪn.kəʊp.ɪŋ/
paint /peɪnt/
palate /ˈpæl.ət/
palatine /ˈpælə,tan/
palliative /ˈpæl.i.ə.tɪv/
pallor /ˈpæl.ər/
palm /pɑːm/
palmar /pælm.ər/
palpation /pælˈpeɪ.ʃən/
palpebral /ˈpæl.pɪ.brəl/
palsy /ˈpɔːl.zi/
pancreatic /ˌpæŋ.krɪˈæ.tɪk/
pancreatitis /ˌpæŋ.kri.əˈtaɪ.tɪs/
panencephalitis /pæn,en.kef.əˈlaɪ.tɪs/

pants /pænts/
Pap smear /ˈpæpˌsmɪərˈ/
papilla pl papillae/pəˈpɪlə/
papilledema /pəˈpɪl.ə.ɪˈdiː.mə/
papillomavirus /ˌpa.pə.ˈləʊ.məˈvaɪə.rəs/
papule /ˈpæpjuːl/
paracentesis /ˌpærəˈ.senˈtiː.sɪs/
parachute /ˈpærəˌʃuːt/
paradoxic /ˌpærəˈdɒksɪk/
parallel /ˈpær.ə.lel/
paralysis /pəˈræl.ə.sɪs/
paramount /ˈpær.ə.maʊnt/
paranasal /ˌpær.əˈneɪ.zəl/ sinus /saɪ.nəs/
paraphimosis /ˌpær.ə.faɪˈməʊ.səs/
parasite /ˈpær.ə.saɪt/
parasitic /ˌpær.əˈsɪt.ɪk/
parasomnia /ˌpar.əˈsɑːm.niː.ə/
paratesticular /ˈpɑːr.ə tesˈtɪk.jə.lər/
paratyphus /ˌpærəˈtaɪfəs/
paravertebral /ˈpɑːr.ə ˈvɜː.tɪ.brəl/
parencephalopathy /ˈpɑːr.ˌen.kef.əˈlɒp.ə.θi/
parenchymal /pəˈreŋ.kə.məl/
parental /pəˈren.təl/
parenteral /pəˈren.tə.rəl/
parenthood /ˈpeərənthʊd/
parenting /ˈpeərəntɪŋ/
parietal /pəˈraɪə.təl/
paronychia /ˌper.ə.ˈni.kiː.ə/
parotid /pəˈrɒt.ɪd/ gland /glænd/
paroxysmal /ˈpær.ɒk.sɪz.məl/
partial /ˈpɑː.ʃəl/
participant /pɑːˈtɪs.ɪ.pənt/
participate /pɑːˈtɪs.ɪ.peɪt/
participation /pɑːˌtɪsɪˈpeɪʃən/
particle /ˈpɑː.tɪ.kl̩/
particularly /pəˈtɪk.jʊ.lə.li/
parvovirus /ˈpɑːr.vəʊ.ˌvaɪ.rəs/
passage /ˈpæs.ɪdʒ/
pat /ˈpæt/
patch /pætʃ/
patchy /ˈpætʃɪ/
patency /ˈpeɪ.tən.si/
patent /ˈpeɪ.tənt/
pathogen /ˈpæθ.ə.dʒən/
pathognomonic /ˌpath.əgˈnɒm.ɒ.nik/
pathway /ˈpɑː.θ.weɪ/
pattern /ˈpæt.ən/

paucity /ˈpɔː.sə.ti/

Pavlik /pɒvˈlɪk/ **harness** /ˈhɑː.nəs/

peak /piːk/ **flow** /fləʊ/

peanut /ˈpiː.nʌt/

pearl /pɜːl/

pebble /ˈpebəl/

pectus excavatum /ˌpek.təs eks.kəˈveɪ.təm/

peddle /ˈpedəl/

pedestrian /pəˈdes.tri.ən/

pediculosis /pi.ˌdi.kjə.ˈləʊ.səs/ **capitis** /ˈkap.ət.əs/

peel /piːl/

peer /pɪər/

penetrance /ˈpe.nə.trəns/

Penrose /ˈpen.ˌrəʊz/ **drain** /dreɪn/

perceive /pəˈsiːv/

percentage /pəˈsen.tɪdʒ/

perception /pəˈsep.ʃən/

perceptual /pəˈseptjʊəl/

percussion /pəˈkʌʃ.ən/

perennial /pəˈreniəl/

perfection /pəˈfekʃən/

perforation /pɜː.fərˈeɪ.ʃən/

perform /pəˈfɔːm/

performance /pəˈfɔː.məns/

performing /pəˈfɔːm.ɪŋ/

perfusion /pəˈfjuː.ʒən/

peri- /ˌperi/

pericarditis /ˌper.ɪ.kɑːdˈaɪ.tɪs/

perioral /ˌper.ɪˈɔː.rəl/

periorbital /ˌper.ɪ.ˈɔːbɪtəl/

periosteum /ˌper.ɪˈɒs.ti.əm/ pl **periostea**

peripheral /pəˈrɪf.ər.əl/

peristalsis /ˌper.ɪˈstæl.sɪs/

peristaltic /ˌper.ə.ˈstɔːl.tik/

peritonsillar /ˌperɪˈtɒns.ələ/

periventricular /ˌper.ɪ.venˈtrɪk.jə.ləʳ/

permanence /ˈpɜːmənəns/

permeability /ˌpɜː.mi.əˈbɪl.ɪ.ti/

permission /pəˈmɪʃ.ən/

permissive /pəˈmɪsɪv/

pernasal /ˈpər.ˈneɪ.zᵊl/

peroxisomal /pəˌrɒksɪˈsəʊməl/

perpetuate /pəˈpetʃ.u.eɪt/

persecution /ˌpɜːsɪˈkjuːʃən/

persist /pəˈsɪst/

persistence /pəˈsɪstəns/

persistent /pəˈsɪs.tənt/

personality /ˌpɜː.sənˈæl.ə.ti/

persuade /pəˈsweɪd/

Perthes /ˈper.ðez/ **disease** /dɪˈziːz/

pertinent /ˈpɜːtɪnənt/

pertussis /pəˈtʌ.sɪs/

petechia /pɪˈtiːkɪ.ə/ pl **petechiae**

petechial /pɪˈtiːkɪ.əl/

phalanx /fælæŋks/ pl **phalanges**

pharyngitis /ˌfær.ɪnˈdʒaɪ.tɪs/

phenomenon /fəˈnɒm.ɪ.nən/ pl **phenomena**

phenylketonuria /ˌfe.nᵊl.ˌkiː.tᵊn.ˈjʊə.rɪə/

pheochromocytoma /fiː.əʊ.krəʊ.məʊs.aɪˈtəʊ.mə/

philtrum /ˈfil.trəm/ pl **philtra** /-trə/

phimosis /faɪ.ˈməʊ.səs/

phobia /ˈfəʊ.bi.ə/

phobic /fəʊbɪk/

phosphate /ˈfɒs.feɪt/

phototherapy /ˈfəʊ.təʊ.θer.ə.pi/

phrase /freɪz/

phrenic /ˈfren.ɪk/

physical /ˈfɪz.ɪ.kəl/

phytate /ˈfaɪ.ˌteɪt/

pica /ˈpaɪ.kə/

pick /pɪk/

pick /ˈpɪk/ **up** /ʌp/

picky /ˈpɪkɪ/

pierce /ˈpɪə.s/

pigment /ˈpɪgmənt/

pigmentation /ˌpɪg.mənˈteɪ.ʃən/

pigmentosa renitis

pilchard /ˈpɪltʃəd/

pillow /ˈpɪl.əʊ/

pilocarpine /ˌpaɪ.lə.ˈkɑːr.ˌpiːn/

pilosebaceous /ˌpaɪ.ləʊ.si.ˈbeɪ.ʃəs/

pimple /ˈpɪm.pl̩/

pin /pɪn/

pincer /ˈpɪnsə/

pinch /pɪntʃ/

pinpoint /ˈpɪn.pɔɪnt/

pitch /pɪtʃ/

pituitary /pə.ˈtʊ.ə.ˌter.i:/ stalk /ˈstɔːk/

pituitary gland /pɪˈtjuː.ɪ.tər.i ˌglænd/

pityriasis /ˌpi.ti.ˈraɪ.ə.səs/

pityriasis /ˌpi.ti.ˈraɪ.ə.səs/ **rosea** /ˈrəʊ.ziː.ə/

pivotal /ˈpɪvətəl/

place /pleɪs/

placental /pləˈsen.təl/ **abruption** /əˈbrʌp.ʃən/

plantar /ˈplænt.ə/ **reflex** /ˈriː.fleks/
plaster /ˈplɑː.stər/
platelet /ˈpleɪt.lət/
play /pleɪ/ **up** /ʌp/
playpen /ˈpleɪˌpen/
pleiotropy /plaɪ.ˈɑː.trə.pi:/
plethora /ˈpleθ.ᵊr.ə/
plethoric /plə.ˈθɔːr.ik/
plot /plɒt/
pluck /plʌk/
plug /plʌɡ/
plunger /ˈplʌn.dʒər/
pneumococcal /ˌnjuː.məˈkɒkəl/
pneumococcus /ˌnuː.moʊˈkɑː.kəs/ pl **pneumococci** /ˌnuː.moʊˈkɒkaɪ/
Pneumocystis /njuːməʊˈsɪstɪs/ **jiroveci** /dʒaɪ.rəʊ.viːˈsaɪ/ (**carinii**) /kæ.raɪ.niːaɪ/
pneumomediastinum /ˌnu.məˌmiː.di.əˈstaɪ.nəm/
pneumonia /njuːˈməʊ.ni.ə/
pneumonitis /ˌnu.məˈnaɪ.tɪs/
point /pɔɪnt/
polio /ˈpəʊ.li.əʊ/
poliomyelitis /poʊ.li.oʊ.maɪ.ə.laɪ.tɪs/
pollen /ˈpɒl.ən/
pollution /pəˈluː.ʃən/
polycystic disease /pɒl.iˌsɪs.tɪk dɪˌziːz/
polycythemia /ˌpɑː.liːˌsaɪ.ˈthiː.miː.ə/
polydipsia /ˌpɒl.ɪˈdɪp.sɪ.ə/
polymyositis /ˌpɒlɪˈmaɪəs aɪtɪs/
polyneuropathy /ˈpɒlɪnjʊˈrɒpəθɪ/
polyp /ˈpɒlɪp/
polyphonic /ˈpɒlɪˈfɒnɪk/
polysyllabic /ˌpɒl.i.sɪˈlæb.ɪk/
polyuria /ˌpɒl.ɪˈjʊə.rɪ.ə/
pontocerebellar /pɒnˈto.ser.e.belˈar/
popliteal /pɑpˈlɪʈ.i.əl/
pore /pɔr/
porosis /ˈpɔːrəsɪs/
port /pɔːt/
Port /pɔːt/ **wine** /waɪn/
portacath /ˈpɔːtəˈkæθ/
portal /ˈpɔː.təl/
pose /pəʊz/
possess /pəˈzes/
post /ˈpəʊst/
postauricular /ˈpəʊst ɔːˈrɪkjʊlə/
postcoital /ˌpəʊstˈkəʊitᵊl/
posterior /pɒsˈtɪə.ri.ər/
postexposure /ˈpəʊst.ɪkˈspəʊ.ʒəʳ/

postictal /ˈpəʊstˈɪkt.əl/
postnasal /ˈpəʊstˈneɪ.zᵊl/
postpone /pəʊstˈpəʊn/
postrenal /ˈpəʊstˈriː.nəl/
postural /ˈpɒstˌʃər.əl/
posture /ˈpɒs.tʃər/
potent /ˈpəʊ.tənt/
pounding /ˈpaʊn.dɪŋ/
pour /pɔːr/
poverty /ˈpɒv.ə.ti/
povidone /ˈpəʊ.vəˌdəʊn / iodine /ˈaɪ.əˌdaɪn/
power /ˈpaʊə/
powerful /ˈpaʊə.fəl/
practicality /ˌpræktɪˈkælɪtɪ/
preach /priːtʃ/
precaution /prɪˈkɔːˌʃən/
precede /prɪˈsiːd/
precipitate /prɪˈsɪp.ɪ.teɪt/
precipitating /prɪˈsɪp.ɪ.teɪt.ɪŋ/
precipitation /prɪˌsɪpɪˈteɪʃən/
precipitator /prɪˌsɪp.ɪˈteɪ.təʳ/
precipitously /prɪˈsɪp.ɪ.təs.li/
precocious /prɪˈkəʊ.ʃəs/
preconceptual /ˌpriː.kənˈsep.tʃu.əl/
predetermined /ˌpriː.dɪˈtɜː.mɪnd/
predicament /prɪˈdɪk.ə.mənt/
predict /prɪˈdɪkt/
predictable /prɪˈdɪk.tə.blˌ/
prediction /prɪˈdɪkʃən/
predictor /prɪˈdɪk.tər/
predispose /ˌpriː.dɪˈspəʊz/
predisposition /ˌpriːdɪs.pəˈzɪʃ.ən/
predominantly /prɪˈdɒmɪnəntlɪ/
predominate /prɪˈdɒm.ɪ.neɪt/
preference /ˈpref.ər.ənt s/
pregnancy /ˈpreg.nən.si/
prelabour /ˌpriːˈleɪ.bəʳ/
prelinguistic /ˌpriː.lɪŋˈgwɪs.tɪk/
premature /ˈprem.ə.tʃər/
prematurity /priː məˈtjʊə.rɪ.ti/
premonitoring /priːˈmɒnɪtərɪŋ/
preoccupation /priːˌɒkjʊˈpeɪʃən/
preoccupied /ˌpriːˈɒk.jʊ.paɪd/
preparation /ˌprepəˈreɪʃən/
preponderance /prɪˈpɒndərəns/
prerenal /prɪˌˈriː.nəl/
preschool /priːˈskuːl/

presentation /ˌprez.ənˈteɪ.ʃən/
presenter /prɪˈzentə/
presenting /prɪˈzent.ɪŋ/ **part** /pɑːt/
preservation /ˌprez.əˈveɪ.ʃən/
preservative /prɪˈzɜːvətɪv/
pressure /ˈpreʃ.ə/
pressure /ˈpreʃ.ə/ **ulcer** /ˈʌl.sər/
presume /prɪˈzjuːm/
presumptive /prɪˈzʌmptɪv/
pretend /prɪˈtend/
prevalence /ˈprevələns/
prevent /prɪˈvent/
preventable /prɪˈven.tə.bl̩/
preventive /prɪ.ventiv/
priapism /ˈpraɪ.əˌpɪz.əm/
primitive /ˈprɪmɪtɪv/
principal /ˈprɪnt.sɪ.pəl/
privilege /ˈprɪvɪlɪdʒ/
probe /prəʊb/
procedure /prəˈsiːdʒə/
proceed /prəˈsiːd/
process /ˈprəʊ.ses/
prodrome /ˈprəʊ.drəʊm/
productive /prəˈdʌk.tɪv/
proficient /prəˈfɪʃənt/
profound /prəˈfaʊnd/
profoundly /prəˈfaʊnd.li/
prognathia /ˈprɒg.nə.θɪ.ə/
prognosis /prɒgˈnəʊ.sɪs/
projectile /prəˈdʒek.taɪl/
prolapsed /prəʊˈlæpst/
prolong /prəˈlɒŋ/
prolyferative /prəˈlɪfərətɪv/
prominence /ˈprɒm.ɪ.nəns/
prominent /ˈprɒm.ɪ.nənt/
prominently /ˈprɒm.ɪ.nənt.li/
promotion /prəˈməʊ.ʃən/
promptly /ˈprɒmpt.li/
proof /pruːf/
prop /prɒp/
property /ˈprɒp.ə.ti/
prophylaxis /ˌprɒf.ɪˈlæk.sɪs/
proposition /ˌprɒpəˈzɪʃən/
proptosis /prɑːp.ˈtəʊ.səs/
prostaglandins /ˌprɒstəˈglændɪnz/
protective /prəˈtek.tɪv/
protein /ˈprəʊ.tiːn/

proteinuria /ˈprəʊ.tiːn.jʊəˈriː.ə/

proton /ˈprəʊtɒn/

protrusion /prəˈtruːʒən/

protuberant /prəˈtjuːbərənt/

provide /prəˈvaɪd/

proximity /prɒkˈsɪm.ɪ.ti/

proxy /ˈprɒksɪ/

prune /pruːn/

pruritus /prʊəˈraɪ.təs/

pseudomonas aeruginosa /suː.dəʊ.məʊnæz e.rɜːdʒi.nəʊsæ/

pseudoseizure /ˌsjuːdəʊˈsiːʒə/

psoriasis /səˈraɪəsɪs/

psychogenic /ˌsaɪ.kəʊˈdʒɛ.nɪk/

psychosis /saɪˈkəʊ.sɪs/

pubis /ˈpjuː.bɪs/

puff /ˈpʌf/

puffy /ˈpʌf.i/

pull /pʊl/

pull /pʊl/ **in** /ɪn/

pulling /pʊl.ɪŋ/

pulmonary /ˈpʊl.mə.nə.ri/

pulsatile /ˈpʌlsəˌtaɪl/ **mass** /mæs/

pulse /pʌls/ **oximetry** /ˈɒk.sɪ.m.ɪ.tri/

punch /pʌntʃ/

puncture / ˈpʌŋk.tʃə/

punish /ˈpʌnɪʃ/

punishment /ˈpʌn.ɪʃ.mənt/

pupillary /pjuː.pɪl.ər.i/

purple /ˈpɜː.plˌ/

purpose /ˈpɜː.pəs/

purposeful /ˈpɜːpəsfəl/

purposefully /ˈpɜːpəsfəlɪ/

purpura /ˈpər.pjə.rə/

purse /pɜːs/

pursue /pəˈsjuː/

purulent /ˈpjʊə.rʊ.lənt/

pus /pʌs/

push /pʊʃ/

pustular /ˈpʌs.tjuːl.ər/

pustule /ˈpʌstjuːl/

pyelonephritis /ˌpaɪ.ə.lə.nɪˈfraɪ.tɪs/

pyloric /paɪˈlɔːr.ik/

pyloromyotomy /ˌpaɪlɔːrˈmaɪə.tə.mɪ/

pylorospasm /paɪˈləʊr.ə.ˌspaz.əm/

pyramidal /pɪˈræm.ɪ.dəl/

pyridoxine /ˌpir.ə.ˈdɑːk.ˌsiːn/

562

Q

quarrel /ˈkwɒrəl/
queasiness /ˈkwiːzɪnɪs/
quieten /ˈkwaɪə.tᵊn/
quietly /ˈkwaɪətlɪ/
quinsy /ˈkwɪnzɪ/

R

radial /ˈreɪ.dɪəl/
radiant /ˈreɪ.di.ənt/
radiograph /ˈreɪ.di.əˌgrɑːf/
raindrop /ˈreɪnˌdrɒp/
raise /reɪz/
raisin /ˈreɪzən/
random /ˈrændəm/
ranula /ˈran.jə.lə/
rapid /ˈræpɪd/
rash /ræʃ/
rasping /ˈrɑːspɪŋ/
rating /ˈreɪ.tɪŋ/
ratio /ˈreɪ.ʃi.əʊ/
rattan /ræˈtæn/
rave /reɪv/
reabsorption /riː.əbˈzɔːp.ʃən/
reach for /riːtʃ/
reactant /riˈæk.tənt/
read /riːd/ **out** /aʊt/
reading /ˈriː.dɪŋ/
realize /ˈrɪə.laɪz/
reappear /ˌriː.əˈpɪər/
reassessment /ˌriː.əˈses.mənt/
reassurance /ˌriːəˈʃʊə.rəns/
rebellion /rɪˈbeljən/
recall / rɪˈkɔːl/
recent /ˈriː.sənt/
receptor /rɪˈsep.tər/
recessive /rɪˈses.ɪv/
recheck /ˌriːˈtʃek/
reciprocal /rɪˈsɪprəkəl/
recognition /ˌrek.əgˈnɪʃ.ən/
recoil /rɪˈkɔɪl/
recollection /ˌrekəˈlekʃən/
reconciliation /ˌrek.ənˌsɪl.iˈeɪ.ʃən/
reconstitute /ˌriːˈkɒn.stɪ.tjuːt/
record /ˈrekɔːd/
recovery /rɪˈkʌv.ər.i/
rectal /ˈrek.təl/

recumbent /rɪˈkʌm.bənt/
recur /rɪˈkɜːr/
recurrence /rɪˈkʌ.rəns/
recurrent /rɪˈkʌ.rənt/
redden /ˈred.ən/
redistribution /ˌriːdɪstrɪˈbjuːʃən/
reduction /rɪˈdʌk.ʃən/
refeeding /rɪˈfiː.dɪŋ/
refer /rɪˈfɜːr/
reference /ˈref.ər.ənt s/
referral /rɪˈfɜː.rəl/
referred /rɪˈfɜːd/
refine /rɪˈfaɪn/
reflect /rɪˈflekt/
reflex /ˈriː.fleks/
refractive /rɪˈfræk.tɪv/
refrigeration /rɪˌfrɪdʒ.əˈreɪ.ʃən/
refugee /ˌrefjʊˈdʒiː/
refuse /rɪˈfjuːz/
regarding /rɪˈɡɑː.dɪŋ/
regimen /ˈredʒ.ɪ.mən/
regression /rɪˈɡreʃ.ən/
regressive /rɪˈɡresɪv/
regular /ˈreɡ.jʊ.lər/
regularity /ˌreɡ.jʊˈlær.ə.ti/
regurgitation /rɪˌɡɜː.dʒɪˈteɪ.ʃən/
reinforcement /ˌriːɪnˈfɔːsmənt/
reinstitution /riːˌɪn.stɪˈtʃuː.ʃ°n/
reject /rɪˈdʒekt/
rejection /rɪˈdʒek.ʃən/
relapse /rɪˈlæps/
relationship /rɪˈleɪ.ʃən.ʃɪp/
release /rɪˈliːs/
reliable /rɪˈlaɪə.b|/
relieve /rɪˈliːv/
religious /rɪˈlɪdʒəs/
reluctant /rɪˈlʌktənt/
rely /rɪˈlaɪ/ **on** /ɒn/
remark /rɪˈmɑːk/
remarkably /rɪˈmɑːkəblɪ/
remarriage /ˌriːˈmærɪdʒ/
remedy /ˈrem.ə.di/
remission /rɪˈmɪʃ.ən/
remit /rɪˈmɪt/
renal /ˈriː.nəl/
renal /ˈriː.nəl/ **tubule** /ˈtjuː.bjuːl/
render /ˈren.dər/

repair /rɪˈpeər/
repeat /rɪˈpiːt/
repetition /ˌrepɪˈtɪʃən/
repetitive /rɪˈpet.ə.tɪv/
replacement / rɪˈpleɪs.mənt/
replication /ˌrep.lɪˈkeɪʃən/
reproducible /ˌriː.prə.djuːsɪ.bḷ/
request /rɪˈkwest/
requirement /rɪˈkwaɪə.mənt/
rescue /ˈreskjuː/
resectability /rɪsektəˈbɪlɪtɪ/
resemble /rɪˈzem.bḷ/
resentful /rɪˈzentfə/
residual /rɪˈzɪd.ju.əl/
residue /ˈrez.ɪ.djuː/
resilience /rɪˈzɪlɪəns/
resilient /rɪˈzɪl.i.ənt/
resistance /rɪˈzɪs.tənt s/
resistant /rɪˈzɪs.tənt/
resolution /ˌrez.əˈluː.ʃən/
resolve /rɪˈzɒlv/
resorption /ˌriː.ˈsɔːrp.ʃən/
respectful /rɪˈspektfəl/
respiratory /ˈre.spə.rə.ˌtɔːr.iː/ distress /di.ˈstres/ syndrome /sin.ˌdrəʊm/ RDS
responsibility /rɪˌspɒn.sɪˈbɪl.ɪ.ti/
responsive /rɪˈspɒn.sɪv/
rest /rest/
restless /ˈrest.ləs/
restlessness /ˈrest.ləs.nəs/
restore /rɪˈstɔːr/
restrain /rɪˈstreɪn/
restraint /rɪˈstreɪnt/
restrict /rɪˈstrɪkt/
restricted /rɪˈstrɪk.tɪd/
retardant /rɪˈtɑː.dᵊnt/
retardation /ˌriː.tɑːˈdeɪ.ʃən/
retention /rɪˈten.ʃən/
reticuloendothelial /rɪˌtɪk.jəˈleˌen.dəʊˈθiː.li.əl/
retina /ˈret.ə.nə/
retinal /ˈret.ɪ.nəl/
retinitis /ˌre.tə.ˈnaɪ.təs/
retinoblastoma /ˌre.tə.nəʊ.ˌbla.ˈstəʊ.mə/
retinoid /ˈre.tə.ˌnɔːid/
retract /rɪˈtrækt/
retraction /rɪˈtræk.ʃən/
retraining /ˌriː.ˈtreɪn.ɪŋ/
retreat /rɪˈtriːt/

retrognathia /ˈreˌtrəʊˈnath.iː.ə/
retrograde /ˈret.rəʊ .greɪd/
retroperitoneal /ˌretrəʊˌperɪˈniːəl/
retropharyngeal /ˌretrəʊˌfærɪnˈdʒiːəl/
Rett syndrome /ˈret sɪndrəʊm/
reveal /rɪˈviːl/
revenge /rɪˈvendʒ/
reversal /rɪˈvɜː.səl/
reward /rɪˈwɔːd/
rhabdomyoma /ˌræbdəʊmaɪˈəʊmə/
rheumatic /ruːˈmætɪk/
rhinitis /raɪˈnaɪtɪs/
rhinorrhoea /raɪ.nəˈriə/
rhonchus /ˈrɒŋkəs/ pl **rhonchi** /ˈrɒŋ.kaɪ/
rhubarb /ˈruːbɑːb/
rhythmic /ˈrɪðmɪk/
rhythmicity /ˈrɪðmɪsə.tiː/
ribbon /ˈrɪbən/
rickets /ˈrɪk.ɪts/
Rickettsiae /rɪˈkɛt.si.ə/
ridge /rɪdʒ/
rigid /ˈrɪdʒɪd/
rigor /ˌrɪg.ə/
ring /rɪŋ/
ringworm /ˈrɪŋˌwɜːm/
rinse /rɪns/
road /rəʊd/ **traffic** /ˈtræf.ɪk/
robust /roʊˈbʌst/
rock /rɒk/
rodent /ˈrəʊ.dənt/
role /rəʊl/ **taking** /teɪk.ɪŋ/
roll /rəʊl/
Romberg /romˈbərg/ **sign** /saɪn/
rooting /ˈruːt ɪŋ/
roseola /rəʊˈziːələ/
rotate /rəʊ ˈteɪt/
rotavirus /ˈrəʊtəˌvaɪrəs/
rough /rʌf/
roughen /ˈrʌfən/
round /raʊnd/
rounded /ˈraʊn.dɪd/
rub /rʌb/
rubber /ˈrʌbə/
rug /rʌg/
running /ˈrʌn.ɪŋ/
runny /ˈrʌn.i/ **nose** /nəʊz/
rupture /ˈrʌp.tʃər/

rural /ˈrʊərəl/
rust /rʌst/

S
salicylate /səˈlɪs.ə.leɪt/
saline /ˈseɪ.laɪn/
salivation /ˈsæl.ɪ.veɪ.ʃən/
salmonella /ˌsæl.məˈnel.ə/ pl **salmonellae**
salute /səˈluːt/
sample /ˈsɑːm.pl̩/
sand /sænd/ **sharp** /ˈʃɑːrp/
sandpaper /ˈsændˌpeɪpə/
sanitation /ˌsæn.ɪˈteɪ.ʃən/
sarcoidosis /ˌsɑr.kɔɪˈdoʊ.sɪs/
sarcoma /sɑːˈkəʊ.mə/
satisfaction /ˌsætɪsˈfækʃən/
saturation /ˌsæt.jʊˈreɪ.ʃən/
saving /ˈlaɪfˌseɪ.vɪŋ/
scabies /ˈskeɪ.biːz/
scale /skeɪl/
scaling /skeɪl.ɪŋ/
scaly /ˈskeɪ.li/
scarf /skɑːf/
scarlet /ˈskɑːlɪt/ **fever** /ˈfiːvə/
scarring /skɑːr.ɪŋ/
scatter /ˈskæt.ər/
schedule /ˈʃedjuːl/
Scheuermann /ˈʃojer.maen/ **disease** /dɪˈziːz/
schizophrenia /ˌskɪt.səˈfriː.ni.ə/
sclera /ˈsklɪə.rə/
scleral /ˈsklɪə.rəl/
sclerosis /skləˈrəʊ.sɪs/ pl **scleroses**
scold /skəʊld/
scoliosis /ˌskɒl.iˈəʊ.sɪs/
score /skɔː/
scraping /ˈskreɪ.pɪŋ/
scratch /skrætʃ/
scribble /ˈskrɪb.l̩/
scrotal /ˈskrəʊ.təl/
scrotum /ˈskrəʊ.təm/ pl **scrotta**
scrutinize /ˈskruː.tɪˌnaɪz/
seafood /ˈsiː.fuːd/
sebaceous /sɪˈbeɪʃəs/
seborrheic /ˌsebərˈriː.ɪk/
seborrhoea /sɪˈb.əˈri.ə/
sebum /ˈsiːbəm/
secretion /sɪˈkriː.ʃən/

secretory /'sek.rə.tər.i/
secure /sɪ'kjʊə/
security /sɪ'kjʊə.rɪ.ti/
sedentary /'sed.ən.tər.i/
sedimentation /ˌsedɪmen'teɪ.ʃən/ **rate** /reɪt/
seed /siːd/
seek /siːk/ **(sought, sought)**
seem /siːm/
seemingly /'siː.mɪŋ.li/
seesaw /'siːˌsɔː/
segment /'seg.mənt/
seizure /'siː.ʒə/
selective /sɪ'lek.tɪv/
self-autonomy /ˌself.ɔː'tɒn.ə.mi/
self-concept /self 'kɒn.sept/
self-confidence /ˌself 'kɒn.fɪ.dəns/
self-control /ˌself.kən'trəʊl/
self-destructive /ˌself dɪ'strʌk.tɪv/
self-esteem /ˌself.ɪ'stiːm/
self-fulfilment /ˌself fʊl'fɪl.mənt/
self-gratification /selfˌgræt.ɪ.frɪ'keɪ.ʃən/
self-induced /ˌself.ɪn'djuːst/
self-limiting /self.'lɪm.ɪ.tɪŋ/
self-locking /ˌself lɒk.ɪŋ/
self-perception /ˌself pə'sep.ʃən/
self-protection /ˌself prə'tek.ʃən/
self-quieting /ˌself 'kwaɪ.ət.ɪŋ/
self-reflective /ˌself rɪ'flek.tɪv/
self-regulating /ˌself.'reg.jə.leɪt.ɪŋ/
self-reliant /ˌself rɪ'laɪ.ənt/
self-resolving /ˌself rɪ'zɒlv.ɪŋ/
self-starvation /ˌself stɑː'veɪ.ʃən/
self-worth /ˌself'wɜːθ/
semipermeable /sem.i 'pɜː.mi.ə.bl/
sensation /sen'seɪ.ʃən/
sensible /'sensɪbəl/
sensitization /ˌsen.sɪ.taɪ'zeɪ.ʃən/
sensitize /'sen.sɪ.taɪz/
sensorimotor /sensɒ.re.məʊ.tər/
sensorineural /sen'sə.riː.nuːr'əl/
sensory / 'sent .sər.i/
sentence /'sen.təns/
separate /'sep.ər.ət/
separation /ˌsep.ə'reɪ.ʃən/
sepsis /'sep.sɪs/
septicaemia /ˌsep.tɪ'siː.mi.ə/
septo-optic /ˌsep.təʊ.op'tik/

septostomy /sepˈtɒstəmɪ/
septum /ˈsep.təm/
sequence /ˈsiː.kwəns/
sequential /sɪˈkwen.ʃəl/
sequestration /ˌsiː.kwesˈtreɪʃᵊn/
serially /ˈsɪə.ri.ə.li/
seroconversion /sɪˈrɒ.kənˈvɜː.ʃᵊn/
serum /ˈsɪə.rəm/ pl **sera**
session /ˈseʃ.ən/
setting /ˈsetɪŋ/
settle /ˈsetəl/ **back** /bæk/
severity /sɪˈver.ɪ.ti/
shade /ʃeɪd/
shadow /ˈʃæd.əʊ/
shaft /ʃɑːft/
shake /ʃeɪk/ (**shook, shaken**)
shallow /ˈʃæləʊ/
shame /ʃeɪm/
shape /ʃeɪp/
share /ʃeə/
sharp /ʃɑːp/
shed /ʃed/
sheet /ʃiːt/
shellfish /ˈʃel.fɪʃ/
shelter /ˈʃel.tər/
shift /ʃɪft/
shin /ʃɪn/
shiny /ˈʃaɪ.ni/
shivering /ˈʃɪv.ər.ɪŋ/
shooting /ˈʃuː.tɪŋ/ **pain** /peɪn/
short tempered /ˌʃɔːtˈtem.pəd/
short-chain /ʃɔːt tʃeɪn/
shortening /ˈʃɔː.tənɪŋ/
shortness /ˈʃɔːt.nəs/
shoulder /ˈʃəʊl.dər/
shout /ʃaʊt/ **at** /ət/
shouting /ˈʃaʊ.tɪŋ/
shrink /ʃrɪŋk/
shrub /ʃrʌb/
shunt /ʃʌnt/
Shwachman syndrome /ʃwaːkmæn ˈsɪndrəʊm/
shyness /ʃaɪnɪs/
sibling /ˈsɪb.lɪŋ/
side /saɪd/ **effect** /ɪˈfekt/
sideways /ˈsaɪdˌweɪz/
sign /saɪn/
silence /ˈsaɪ.ləns/

simultaneously /ˌsɪm.əlˈteɪ.ni.əs.li/

single-parent /ˈsɪŋɡəl ˈpeə.rənt/

single-parenting /ˈsɪŋɡəl.ˈpeərəntɪŋ/

sink /sɪŋk/

sinus /ˈsaɪ.nəs/ pl **sinuses**

sinusitis /ˌsaɪˌnəˈsaɪ.tɪs/

skeletal /ˈskel.ɪ.təl/

skim /skɪm/

skin /skɪn/

skin fold /ˈskin.ˌfəʊld/

skinfold /ˈskin.ˌfəʊld/

skin-prick /skɪn prɪk/

slam /slæm/

slant /slɑːnt/

slate /sleɪt/

sleepiness /ˈsliː.pɪ.nəs/

sleepwalk /ˈsliːpˌwɔːk/

slide /slaɪd/ **(slid, slid)**

slim /slɪm/

slip /slɪp/

slit-lamp /slɪt læmp/

smack /smæk/

small /smɔːl/ **bowel** /ˈbaʊ.əl/

smallpox /ˈsmɔːl.pɒks/

smell /smel/

smooth /smuːð/

smother /ˈsmʌð.ər/

snake /sneɪk/

snap /snæp/

sneeze /sniːz/

sneezing /sniːz.ɪŋ/

sniffing /snɪf.ɪŋ/

snore /snɔːr/

sodium /ˈsəʊ.di.əm/ **chloride** /ˈklɔː.raɪd/

soft /sɒft/ **palate** /ˈpæl.ət/

softener /ˈsɒfənə/

sole /səʊl/

solvent /ˈsɒl.vənt/

somatic /səˈmæt.ɪk/

somatization /səʊˈmæ.taɪ.zeɪʃən/

somnolence /ˈsɒm.nəl.əns/

sorbitol /səʊrˈbi.tol/

sore /sɔː/ **throat** /θrəʊt/

sorrow /ˈsɒrəʊ/

spare /ˈspeə/

sparing /ˈspeə.rɪŋ/

spasm /ˈspæz.əm/

spasmodic /spæzˈmɒd.ɪk/
spasticity /spæsˈtɪs.ə.ti/
species /ˈspiː.ʃiːz/
specific /spəˈsɪf.ɪk/
specimen /ˈspes.ə.mɪn/
spectroscopy /ˈspektrəˌskə.pɪ/
speech /spiːtʃ/ **therapist** /ˈθer.ə.pɪst/
spell /spel/
spending /spendɪŋ/
sperm /spɜːm/
spermatogenesis /spər.mat.əˈdʒen.ə.səs/
sphenoid /sfiːn.ɒ.ɪd/
spherocytosis /ˌsfɪərəʊsaɪˈtəʊsɪs/
sphincter /ˈsfɪŋk.tər/
sphygmomanometer /ˌsfɪg.məʊ.mɪ.tər/
spider /ˈspaɪ.dər/
spina bifida /ˌspaɪ.nəˈbɪf.ɪ.də/
spinach /ˈspɪn.ɪtʃ/
spinal /ˈspaɪ.nəl/ **cord** /kɔːd/
spirit /ˈspɪr.ɪt/
spiritual /ˈspɪr.ɪ.tju.əl/
spirometry /spaɪˈrɒ.m.ɪ.tri/
spit up /spɪt ʌp/
spite /spaɪt/
spleen /spliːn/
splenectomy /spləˈnek.tə.mi/
splenomegaly /ˌspliː.nəʊˈmɛg.ə.lɪ/
splint /splɪnt/
splinter /ˈsplɪn.tər/
split /splɪt/
spondylolisthesis /spɒnˈdl.əʊ.lɪs.thiːˈ.sɪs/
spondylosis /ˌspɒn.dɪˈləʊ.sɪs/
sporadic /spəˈrædɪk/
spore /spɔːr/
spot /spɒt/
spouse /spaʊs/
sprain /spreɪn/
spread /spred/
spring /sprɪŋ/
spurt /spɜːt/
sputum /ˈspjuː.təm/ pl **sputa**
spying /spaɪ.ɪŋ/
squeak /skwiːk/
squint /skwɪnt/
stable /ˈsteɪ.bl̩/
stage /steɪdʒ/
stain /steɪn/

stance /stɑːns/
startle /ˈstɑː.tl̩/
starvation /stɑːˈveɪ.ʃən/
state /steɪt/
stature /ˈstætʃ.ər/
status /ˈsteɪ.təs/
steadily /ˈsted.ɪ.li/
steal /stiːl/
steatohepatitis /ˌstɪətəˌhe.pəˈtaɪ.təs/
steatorrhea /ˌstɪətəˈrɪə/
stem /stem/ **cell** /sel/
stenosis /steˈnəʊ.sɪs/
stent /stent/
step /step/
steplike /ˈstep.laɪk/
stepparent /ˈstepˌpeərənt/
stepping /step.ɪŋ/
sternal /ˈstɜː.nəl/
sternum /ˈstɜː.nəm/
stertor /ˈstɜr.tər/ c
stethoscope /ˈsteθ.ə.skəʊp/
stick /stɪk/ **(stuck, stuck)**
sticky /ˈstɪk.i/
stiffness /ˈstɪf.nəs/
stigmata /stɪgˈmɑː.tə/
stillbirth /ˈstɪlˌbɜːθ/
stillborn /ˈstɪl.bɔːn/
stimulation /ˌstɪm.jʊˈleɪ.ʃən/
stimulus /ˈstɪm.jʊ.ləs/ pl **stimuli**
sting /stɪŋ/
stockinette /ˌstɒk.əˈnɛt/
stool /stuːl/
storage /ˈstɔː.rɪdʒ/
stow /stəʊ/
strabismus /strəˈbɪz.məs/
straighteners /ˈstreɪ.tᵊn.əz/
straining /streɪn.ɪŋ/
stranger /ˈstreɪn.dʒər/
strangulation /ˌstræŋ.gjʊˈleɪ.ʃən/
strawberry /ˈstrɔː.bər.i/
stream /striːm/
stress /stres/
stretch /stretʃ/
stridor /straɪd.ər/
string /strɪŋ/
string /strɪŋ/ **bean** /biːn/
strip /strɪp/
strive /straɪv/

stroke /strəʊk/

struggle /ˈstrʌɡəl/

stuffed /stʌft/

stuffy /ˈstʌfɪ/

stupor /ˈstjuː.pər/

sturdy /ˈstɜːdɪ/

stuttering /ˈstʌtərɪŋ/

stye /staɪ/

subaponeurotic /ˌsəb.ˌap.ə.ˌnjʊə.rəʊ.tɪk/

subarachnoid /ˌsʌb.əˈræk.nɔɪd/

subclavian /sʌbˈkleɪv.ɪ.ən/

subclavicular /sʌbˈ.kləˈvɪk.jə.ləʳ/

subclinical /sʌbˈklɪn.ɪ.kəl/

subconjunctival /ˌsʌbˌkɒn.dʒaŋk.ˈtɪ.vəl/

subcutaneous /ˌsʌb.kjʊˈteɪ.ni.əs/

subcutaneously /ˌsʌb.kjʊˈteɪ.ni.əs.li/

subdural /sʌbˈdjʊ.ə.rəl/

subgaleal /ˌsʌb.geɪ.lɪ.əl/

subjective /səbˈdʒek.tɪv/

sublingually /ˌsʌbˈlɪŋ.gwəli/

submission /səbˈmɪʃ.ən/

submucous /ˌsʌb.ˈmjuː.kəs/

suboccipital /ˌsʌb.ɒkˈsɪp.ɪ.təl/

subsequent /ˈsʌb.sɪ.kwənt/

subsequently /ˈsʌb.sɪ.kwənt.li/

substandard /sʌbˈstændəd/

substernal /sʌbˈstɜː.nəl/

substitute /ˈsʌb.stɪ.tjuːt/

subtle /ˈsʌt.əl/

subungual /sʌbˈʌŋgwəl/

succedaneum /sʌkse.deɪniː.um/

succession /səkˈseʃ.ən/

successive /səkˈsesɪv/

suck /sʌk/

sucrase /ˈsuːkreɪz/

suction /ˈsʌk.ʃən/

suddenness /ˈsʌdənnɪs/

sufasalazine /sulfaː.sal.aː.ziːn/

suffocate /ˈsʌf.ə.keɪt/

suggestive /səˈdʒes.tɪv/

suicide /ˈsuː.ɪ.saɪd/

suitable /ˈsj uː.tə.bl̩/

sulcus /ˈsʌl.kəs/ pl sulci

sulfite /ˈsʌl.faɪt/

sultana /sʌlˈtɑː.nə/

summarize /ˈsʌm.ər.aɪz/

summon /ˈsʌm.ən/

superimposed /ˌsuːpərɪmˈpəʊzd/
superior /suːˈpɪə.ri.ər/ **vena cava** /ˌviː.nəˈkeɪ.və/
superiority /suːˌpɪərɪˈɒrɪtɪ/
supernatural /ˌsuːpəˈnætʃrəl/
supinate/ˈsuː.pɪn.eɪt/
supine /ˈsuː.paɪn/
supplement /ˈsʌp.lɪ.mənt/
supplemental /ˌsʌp.lɪˈmen.təl/
support /səˈpɔːt/
supportive /səˈpɔː.tɪv/
suppress /səˈpres/
suppression /səˈpreʃən/
suppurative /ˈsʌpjʊrə.tɪv/
suprapubic /ˌsuː.prəˈpjuː.bɪk/
suprasternal /ˌsuː.prə.ˈstɜː.nəl/
surface /ˈsɜː.fɪs/
surfactant /sərˈfak.tənt/
surgery /ˈsɜː.dʒər.i/
surgical /ˈsɜː.dʒɪ.kəl/
surrender /səˈrendə/
surrogate /ˈsʌr.ə.gət/
surveillance /səˈveɪ.ləns/
survive /səˈvaɪv/
survivor /səˈvaɪ.vər/
susceptibility /səˌsep.tɪˈbɪl.ɪ.ti/
susceptible /səˈsep.tɪ.bl̩/
suspected /səˈspek.tɪd/
suspend /səˈspend/
suspension /səˈspen.ʃən/
suspicion /səˈspɪ.ʃən/
suture /ˈsuː.tʃər/
swab /swɒb/
swaddle /ˈswɒdəl/
swallow /ˈswɒl.əʊ/
sweat /swet/
sweatiness /ˈswe.tiː.nəs/
sweating /swet.ɪŋ/
swelling /ˈswel.ɪŋ/
swish /swɪʃ/
Sydenham /sidʼen.ham/ **chorea** /kɒˈrɪə/
sympathetic /ˌsɪm.pəˈθe.tɪk/
symphysis /ˈsɪm.fɪ.sɪs/ **pubis** /ˈpjuː.bɪs/
synchronous /ˈsɪŋ.krə.nəs/
syncitial virus /sin.ˈsi.ʃiː.əl ˈvaɪ.rəs/
syncope /ˈsɪŋ.kə.pi/
synovitis /saɪˈnəʊ.vaɪ.tɪs/
syntactic /sɪnˈtæktɪk/

synthesize /'sɪnθɪˌsaɪz/
syphilis /'sɪf.ɪ.lɪs/
syringe /sɪ'rɪndʒ/
syringomyelia /sə.rɪŋ'gəʊ.maɪ.iː'liː.ə/
syrup /'sɪr.əp/

T
tachycardia /ˌtæk.ɪ'kɑː.di.ə/
tachypnoea /ˌtæk.ɪ.'pnɪə/
tactile /'tæk.taɪl/
tag /tæg/
take /'teɪk/ **a history** /'hɪs.tər.i/
talcum powder /'tælkəm'paʊdə/
talipes /tal.ə.piːz/
tamponade /tæm.pə'neɪd
tangible /'tæn.dʒə.bļ/
tannin /'tænɪn/
tantrum /'tæntrəm/
tape /teɪp/
tar /tɑː/
target /'tɑː.gɪt/
tarry /'tær.i/
tarsus /'tɑː.səs/ pl **tarsi**
tattoo /tə'tuː/
taurine /'tɔː.riːn/
taxi /'tæksɪ/
Tay Sachs /ˌteɪ'sæks/ **hypertonia** /ˌhaɪpə'təʊnɪə/
tearful /'tɪə.fəl/
tearing /teər.ɪŋ/
tease /tiːz/
teat /tiːt/
teenage /'tiːnˌeɪdʒ/
teething /tiːθɪŋ/
telangiectasia /tɪˌlændʒiek'teɪ.zɪə/
temper /'tem.pər/
temperate /'tempərɪt/
temporal /'tem.pər.əl/
temporarily /'tem.pər.er.ɪ.li/
temporary /'tem.pər.ər.i/
temporomandibular /ˌtem.pər.ə.mæn.'dɪ.bjʊ.lə/
temptation /temp'teɪʃən/
tend to /tend/
tenderness /'ten.də.nəs/
tense /tens/
tension /'ten.ʃən/
term /tɜːm/ **infant** /'ɪn.fənt/
terminate /'tɜː.mɪ.neɪt/

termination /ˌtɜː.mɪˈneɪ.ʃən/
terror /ˈterə/
test /test/ strip /strɪp/
testicle /ˈtes.tɪ.kļ/
testicular /tesˈtɪk.jə.lər/
tetanus /ˈtet.ən.əs/
tetany /ˈtet.ən.i/
tetralogy /teˈtræ.lə.dʒɪ/
tetralogy /teˈtræ.lə.dʒɪ/ of Fallot
texture /ˈteks.tʃər/
thalassemia /ˌθæl.əˈsiː.mi.ə/
theraband /ˌθer.əˈ.bænd/
thick /θɪk/
thickness /ˈθɪk.nəs/
thigh /θaɪ/
thin /θɪn/
thinness /θɪnnɪs/
thoracic /θəˌræs.ɪk/
thought /θɔːt/
thrash /θræʃ/
threat /θret/
threaten /ˈθret.ən/
threshold /ˈθreʃ.h əʊld/
thrive /θraɪv/
throat /θrəʊt/
throat /θrəʊt/ swab /swɒb/
thrombocytopenia /ˌθrɒm.bəʊ.saɪt.əˈpiː.ni.ə/
thrombocytopenic /ˌθrɒm.bəʊˌsaɪt.əʊˈpiː.nik/
thromboembolism /ˌθrɒmbəʊˈembəˌlɪzəm/
throw /θrəʊ/ (threw, thrown)
thymic /ˈθaɪ mɪk/
thyroid /ˈθaɪə .rɔɪd/
tibia /ˈtɪb.i.ə/ pl tibiae
tibial /ˈtɪb.i.əl/
tick /tɪk/
tie /taɪ/
tied /taɪd/
tightness /ˈtaɪt.nəs/
tile /taɪl/
tilt /tɪlt/
time /taɪm/ out /aʊt/
timing /ˈtaɪ.mɪŋ/
tip /tɪp/
tire /taɪər/
tissue /ˈtɪʃ.uː/
titrate /ˈtaɪ.treɪt/
titre /ˈtaɪ.tə/

tolerance /ˈtɒl.ər.əns/

tone /təʊn/

tonsil /ˈtɒnt.səl/

tonsillar /ˈtɒnt.səl.ər/

tonsillectomy /ˌtɒn.səˈl.ek.tə.mi/

tonsillitis /ˌtɒnsɪˈlaɪ.tɪs/

toothache /ˈtuːθˌeɪk/

tooth-brushing /ˈtuːθ brʌʃɪŋ/

topical /ˈtɒp.ɪ.kəl/

torsion /ˈtɔː.ʃən/

torticollis /tɔː.tɪˈkɒl.ɪs/

Tourette syndrome /tʊəˈrets ˌsɪn.drəʊm/

tourniquet /ˈtʊə.nɪ.keɪ/

toxocariasis /ˌtɑː.k.sə.kə.ˈraɪ.ə.səs/

toxoplasma /ˌtɒksəʊˈplæzmə/

toxoplasma gondii /tokˈsəʊ.plazˈmæ gonˈdiːaɪ/

toxoplasmosis /ˌtɒk.səʊ.plæzˈməʊ.sɪs/

trace /treɪs/

trachea /trəˈkiː.ə/

tracheitis /treɪ.kiː.aɪˈtis/

tracheo-bronchomalacia /ˈtreɪkɪəʊˈbrɒnkə məˈleɪ.ʃɪə/

tracheooesophageal /træk.iˈɒ ɪˌsɒf.əˈdʒi.əl/

tracheostenosis /træk.iˈɒ.stɪˈnəʊ.sɪs/

tracheostomy /ˌtræk.iˈɒst.ə.mi/

traction /ˈtræk.ʃən/

trait /treɪt/

transcutaneous /trænzˌkjuːˈteɪ.ni.əs/

transduction /trænzˈdʌkʃən/

transepidermal /trænz.ˌep.ə.ˌdər.mæl/

transglutaminase /tranzˈgluːtə.ˈmɪn.eɪs/

transient /ˈtræn.zi.ənt/

transition /trænˈzɪʃ.ən/

transitional /trænˈzɪʃənəl/

translocation /ˌtrænz.ləʊˈkeɪ.ʃⁿn/

transmission /trænzˈmɪʃ.ən/

transmitted /trænzˈmɪt.ɪd/

transposition /ˌtrænspəˈzɪ.ʃən/

trap /træp/

treat /triːt/

treatment /ˈtriːt.mənt/

tree /triː/ **nut** /nʌt/

tremendous /trɪˈmen.dəs/

tremor /ˈtrem.ər/

tricuspid /traɪˈkʌs.pɪd/

trigeminal /traɪˈdʒem.ɪ.nəl/

trigger /ˈtrɪg.ər/

trim /trɪm/

trip /trɪp/
triple /'trɪp.l̩/
tripod /'traɪ.pɒd/
truancy /'truː.ənsɪ/
trust /trʌst/
tube /tjuːb/
tuberculin /tjuː'bɔː.kjə.lɪn/
tuberculous /ˌtjʊˌbɜːkjʊ'ləs/
tuberous /'tʃuː.bə.rəs/ **sclerosis** /sklə'rəʊ.sɪs/
tubing /'tjuː.bɪŋ/
tubular /'tjuː.bjʊ.lər/
tuck /tʌk/
tuft /tʌft/
tug /tʌg/
tumour /'tjuː.mər/
tunnel /'tʌn.əl/
turbinate bone /'təːbɪnɪt'bone/
turgor /'tɜːgə/
turmoil /'tɜː.mɔɪl/
turnip /'tɜː.nɪp/
twitch /twɪtʃ/
twitching /twɪtʃ.iŋ/
typhus /'taɪfəs/
tyrosinemia /ˌtaɪ.rəʊ.sɪ'niː.mɪə/

U

ulcer /'ʌl.sər/
ulceration /ˌʌl.sər'eɪ.ʃən/
ulcerative /'ʌl.sər.ə.tɪv/ **colitis** /kəʊ 'laɪ.təs/
ultimately /'ʌl.tɪ.mət.li/
ultrafiltration /'ʌl.trə.fɪl'treɪ.ʃən/
ultrasound /'ʌl.trə.saʊnd/
umbilical /ʌm'bɪl.ɪ.kəl/
umbilical /ʌm'bɪl.ɪ.kəl/ **hernia** /'hɜː.ni.ə/
umbilicus /ʌm'bɪl.ɪ.kəs/
unaccustomed /ˌʌnə'kʌstəmd/
unaffected /ˌʌn.ə'fek.tɪd/
unaware /ˌʌn.ə'weər/
unbiased /ʌn'baɪəst/
uncircumcised /'sɜː.kəm.saɪzd/
unclamp /ʌn'klæmp/
uncluttered /ʌn'klʌtəd/
unconjugated /'kɒn.dʒə.geɪt.ɪd/
uncooperative /ˌʌn.kəʊ'ɒp.ər.ə.tɪv/
under /'ʌn.dər/
underachievement /ʌn.də.rə'tʃiː.v.mənt/
underestimate /ˌʌn.də'res.tɪ.meɪt/

underinvolved /ˌʌn.dəˈɪnˈvɒlvd/
underlying /ˌʌn.dəˈlaɪ.ɪŋ/
undermine /ˌʌndəˈmaɪn/
underpin /ˌʌndəˈpɪn/
understanding /ˌʌn.dəˈstæn.dɪŋ/
undertake /ˌʌn.dəˈteɪk/
undescended /ˌʌn.dɪˈsen.dɪd/
undifferentiated /ˌʌndɪfəˈren.ʃi.eɪ.tɪd/
undue /ʌnˈdjuː/
unduly /ʌnˈdjuːlɪ/
unequal /ʌnˈiː.kwəl/
unexpected /ˌʌn.ɪkˈspek.tɪd/
unfamiliar /ʌn.fəˈmɪl.i.ər/
unfocused /ʌnˈfəʊkəst/
unhurried /ʌnˈhʌrɪd/
unintentional /ˌʌnɪnˈtenʃənəl/
unique /juːˈniːk/
unite /juːˈnaɪt/
unpleasant /ʌnˈplez.ənt/
unpredictable /ˌʌn.prɪˈdɪk.tə.bl̩/
unreasonable /ʌnˈriː.zən.ə.bl̩/
unrefined /ˌʌn.rɪˈfaɪnd/
unrelated /ˌʌn.rɪˈleɪ.tɪd/
unreliable /ˌʌn.rɪˈlaɪə.bl̩/
unresponsive /ˌʌn.rɪˈspɒnt.sɪv/
unrest /ʌnˈrest/
unsafe /ʌnˈseɪf/
unsteadiness /ʌnˈsted.i.nəs/
unsuccesful /ʌn.səkˈses.fʊl/
unsuitable /ʌnˈsuːtəbəl/
unsuspected /ʌnˈsə.ˈspekt.ɪd/
unused /ʌnˈjuːzd/
unusually /ʌnˈjuːʒʊəl.i/
update /ʌpˈdeɪt/
upholstered /ʌpˈhəʊlstəd/
upright /ˈʌp.raɪt/
uproot /ʌpˈruːt/
upset /ʌpˈset/
upsetting /ʌpˈsetɪŋ/
uptake /ˈʌp.teɪk/
upturned /ʌpˈtɜːnd/
uraemic /ˌjʊəˈriː.mɪk/
urban /ˈɜːbən/
ureter /jʊəˈriː.tər/
urethra /jʊəˈriː.θrə/
urethral /jʊəˈriː.θrəl/
urethritis /ˌjʊə.rɪːˈθraɪ.tɪs/

urge /ɜːdʒ/
urgency /ˈɜː.dʒən.si/
urinalysis /ˌjʊə.rɪˈnæl.ə.sɪs/
urination /ˌjʊə.rɪˈneɪ.ʃən/
urodynamics /ˌjʊə.rəʊ.daɪˈnæm.ɪks/
urosepsis /jʊə.rəʊˈsep.sɪs/
urticaria /ˌɔː.tɪˈkeə.ri.ə/
uterus /ˈjuː.tər.əs/ pl **uteri**
utility /juːˈtɪl.ə.ti/
utilization /ˌjuːtɪlɪˈzeɪʃən/
utter /ˈʌtə/
utterance /ˈʌtərəns/

V

vacuole /ˈvækjʊˌəʊl/
vacuum /ˈvæk.juːm/ cleaner /ˈkliː.nər/
vagal /ˈveɪ gəl/
vaginal /vəˌdʒaɪ.nəl/
vague /veɪg/
validate /ˈvælɪˌdeɪt/
value /ˈvæl.juː/
valve /vælv/
valvular /ˈvælv.jə.lər/
vaporizer /ˈveɪpəˌraɪzər/
variability /ˌveərɪəˈbɪlɪtɪ/
variant /ˈveərɪənt/
variation /ˌveə.riˈeɪ.ʃən/
varicella /ˌvær.ɪˈsel.ə/ **zoster** /zɒ.stər/
varicocele /ˈvær.ɪ.koʊˌsil/
varix /ˈveə.rɪks/ pl **varices** /ˈvær.ɪ.siːz/
varus /ˈveə.rəs/
vary /ˈveə.ri/
vas /væs/
vasculitis /væskjʊˈlaɪ.tɪs/
vasodepressor /ˌvəɪzəʊ dɪˈprəsə/
vasodilator /ˌveɪ.zəʊ.daɪˈleɪ.tər/
vaso-occlusion /veɪˈzəʊ.əˈkluː.ʒən/
vaso-occlusive /veɪˈzəʊ.əˈkluː.sɪv/
vasopressor /ˌveɪzəʊˈpresər/
vasovagal /ˌveɪ.zəʊˈvæg.əl/
vector /ˈvek.tər/
vehicle /ˈviː.ɪ.kl/
venepuncture /viːˈnɪ.pʌŋk.tʃə/
venom /ˈvenəm/
venous /ˈviː.nəs/
vent /vent/
venter / vent.ə/

ventilate /ˈven.tɪ.leɪt/
ventilation /ˌven.tɪˈleɪ.ʃən/
ventilator /ˈven.tɪ.leɪ.tər/
ventouse /ven.tuːˈs/
ventral /vent.rəl/
ventrical /ˈventrɪkəl/
ventricle /ˈven.trɪ.kl̩/
ventriculo-peritoneal /ven.ˌtrik.jə.ləʊ ˌper.ɪ.təˈni.əl/ **shunt** /ˈʃənt/
verbalize /ˈvɜːbəˌlaɪz/
vernix caseosa /vɜːrˈniks kasˈiː.əʊˈsə/
verruca /vəˈruː.kə/ pl **verrucae**
vertebra /ˈvɜː.tɪ.brə/ pl **vertebrae** /ˈvər.tə.ˌbreɪ/
vertebral /ˈvɜː.tɪ.brə/
vertical /ˈvɜː.tɪ.kəl/
vertically /ˈvɜː.tɪ.kəl.i/
vertigo /ˈvɜː.tɪ.gəʊ/
vesicle /ˈves.ɪ.kəl/
vesicoureteral /ˈves.ɪ.kə jʊr.əˈter.əl/
vesicoureteric /vesɪ.kəʊ.jʊˈriː.tər.ɪk/
vesicular /vəˈsɪk.jəˌlər/
vessel /ˈves.əl/
vestibular /vesˈtɪb.jə.lər/
vial /vaɪl/
vibration /vɑɪˈbreɪ.ʃən/
vibratory /ˈvaɪ.brə.tɜːri./
vice versa /ˈvaɪsɪ ˈvɜːsə/
victim /ˈvɪk.tɪm/
viewpoint /vjuː.pɔɪnt/
vigilance /ˈvɪdʒ.ɪ.ləns/
vigor /ˈvɪgə/
vigorous /ˈvɪg.ər.əs/
villus /ˈvɪl.əs/ pl **villi** /ˈvɪl.aɪ/
violence /ˈvaɪə.ləns/
violent /ˈvaɪə.lənt/
viraemic /vaɪˈri.mik/
virilization /ˌvɪrɪlaɪˈzeɪʃən/
virology /vaɪˈrɒl.ə.dʒɪ/
virtually /ˈvɜː.tju.ə.li/
virus /ˈvaɪ.rəs/
viscous /ˈvɪs.kəs/
vitiligo /ˌvɪt.ɪˈlaɪ.gəʊ/
vocal /ˈvəʊkəl/ **cords** /kɔːdz/
vocalization /ˌvəʊ.kəl.aɪˈzeɪ.ʃⁿn/
vocational /vəʊˈkeɪ.ʃə.nəl/
void /vɔɪd/
volume /ˈvɒl.juːm/
voluntarily /ˈvɒl.ən.tər.i.li/

voluntary /ˈvɒl.ən.tər.i/
volvulus /ˈvɒlvjʊləs/
von Willebrand disease (vWD) /fɒn wɪlˈə.brænd dɪˈziːz/
vulnerable /ˈvʌl.nər.ə.bļ/
vulval /vʌlˈvᵊl/
vulvitis /vʌlˈvaɪ.tɪs/

W

wake /weɪk/
wallpaper /ˈwɔːl.peɪpə/
wart /wɔːt/
washcloth /ˈwɒʃ.klɒθ/
washout /ˈwɒʃ.aʊt/
wasp /wɒsp/
waste /weɪst/
wave /weɪv/
weakness /ˈwiː.k.nəs/
weal /wiːl/
wealth /welθ/
wean /wiːn/
web /web/
wedge /wedʒ/
weed /wiːd/
well-being /ˌwelˈbiː.ɪŋ/
wheat /wiːt/
wheelchair /ˈwiːl.tʃeər/
wheeze /wiːz/
whine /waɪn/
whispering /ˈwɪs.pər.ɪŋ/
whole /həʊl/
wholemeal /ˈhəʊlˌmiːl/
whoop /wuːp/
whooping cough /ˈhuː.pɪŋˌkɒf/
wicker /ˈwɪkə/
widen /ˈwaɪ.dən/
widespread /ˌwaɪdˈspred/
willingness /ˈwɪl.ɪŋ.nəs/
Wilms' /wɪlmz/ **tumour** /ˈtjuː.mər/
Wilson /wilˈsɒn/ **disease** /dɪˈziːz/
Wiskott-Aldrich syndrome /wɪsˈkɒt-ɔːlˈdrɪch ˈsɪndrəʊm/
withdraw /wɪðˈdrɔː/
withstand /wɪðˈstænd/
witness /ˈwɪt.nəs/
wobbly /ˈwɒblɪ/
woollen /ˈwʊlən/
worry /ˈwʌr.i/
wrapping /ˈræp.ɪŋ/

wring /rɪŋ/
wry /raɪ/

X
xerotic/ zɪˈrɒtɪk/
X-ray /ˈeks.reɪ/

Y
yawn /jɔːn/
yeast /jiːst/

Z
zygote /ˈzaɪ.gəʊt

Literature

1. **Fenwick**, Elizabeth: The complete Book of mother and baby care. London, Dorling Kindersley 2011. New fully updated Ed. 264 p.
2. **Glasper**, Edward – **Richardson**, James: A Textbook of Children's and Young People's Nursing. Churchill Livingstone 2005. 1st Ed. 832p.
3. **Lissauer**, Tom – **Carroll**, Will: Illustrated Textbook of Paediatrics. Elsevier 2017. 5th Ed. 600 p.

INDEX

Signs of stress or fatigue in neonates;
Specific bacterial infections;
Stages in development of language;
Strategy for meal refusal;
The child with disturbance of oxygen and carbon dioxide exchange;
The child with gastrointestinal dysfunction
The child with renal dysfunction
The child with respiratory dysfunction;
The high-risk newborn and family;
The neurocutaneous syndromes;
Thyroid disorders;

www.ingramcontent.com/pod-product-compliance
Lightning Source LLC
Chambersburg PA
CBHW021347210526
45463CB00001B/4